SUBSTANCE USE AND ABUSE

SUBSTANCE USE AND ABUSE

Everything Matters

Rick Csiernik

Second Edition

Canadian Scholars' Press
Toronto, Ontario

Substance Use and Abuse: Everything Matters, Second Edition
by Rick Csiernik

First published in 2016 by
Canadian Scholars' Press Inc.
425 Adelaide Street West, Suite 200
Toronto, Ontario
M5V 3C1

www.cspi.org

Library and Archives Canada Cataloguing in Publication

Csiernik, Rick, author
      Substance use and abuse : everything matters / Rick Csiernik. -- Second
edition.

Includes bibliographical references and index.
Issued in print and electronic formats.
ISBN 978-1-55130-891-3 (paperback).--ISBN 978-1-55130-892-0 (pdf).-- ISBN 978-1-55130-893-7 (epub)

1. Substance abuse--Canada. 2. Substance abuse--Treatment--Canada. 3. Drug abuse--Canada. 4. Drug abuse--Treatment--Canada. 5. Psychotropic drugs. I. Title.

HV5840.C3C75 2016   362.290971   C2015-907237-9   C2015-907238-7

Text design by Aldo Fierro
Cover design by Em Dash Design

Printed and bound in Canada by Marquis

Canada

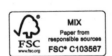

CONTENTS

PREFACE

The preface of the first edition of *Substance Use and Abuse: Everything Matters* began with this statement to contextualize drug use in our society:

Select any day of any week, of any month, of any year and read any major media source on any continent and you will find at least one article, typically within the first three pages, or first five minutes of a broadcast, pertaining to psychoactive drugs:

Addict's body to be exhumed for new tests
   —*The Guardian*, Manchester, United Kingdom, Saturday, February 14, 2004
'War on drugs' not meant to be won
   —*Norwich Bulletin*, Connecticut, United States, Monday, June 6, 2005
West Africa new hub for drug-trafficking networks
   —*Mail and Guardian*, Johannesburg, South Africa, Saturday, May 13, 2006
Prince uses speech to talk about his alcohol problem
   —*The Japan Times*, Tokyo, Japan, Sunday, July 8, 2007
Authorities smash drug ring with Hezbollah ties
   —*Colombia Reports*, Medellin, Colombia, Tuesday, October 21, 2008
Australians arrested in global drug swoop
   —*Sydney Morning Herald*, Sydney, Australia, Thursday, April 9, 2009
Quebec's landmark heroin study in jeopardy
   —*The Globe and Mail*, Toronto, Ontario, Wednesday, August 26, 2009

Unfortunately, the same can be done just as easily for this second edition:

Nigeria: Still on the Tobacco Control Bill
   —*All Africa*, Johannesburg, South Africa, Sunday, March 15, 2015
Saudi Arabia beheads four men for smuggling drugs
   —*Al Jazeera*, Doha, Qatar, Monday, August 18, 2014
Drug treatment court is proof people care
   —*The Spectator*, Hamilton, Ontario, Tuesday, February 17, 2015

Senate bill would end federal prohibition on medical marijuana
    —*The Washington Post*, Washington, United States, Wednesday, March 11, 2015
Ban alcohol firms from sponsoring sports clubs and events, doctors urge
    —*The Guardian*, London, England, Thursday, December 25, 2014
Drugs bound for Future Music Festival seized by Queensland anti-bikie squad
    —*The Sydney Morning Herald*, Sydney, Australia, Friday, March 6, 2015
Ottawa rejects marijuana firm CEN Biotech's licence application
    —*The Globe and Mail*, Toronto, Ontario, Saturday, February 14, 2015

When it comes to addiction, everything does truly matter. Everything is connected and thus has an impact on the drugs we use, misuse, and abuse. The "everything" includes our physiology and biological makeup, our psychological well-being, our connections to our immediate environment, how much money our parents earned in the labour market, if we were raised in a single-parent family, the immediate community in which we live and work, and even the continent of our birth. All these items and more factor into what we deem to be appropriate, legal, licit, functional, and necessary when it comes to taking or avoiding psychoactive substances. Psychoactive drugs are an integral part of the human experience. They were in use before we as a species even had any formal written language, and once we learned to read and write, their use became a topic as prominent in literature and media as aggression and sexuality. Drugs define us in so many ways but extend even beyond the scope of humanity, as illustrated by the infamous YouTube video of a drunken elephant (www.youtube.com/watch?v=AmQPwgV-WbQ) and, closer to home, drunken squirrels (www.youtube.com/watch?v=0so5er4X3dc).

As evidenced by the sample of newspaper headlines above, taken from every continent save Antarctica, psychoactive drugs are a global phenomenon. The issue of addiction, even though the concept is relatively new for helping professionals, predates recorded history. Every culture we know of has had or does have a very specific relationship with one or more psychoactive drugs, and most include some level of tragedy directly related to the use of these substances. The contemporary global drug trade keeps some national economies afloat. In some developed nations, significant economies have evolved around both rehabilitation and incarceration. Historically, drugs have been a component of the slave trade, responsible for the creation of national boundaries, and instrumental in the creation of cultural identities. Psychoactive substances sustain us. They provide us with euphoria. They are integral to our concepts of recreation and celebration. And they ease the pain of our loved ones when they are terminally ill, yet can shorten our lifespan such that issues of aging are never even a consideration. Thus, what can our response be in the 21st century to something as integrated into our lives and culture as is the use of drugs?

In forming our response, our first step must be to enhance our knowledge of this global phenomenon. This book attempts to provide a fundamental working knowledge of the world of psychoactive drugs. *Substance Use and Abuse: Everything Matters* will introduce you to the foundational knowledge you need to understand the bio-psycho-social phenomenon that is addiction, its prevalence, why it arises, and the range of psychoactive drugs ingested and how they affect the users and the users' environment. The range of treatment options, from pharmacological treatments, to harm reduction, to self-help mutual aid, are discussed, followed by an examination of treatment resources required to comprehensively and holistically assist those with addiction issues. Ideas concerning best practices in prevention precede a review of legal, ethical, and competency issues of which those working in the addiction field need to be cognizant. The book concludes with two appendices, with one tracing the history of drug use in Canada. The other looks at global events ranging from 50,000 BCE, when soil samples indicate that Neanderthals living in Northern Iraq were already using plants with amphetamine-like effects, to 2015 CE, when David Wilks, MP for the riding of Kootenay-Columbia, rose in the House of Commons and became the first MP in Canadian history to publically acknowledge his history of drug abuse and recovery. Throughout the book, you will be introduced not only to how everything matters when it comes to the process of developing an addiction, but also to how everything matters with regard to how we respond to the issues raised by this process.

Rick Csiernik
Hamilton, Ontario
September 2015

ACKNOWLEDGEMENTS

I would like to begin by acknowledging all of you who have the desire to do this difficult work in a field and with a population that remains marginalized and oppressed even in the most open of societies. I want to thank Dr. Susan Silva-Wayne for her ongoing support of my work in this area of practice, along with all the staff at Canadian Scholars' Press for turning thoughts and ideas into substance, especially Daniella Balabuk, Nicholas Cameron, Caley Clements, Emma Johnson, Emma Waghorn, and Natalie Garriga. I would also like to thank the reviewers of the first edition, Kristen Buscaglia, Phil Durrant, and Heidi Stanley, who provided feedback and insight to enhance and refine the manuscript, along with Derek Chechak for his assistance with revisions to the second edition, and, of course, Deborah, Alex, and Ben for giving me the space and time to do the work and for their ongoing, unintended inspiration.

> We are all insecure at times…
> We are all afraid at times…
> However, it is what we do with our insecurities and with our fears that defines us and allows us to make the impact upon the world that we all need to so that our labours, our lives, have meaning…

LET US ADVANCE NOT BY RUNNING FROM FEAR BUT RATHER BY
PURSUING HOPE.

d.p.

Chapter 1

FUNDAMENTAL CONCEPTS

Drugs may be employed not only to treat pathological conditions; reduce pain, suffering, agitation and anxiety, but also to enhance the normal state—increase pleasure, facilitate learning and memory, reduce jealousy and aggressiveness. Hopefully, such pharmacological developments will come about as an accompaniment of, and not as a substitute for, a more ideal society.

—Stanley Jarvik, 1967

Are you the fish that can see the water that you swim in?

Do we live in a drug culture? This question is moot, for if one examines the history of humanity, we as a species have so incorporated psychoactive drugs into every aspect of our civilization—celebration, medicine, escapism, sport, entertainment, survival, relaxation, day-to-day living—that to ask if there is a drug culture is synonymous with asking if there is a human culture. So are you the fish that can see the water that you swim in?

The United Nations Office on Drugs and Crime (2011) estimates that the annual illicit drug trade is worth $870 billion, which is equivalent to 1.5 percent of global gross domestic product (GDP), with the cocaine trade alone accounting for $85 billion. This US dollar amount is greater than the annual revenues of all but 15 national economies. This means that the drug trade produces more revenue than the paid work in Argentina, Saudi Arabia, Nigeria, or Switzerland and is far greater than the revenue produced by the world's largest multinationals, such as Nestlé, Procter & Gamble, or Sony. In the United States alone, more than $65 billion worth of illegal drugs are sold every year, yet only a tiny fraction is intercepted and seized by law enforcement agents. This has led the director of the National Drug Control Policy, Michael Botticelli, to state that the United States can no longer attempt to arrest itself out of its drug problem (Lopez, 2014).

Herein lies the core problem. As a species, humans have a fascination with any psychoactive agent that alters our basic perception of our environment— our interactions with and reactions to the external world and thus to our own internal world. Anthropologists have postulated that a primary motivation for the shift from hunting and gathering societies to agrarian-based cultures was to allow for the regular and systematic cultivation of intoxicating beverages. Archaeological evidence in multiple sites indicates that the regular use of psychoactive substances dates back 10,000 years (Hayen, Canuel, & Shanse, 2013; Merlin, 2003). In ancient Egypt, hieroglyphics illustrate gods holding and using different hallucinogenic drugs (Bertol, Fineschi, Karch, Mari, & Riezzo, 2004). Unfortunately, the use, misuse, and abuse of these psychoactive substances has an indisputable cost in terms of individual suffering—not only financially, but also personally—and to us all as a society and a species (Nutt, King, Saulbury, & Blakemore, 2007).

Psychoactive drug use is not a strange anomaly of the 21st century but rather a historical part of human civilization.[1] Societies have regularly used, misused, and abused mind-altering drugs of some type for various reasons. Despite the perpetual historic discouragement of drug use, this behaviour has become an integral part of cultures worldwide, and it is unlikely that it will subside in the near future, if ever. A more realistic and pragmatic goal is a move toward wellness, harm reduction, and the abatement of abuse in lessening the extent to which persons are harmed and cause harm to others because of psychoactive drugs.

1.1 CONCEPTUALIZING ADDICTION
Psychoactive Drug
Addiction
Dependency
What Is Not an Addiction

Psychoactive Drug

To a pharmacologist, a psychoactive drug is either a chemical not naturally found in the body or is a body chemical administered in a larger dose than is normal to the body. A specific person, via some mode of administration (see Table 1.1), takes the substance in a given amount (the dose level) on a particular frequency (the schedule of use) for a certain period of time. It is administered with the intent of producing a change in behaviour by specifically altering the central nervous system (CNS), but also has a profound effect on the larger peripheral nervous system, particularly the autonomic nervous system (ANS). The Le Dain Commission (1973), who produced the landmark body of work examining drugs in a scientific manner for the first time in Canada, defines a psychoactive drug as any substance, natural or synthesized, that by its chemical nature alters structure or function of the body or mind in the living organism. The more recent Canadian parliamentary Special Committee on Non-Medical Use of Drugs (2002) further defines a psychoactive drug as a substance that, when ingested, alters mental processes such as cognition or affect. Psychoactive drugs are substances that alter brain functioning by increasing, decreasing, or disrupting CNS activity. This in turn produces changes in mood, perception, sensation, need, consciousness, and other psychological functions and ultimately produces changes in behaviour. In addition, these substances influence a great number of physiological functions mediated by the ANS that are outside the realm of conscious control, such as respiration, cardiovascular function, hormonal balance, sexual arousal, and the fight/flight response. Psychoactive agents are used for both medical and non-medical purposes and may be either licit or illicit, depending on the place and time they are being used.

Associated with psychoactive drugs are the concepts of both drug misuse and drug abuse. "Drug misuse" refers to the periodic or occasional improper or inappropriate use of either a social or a prescription drug. The term "drug abuse" has been used in a broader social context to define any instance of drug administration that is disapproved of by the society in which it occurs. According to the medical model (see Chapter 2), the term "drug abuser" is limited to individuals who persistently consume a substance to such an extent that they are impairing their quality of life in some way. Adverse effects can include medical complications, behavioural alterations, difficulties with social relationships, and medical, legal, and vocational issues. Thus, in this context, "abuse" refers to the use of any drug to the extent that it interferes with a person's health or with economic or social adjustment. However, both legal and illegal drugs are employed for a range of reasons without the user ever developing a dependency or an addiction. This can range from the occasional and recreational use of alcohol, cannabis, ecstasy, or khat, to the therapeutic use of Valium, Ritalin, or morphine, to the functional use of coca leaves to help with strenuous labour in the Andes, to the use of opium to counteract the effects of dysentery and hunger in the Middle East.

Addiction

There is a story of a Greek slave named Addictus, who, after a long period of servitude, was finally set free by his master. However, Addictus had become used to being chained and to following his master's commands. Even though he was now allowed to remove what had bound him throughout his life, he had become so accustomed to the pain that, when the chains were unlocked, he could not bring himself to remove them.

The word "addiction" has been used so casually in so many ways and in so many different contexts that in practical terms it has lost its actual meaning. Many definitions begin by observing that addiction is the behaviour engaged in by compulsive drug users in search of their substance(s) of choice. The term itself derives from the Latin word *addicto*, meaning "bound or devoted or bondage to a practice." The idea of addiction in many people's minds relates to the exhibition of either physical or psychological dependence on a chemical agent. This idea implies an inability to resist using a substance, with increased use leading eventually to compulsive use in terms of dosage and/ or frequency.

At the turn of the 20th century, the term "addiction" had a behavioural meaning. It referred to compulsive drug seeking and the loss of personal control to drugs. It also involved a breakdown in lifestyle, including family, work, and leisure activities. In the 1950s and 1960s, addiction became more closely associated with the unpleasant physical reactions that occurred with the stoppage of drug administration, the physical component of the phenomenon. Those who were labelled as addicted continued to take the drug to avoid the negative bodily reactions that occurred when the drug cleared the system, that is, the withdrawal process. In 1964, the World Health Organization (WHO) moved away from the increasingly nebulous term "addiction" and began to use the more precise and narrower concept of "dependence," categorizing it by distinct physical and psychological components. However, the standpoint provided by one's education also plays a vital role in how an idea is conceptualized. The classic example is the American Society of Addiction Medicine (2011), whose very detailed definition of addiction is still enveloped in a unidimensional standpoint:

> Addiction is a primary, chronic disease of brain reward, motivation, memory, and related circuitry. Dysfunction in these circuits leads to characteristic biological, psychological, social, and spiritual manifestations. This is reflected in an individual pathologically pursuing reward and/or relief by substance use and other behaviors.
>
> Addiction is characterized by inability to consistently abstain, impairment in behavioral control, craving, diminished recognition of significant problems with one's behaviors and interpersonal relationships, and a dysfunctional emotional response. Like other chronic diseases, addiction often involves cycles of relapse and remission. Without treatment or engagement in recovery activities, addiction is progressive and can result in disability or premature death.

This definition misses a crucial element inherent in the holistic nature of addiction. Noted psychologist, addiction theorist, and pundit Stanton Peele (1983, 1985, 1989) has been among the most vigorous opponents of any strictly medical definition of addiction. Peele claims that addiction is not a chemical reaction, rather it is a social experience that in and of itself can bring about dependency to a substance in an otherwise healthy individual. People become dependent to a particular state of body and mind. According to Peele, no substance is inherently addictive, nor is substance addiction a single phenomenon. It occurs along a continuum, and even those at the extremes of addictiveness show the capacity to act in other than an addicted way under the right circumstances.

Anthropologists state that drinking alcohol is generally a social act that is performed in a socially recognized setting. Human geographers illustrate that the consumption of alcohol typically takes place at a specific time and in a specific place, with the affective potential of bringing people together in urban places in the evenings and at night (Oksanen, 2013). A dramatic 20th-century example of the importance of the social dimension of addiction involved conscripted American soldiers fighting communist forces in Vietnam as part of the ongoing Cold War conflict between the United States and Russia. As the outcome of a 1971 congressional visit to Vietnam, the United States Department of Defense set up a urine-screening program to detect heroin use in all combat troops at the time of their departure from Vietnam. These veterans, most of whom were still under the age of 21, were then to be detoxified. In one study, 75 percent of ground troops who engaged in combat and who tested positive for heroin use claimed they became addicted in Vietnam. One-third of these soldiers continued using, but less than 10 percent showed signs of what could be classified as dependency on returning to the United States (Roffman, 1976).

A second follow-up study of Vietnam veterans was also commissioned to determine the long-term consequences of their heroin use. Eight to twelve months after their return from Southeast Asia, interviews were conducted with approximately 900 males who had seen active combat duty. The sample was randomly selected from the 14,000 army-enlisted men who returned to the United States in September 1971, the first month in which the urine-screening and detoxification system was operating uniformly throughout Vietnam. Men who had been detected as drug-positive at departure were oversampled, so the full sample included a large number of men who would be at high risk after their return. In 1974, 617 former soldiers with an average age of 24 were re-interviewed. In this follow-up group, it was discovered that the sample was no more likely to be using heroin regularly or daily, if at all, than either marijuana or amphetamines. Despite their initial addiction, the majority of former soldiers had managed to quit on their own. As well, some were even able to return to casual use without becoming dependent again. While treatment was certainly vital in aiding some individuals to become abstinent, these studies clearly indicated there were other factors involved in addiction. The importance of environmental and social factors that precipitate and support drug use were clearly demonstrated. A major difference in this sample and clinical samples of heroin users from the United States entering treatment was not only that the Vietnam group had been exposed to a far more generous supply and superior quality of the drug for one year, but also that the exposure was in an extraordinary setting that featured the constant threat of death. Further, for those veterans who continued to use heroin in the United States two to three years after returning from active duty in Vietnam, only one in six came to treatment (Robins, Helzer, Hesselbrock, & Wish, 2010).

Drugs produce societal harm in multiple ways: through damage to family and social life; through additional costs to the health, social services, and criminal justice systems; through decreased workplace productivity; through property damage; and, of course, through violence and the costs of organized crime (Nutt, King, Saulbury, & Blakemore, 2007). For Peele and Brodsky (1992), the social context for addiction required

- a readily available substance;
- stress in a severe form including misery, danger, and discomfort;
- alienation;
- emotional and/or vocational deprivation; and
- a lack of control over one's life.

When considering what addiction entails, the larger social, environmental, and cultural factors that surround an individual need to be considered, for we human beings are fundamentally social creatures (Oksanen, 2013). This concept was further underscored by the longitudinal work done by Hallam Hurt and her colleagues beginning in 1989 at the height of the "crack baby" epidemic. They followed a cohort of children exposed to cocaine while in utero, along with a comparison group of children exposed to non-gestational cocaine who also lived in the inner city of a large American urban centre and came from low-income, predominantly African-American, single-parent-led families. Over time, they found no difference in school performance, grade point average, reading level, or standardized reading and math test scores between the two groups. Nor were there differences in IQ, executive brain functioning, or general cognitive abilities. However, both groups had lower scores than the average for American children their age across all of the variables. Ongoing evaluations examining environmental factors of all participants found that 81 percent of the children had seen someone arrested; 35 percent had seen someone shot; and 19 percent had seen a dead body in their neighbourhood by the age of seven. Those children who reported a high exposure to violence were also the most likely to have symptoms of depression and anxiety, and to have lower self-esteem. Hurt's conclusion was that poverty was a far more powerful influence on the academic outcomes of inner-city children than gestational exposure to cocaine (Avants et al., 2007;

Farah et al., 2008; Hurt, Brodsky, Roth, Malmud, & Giannetta, 2005; Hurt, Giannetta et al., 2008; Hurt, Malmud et al., 1997; Hurt, Malmud, Betancourt, Brodsky, & Giannetta, 2001).

Dr. Robert DuPont (1994), then head of the Institute for Behavioural Health in Rockville, Maryland, stated that addiction needs to be considered in terms of how it disorganizes and creates crises in individuals' lives. Recently the term "addiction" has finally begun to encompass a greater social orientation rather than a purely biomedical or bio-psycho one. When one views pharmacological data and literature in the light of its social and legal history, the tendency by the medical community to explain drug abuse and addiction becomes, at best, suspect. Addiction may well be a dependent state acquired over an extended period of time by a predisposed person in an attempt to correct a chronic stress condition in a conscious, deliberate, self-satisfying, selective manner; however, there is also extensive evidence that psychological, social, economic, and situational factors play key roles in initiating addiction (Kallant, 2009). Thus, addiction needs to be viewed in a holistic manner and as a process that integrates three constituent components: biological, psychological, and social. Or, to properly and holistically conceptualize it: addiction is a bio-psycho-social phenomenon.

Dependency

When considering both addiction and its sub-component, dependency, it is useful to specify what it is that is being depended on and for what reasons, and then to identify the consequences of its presence or absence. The social and moral significance of dependency changes considerably if the drug is relied on for a societally deemed legitimate reason, such as, taking Dilaudid for pain relief from cancer, as opposed to using the same drug for escape from an unpleasant or intolerable social situation, such as violence in an interpersonal relationship. Psychoactive drug-related problems tend to arise because of both a psychological and physical dependence on a certain drug.

Physical Dependency

Physical dependence is a physiological state of cellular adaptation that occurs when the body becomes so accustomed to a drug that it can only function normally when the drug is present. Without the drug, the user will experience physical disturbances or illness, known as withdrawal. Withdrawal symptoms can be prevented or promptly relieved by the administration of a sufficient quantity of the original drug or, often, by one with similar pharmacological properties, such as a benzodiazepine like Valium in place of alcohol. However, in the latter case, in which one psychoactive drug is used to prevent withdrawal symptoms from another, cross-dependence to the new drug can easily develop.

The development of physical dependence is important in the maintenance of drug taking, not only because of its negative reinforcement, but also because administration, either to alleviate or to prevent withdrawal, can lead to additional positive reinforcement. Instead of a return to a neutral body state, or homeostasis, there may be an overshooting effect, resulting in further positive reinforcement. Physical dependence is usually preceded by serious personal, psychological, social, and even physiological complications. Physical dependence can occur with chronic use of most depressants, opioids, and stimulants. Among the hallucinogens, physical dependence has not yet been demonstrated, except with cannabis.

Psychological Dependency

Psychological dependence can also be referred to as behavioural or emotional dependence. Psychological dependence occurs when a drug becomes so important to a person's thoughts or activities that the person believes that he or she cannot manage without the substance. Psychological dependence may range from a mild wish to a compelling emotional need for periodic or continuous use of a drug, and may escalate to feelings of loss or desperation if the drug is unattainable. In the case of psychological dependence, a person begins to feel and eventually believes that she or he needs the drug effect to cope with a variety of life situations. The feelings of either relaxation or arousal become required because an individual believes he or she cannot get through a day or a situation without these affects.

In many instances, the psychological aspects are considerably more important than physical dependence in maintaining chronic drug use and can last far longer. While physical withdrawal can be managed in weeks or even days, psychological cravings can lead to drug use months and even years after the last actual administration. Subtle yet persistent psychological and social factors are more than adequate to maintain the behaviour of drug consumption even after a successful detoxification process.

In the fourth edition of the American Psychiatric Association's *Diagnostic and Statistical Manual of Mental Disorders* (DSM-IV; 2000), dependence was defined as a maladaptive pattern of substance use leading to clinically significant impairment or distress. However, in the fifth edition (DSM-V; 2013), a new conceptualization relating to alcohol and other psychoactive drugs was created. Problems relating to psychoactive drug use have now been classified as substance-related disorders with separate listings for alcohol, caffeine, cannabis, hallucinogens, inhalants, opioids, sedative-hypnotics (benzodiazepines and barbiturates), stimulants, and tobacco, with a final category entitled "other or unknown." As well, at the very end of the section one new area was added: non-substance-related disorders, which has only one subtype—gambling.

In the development of DSM-V, the working group had extensive discussions regarding the use of the term "addiction." There had been general agreement that dependence as a label for compulsive, out-of-control drug use had been problematic and that the idea had confused many physicians and psychiatrists. This confusion resulted in patients with normal tolerance and withdrawal being labelled with the stigmatizing and oppressive term "addict." This also resulted in the withholding of adequate doses of opioids from patients suffering severe pain because of fear of producing addiction on the part of the physician. Thus, the term "dependence" was removed, and in its place, each of the drugs, including the "other" grouping, is now described in detail under the following headings: use, intoxication, and withdrawal.

What Is Not an Addiction

Toward the end of the 20th century, an evident shift toward the medicalization of behaviour occurred, with non-medical problems becoming defined and treated as such (Szasz, 2007). These newly medicalized behaviours simultaneously became intertwined with both the creation and manufacturing of mental illness, partially because, in the United States, insurance companies would pay for medical or psychiatric treatment only if the situation could be medically framed. No DSM diagnosis, no treatment, and thus everything becomes an addiction (Greenberg, 2010; Watters, 2010). Life problems were increasingly transformed into pathologies, with "addiction" becoming one of the most popular incorrectly and overused medical terms. This has further allowed pharmaceutical companies to market not drugs, but behaviours (Conrad, 2007). Thus, it is not surprising that the popular though problematic label of addiction has been placed on these behavioural issues.

Compulsive Behaviours

Compulsive behaviours, or simply compulsions, are most commonly referenced in the anxiety literature, particularly in the obsessive-compulsive section. In the purest sense, compulsions are repetitive behaviours performed in an effort to control or prevent an obsessive thought, which may or may not be related to the behaviour. For instance, a person may repeatedly wash their hands because of an obsessive fear of germs or because they feel that the action is necessary to prevent some unrelated harm. In Goodman's (1990) early conceptualization of addiction, compulsions are an integral component, along with reward-seeking behaviour, designed to evade or avoid internal discomfort. Everitt and Robbins (2005) view addiction as a progression from a loss of control, to a developed habit, to an eventual compulsion. Although their conceptualization emphasizes the change in the brain that can foster an actual addiction to psychoactive drugs, the end point of compulsion recognizes the dependent nature, and not necessarily goal-directed state, of the process. For instance, a compulsive Internet gamer is not playing just to win but also simply to avoid other life issues. They are gaming for the action, excitement, or emotional high (Nakken, 1996). Whereas a habit develops as people become accustomed to using a psychoactive substance, the compulsion defines the continuous and often escalating drug-seeking behaviours (Everitt & Robbins, 2005). Pickard (2012) defines compulsion as "an urge, impulse or desire that is irresistible: so strong that it is impossible for it not to lead to action" (p. 41). This lack of choice, however, is disputed by Dingela, Hammer, Ostergren, McCormick, and Koenig (2012). They argue that no matter how strong the impulse to act is, there is always an element of choice involved, even if it only occurs at the initiation phase.

Compulsive behaviours referenced in the addiction literature include: eating/food (Pelchat, 2002); exercising (Landolfi, 2013); gambling (Blaszczynski, 2010); hoarding (Frost & Steketee, 2014); kleptomania and pyromania (Grant, Schreiber, & Odlaug, 2013); sex (Carnes, 1996); shopping/buying (Schlosser, Black, Repertinger, & Freet, 1994); ultraviolet indoor tanning (Reed, 2015); work (Van Wijhe, Schaufeli, & Peeters, 2010); and video games (Hellman, Schoenmakers, Nordstrom, & Van Holst, 2013) or Internet use (Thorsteinsson & Davey, 2014), particularly involving pornography (Short, Black, Smith, Wetterneck, & Wells, 2012), and even social media or Facebook (Karaiskos, Tzavellas, Balta, & Paparrigopoulos, 2010). Compulsive behaviours do share characteristics with an addiction, such as an inability to resist an urge or drive that harms oneself (Grant et al., 2013). However, they require distinct treatment, the development of unique treatment systems and policies pertaining to their discrete causes and outcomes primarily because of what they do not share with an addiction—the biological domain.

Benson and Eisenach (2013) provide a clear distinction between a compulsive behaviour and an addiction in their discussion of overshopping or compulsive buying. They begin by citing the standardized criteria first presented by McElroy, Keck, Pope, Smith, and Strakowski (1994), which defined the disorder as a maladaptive preoccupation with buying or shopping, whether impulses or behaviour, that either (a) is irresistible, intrusive, and/or senseless, or (b) results in frequent buying of more than can be afforded, frequent buying of items that are not needed, or shopping for longer periods of time than intended. First documented early in the 20th century by psychiatrists Emil Kraepelin and Eugen Bleuler, whose primary focus was on studying schizophrenia, the underlying issue is preoccupation with shopping and then impulse buying that leads to feelings of distress and that interferes with social and/or occupational functioning. As well, the behaviour can lead to significant debt, family issues, and feelings of shame, guilt, depression, hopelessness, and anger. Benson and Eisenach (2013) also underscore that this is not a behaviour that only arises in cultures with widely accessible credit and unlimited buying opportunities. However, unlike an addiction, there is no distinct biological dimension, no chemically induced change to the central nervous system, no change to the brain itself as occurs with psychoactive drugs, and none of the secondary effects to the autonomic nervous system.

Eating Disorders

Eating disorders are complex psychiatric diagnoses whose etiologies are poorly understood. Generally speaking, they involve either insufficient or excessive food intake, which is detrimental to both physical and psychological health. They are divided into three categories: anorexia nervosa, bulimia nervosa, and atypical (Fairburn & Harrison, 2003). Only about 10–15 percent of people with eating disorders are male (Grogan, 1999). In the anorexic type, patients usually undergo extreme food restriction intake or engage in excessive exercise to maintain a low body weight. In bulimic types, excessive food consumption is often counteracted with some method of purging (Heller, 2003).

In the mid-20th century in the United States, medical thought regarding obesity reinterpreted being overweight and obese as the consequence of addiction because of the psychodynamic theory (see Chapter 2) principle of oral fixation, a psychological defect. This idea quickly became popular, enhancing the stigma and oppression associated with weight gain that produced negative physical effects. As overeating is not an addiction, given that eating is necessary to sustain life, the application of the addiction concept contributed to an ineffective policy response to the epidemiological findings regarding obesity's consequences. In turn, public health initiatives became more focused on correcting individual eating behaviour among obese people by encouraging self-help in lay groups similar to Alcoholics Anonymous and thus missing the vital contribution of population-level interventions (Rasmussen, 2014).

The level of co-morbidity between eating disorders and substance dependence as well as depression appears to be high, but more so with the bulimic than anorexic classifications (Gadalla & Piran, 2009; Holderness, Brooks-Gunn, & Warren, 1994). In one study that examined the sequencing of health issues, it was observed that eating disorders regularly preceded substance abuse (Wiseman et al., 1999). Similarly, Davis and Claridge (1998) found that people with eating disorders scored high on the Addiction Scale of the Eysenck Personality Questionnaire. They presented their findings within the context of the auto-addiction opioid theory—the theory that the body becomes addicted to its own naturally produced opioids, which are increased and reinforced through self-starvation. This neurobiological perspective is strongly opposed by Wilson (2000), who notes that "neither tolerance nor withdrawal reactions to food have been demonstrated" (p. 87). Even the so-called "carbohydrate craving" theory is lacking in evidence. One trait that has been implicated in both substance abuse and eating disorders, which is also observed in the range of compulsive behaviours, is impulsivity, which encapsulates both the pursuit of rewards and the personality dimension (Dawe & Loxton, 2004). People with this trait may be more likely to develop primarily binge eating and substance use disorders.

Though not at all related to the psychiatric diagnosis of an eating disorder, the concept of "food addiction" has garnered attention in recent years and requires examination. The premise that food produces an addiction has been perpetuated and advanced by recent neurobiological findings regarding how sugary foods are processed in the brain. In 2009, a symposium was held to evaluate the notion of food addiction. The conclusion was that although highly palatable foods can promote changes to the body under the right conditions, they are not addictive. However, food consumption is certainly subject to a binge pattern of consumption that is also apparent in addiction, and thus there have been arguments made that treatment patterns should be similar (Corwin & Grigson, 2009). Specifically, binge eating disorder, which was a provisional diagnosis in the DSM-IV, and was retained and enhanced in the DSM-V, involves excessive consumption of food but without the purging behaviours involved in bulimia (Gearhardt, White, & Potenza, 2011). Some authors have noted marked similarities between binge eating disorder and substance dependence disorders, including issues of tolerance and withdrawal (Cassin & von Ranson, 2007), and this is also noted in the DSM-V. However, the major distinction between the two is that food is essential for survival whereas psychoactive drugs are not, and while relapse to drugs indicates a return to previous drug use, what does relapse to eating entail?

Problem Gambling

As Blaszczynski and Nower (2002) note, "There is no single conceptual theoretical model of gambling that adequately accounts for the multiple biological, psychological and ecological variables contributing to the development of pathological gambling" (p. 487). In part, this is because of imprecise definitions of problem gambling. Petry (2005) notes that the current understanding of distressed gambling as a disorder is rooted in biological, neurological, developmental, and environmental factors. Most notably, the character trait of impulsivity has been studied, especially with adolescents (Clarke, 2006; Derevensky, Gupta, & Csiernik, 2010; Lawrence, Luty, Bogdan, Sahakian, & Clark, 2009).

Models of problematic gambling that have emerged over time are based on a wide range of theories: behavioural (Anderson & Brown, 1984; McConaghy, Armstrong, Blaszczynski, & Allcock, 1983); cognitive (Sharpe & Tarrier, 1993; Ladouceur & Walker, 1996); psychobiological (Blaszczynski, Winter, & McConaghy, 1986; Carlton & Goldstein, 1987; Comings, Rosenthal, Lesieur, & Rugle, 1996; Lesieur & Rosenthal, 1991; Rugle, 1993); psychodynamic (Bergler, 1958; Rosenthal, 1992; Wildman, 1997); and sociological (Rosecrance, 1985; Ocean & Smith, 1993). The perspectives are not mutually exclusive, but reflect the different authors' attempts to classify this unique and non-substance-related form of pathology. Authors have also attempted to classify types of distressed gambling. For instance, Blaszczynski and Nower (2002) describe three categories: (1) behaviourally conditioned, (2) emotionally focused, and (3) antisocial-impulsivist. People who comprise each category may vary on coping skills/styles, co-morbid mental health conditions, and thrill-seeking/arousal. All groups are influenced by various ecological factors, such as availability and accessibility, but there is substantial variation in terms of biological, emotional, and personality traits. As well, unlike with addiction, there is no direct biological trigger with problem gambling nor direct health risks that arise with excessive gambling, and no risk of overdose or physical harm from withdrawal, which is a major issue with addiction to psychoactive drugs.

1.2 PHARMACOLOGICAL FOUNDATIONS
Drug Groups
Neurophysiology
Neurotransmitters
Pharmacodynamics

Drug Groups[2]
Depressants
Depressants produce a reduction of arousal and activity in the central nervous system. These drugs are used therapeutically as anaesthetics, aids for sleeping, anti-anxiety agents, and sedatives. For the most part, the non-medical use of these agents results from their ability to produce disinhibition and to artificially relieve feelings of anxiety.

Opioids
Opioids, also termed opiates, are a specific subgroup of CNS depressants. The distinct attribute that differentiates these psychoactive agents from other CNS depressants is their ability to mask pain and also to suppress cough. While depressants initially affect the neurotransmitter, gamma-aminobutyric acid (GABA) opioids mimic endorphin neurotransmitters found in the brain.

Stimulants
Stimulants produce a general increase in the activity of the cerebral cortex, creating mood elevation, increased vigilance, and the postponement of fatigue. Some stimulants are also used as appetite suppressants and decongestants, and to treat attention-deficit/hyperactivity disorder (ADHD). These drugs produce changes through their effect on dopamine.

Hallucinogens
This family of psychoactive agents works in a different manner on the central nervous system than do depressants and stimulants. Hallucinogens produce a generalized disruption in the brain, especially of perception, cognition, and mood. Several, such as ecstasy, have secondary CNS stimulant effects.

The most frequently used hallucinogen, cannabis, has an associated phar-macological effect more closely associated with CNS depressants, as do the dissociative anaesthetics PCP (phencyclidine) and Ketamine. Hallucinogens primarily affect serotonin, though cannabis has its own unique neurotrans-mitter, the endocannabinoids, particularly anandamide.

Psychotherapeutic Agents

These substances are most frequently used to treat people with specific forms of mental illness: depression, bipolar disorder, and psychosis. Many produce unpleasant side effects in persons without the condition as well as in those with a mental health issue. Thus, compliance has historically been of greater concern than misuse, though more recently synthesized members of this group of psychoactive drugs tend to have fewer negative side effects. As well, as these psychoactive drugs do not produce a rapid state of mood enhance-ment in users, they are not generally subject to non-medical use. More recent additions to this category, though, such as the Selected Serotonin Reuptake Inhibitors (SSRIs), an example of which is Prozac, have raised new controver-sies and concerns.

Neurophysiology

In order to gain an understanding of how psychoactive agents affect the cen-tral nervous system, one must have a basic understanding of the process that underlies the functioning of the brain and spinal cord. This field is known as neurophysiology. Of the billions of cells of which the brain is composed, it is only the neuron, or nerve cell, that processes information. Messages travel within each cell as electrical transmissions, but as one neuron has no direct physical contact with another, electrical transmission between cells cannot occur. Thus, information between nerve cells must be communicated chemi-cally. A neuron consists of the cell body, or soma, where metabolic activity occurs featuring the nucleus and dendrites. Dendrites are the extension of the soma that receive messages from the axons of adjoining cells. The axon is the part of the neuron along which signals are transmitted to adjoining cells that terminate in axon terminals. It is in the axon terminals where the various neurotransmitters such as dopamine, endorphins, and serotonin are found. The gap across which the neurotransmitters must travel is referred to as the synaptic cleft. The synaptic cleft is typically 10–20 nanometres across. This is such a tiny space that it takes only 0.1 milliseconds for a neurotransmitter to drift, or diffuse, across the gap to the next axon (see Figure 1.1).

During early brain development, which occurs from the third trimester of pregnancy to the third year of life, there is an overproduction of neuronal tissue. As well, during adolescence, many synapses and neurons are altered and even eliminated in a second reshaping of the brain. These processes are partially influenced by interactions with the environment, with substance use or abuse being one of the most critical. The most powerful alterations occur in the frontal lobes, responsible for higher order thinking, which are still maturing until a person is in their early 20s. The temporal lobes, which are critically involved in memory formation, reach their maximum grey matter volume slightly earlier, at the age of 16 to 17. Thus, due to these maturation processes, adolescents are more vulnerable to the effects of many psychoactive drugs than are older adults (White, Altmann, & Nanchahal, 2002).

FIGURE 1.1: A NEURON

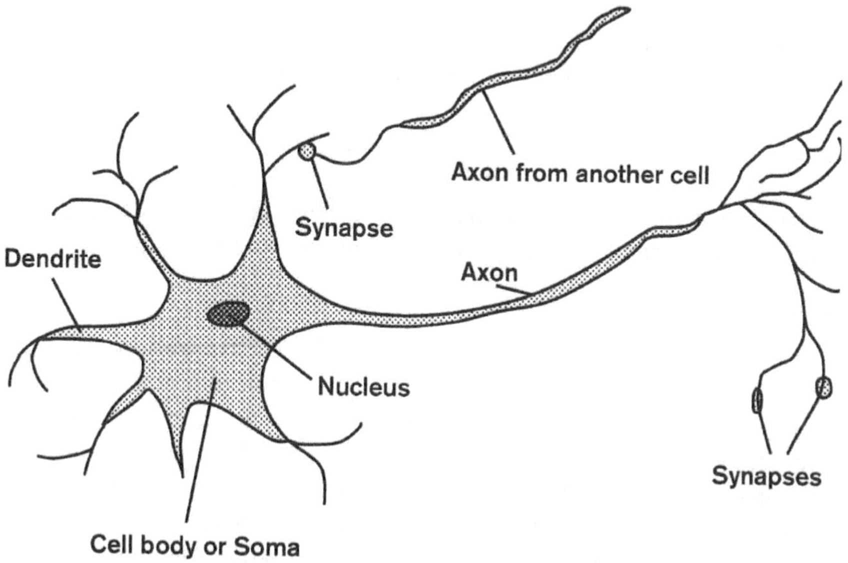

Neurotransmitters

Neurotransmitters are chemicals found in the brain that are used to relay, amplify, and modulate signals between a neuron and another cell. There are over 50 known neurotransmitters that carry chemical information between cells. Despite the fact that different psychoactive drugs affect different neurotransmitters, most drugs of misuse have been linked to their ability to directly or indirectly increase dopamine activity, particularly within the mesolimbic dopaminergic system, which is the key component of the reward system portion of the brain (European Monitoring Centre for Drugs and Drug Addiction, 2009b). Along with dopamine, the most prominent neurotransmitters include endocannabinoids, endomorphins, GABA, glutamate, norepinephrine, and serotonin.

Dopamine

This neurotransmitter is a member of the monoamine catecholamine family of neurotransmitters, which also includes epinephrine and norepinephrine. Dopamine stimulates the nerve receptors in the brain, creating sensations of power, energy, and, most importantly, euphoria. Dopamine has a specific function in terms of regulating mood and affect and also plays a prominent role in motivation and reward processes. There are several dopamine systems in the brain. However, the mesolimbic dopamine system appears to be the most important for motivational processes and the system on which most psychoactive drugs produce their behavioural effects. CNS stimulants such as amphetamines, cocaine, and nicotine act directly on the dopamine systems in the brain.

Endocannabinoids

Cannabis acts on two specific receptors in the brain, CB_1 and CB_2. It is believed that cannabis affects neuronal function by causing the psychoactive component of the drug, tetrahydrocannabinol (THC), to bind to CB_1 receptors that are located primarily in the cerebral cortex, cerebellum, and hippocampus. It is thought to be responsible for the euphoria, time distortion, and hallucinogenic effects. As well, when THC binds to THC-specific receptors on a neighbouring terminal of a dopaminergic neuron, this sends a signal to the dopamine terminal to release more dopamine into the synaptic cleft.

Endorphins

Natural endorphins in the body are mimicked in nature and through synthesis by the opioid family of psychoactive drugs. Endorphins bind to opioid receptors, which are located on post-synaptic cells as well as on the terminals of other neurons. Endorphins, along with blocking the perception of pain, modulate dopamine transmission in the brain. Thus, users not only have the sensation of pain masked by taking drugs such as Demerol, OxyContin, and heroin, but they also obtain an artificially induced sense of euphoria.

Gamma-aminobutyric Acid (GABA)

GABA is an amino acid that acts as a depressant transmitter countering feelings of anxiety in the brain that create awareness of danger or threat in a person's environment. It works by occupying receptor sites and preventing their stimulation. The message that GABA transmits is an inhibitory one: it tells the neurons that it contacts to slow down or stop firing. As approximately 40 percent of the millions of neurons throughout the brain respond to GABA, this means that GABA has a general quietening influence on the entire brain, working as the body's natural calming agent. As well, when GABA molecules are inhibited by CNS depressants such as alcohol, barbiturates, and benzodiazepines, an increased amount of dopamine is released, which produces the sensation of euphoria.

Glutamate

Glutamic acid or glutamate is an excitatory neurotransmitter. It is the base chemical from which GABA, an inhibitory neurotransmitter, is synthesized. Thus the two balance each other. Glutamate itself is linked to memory and learning, and an association has been made between glutamate modulation and the development of attention-deficit/hyperactivity disorder (Petroff, 2002).

Norepinephrine

Norepinephrine is also a monoamine catecholamine. It is released by the adrenal gland and acts not only as a neurotransmitter, but also as a hormone. In its hormonal form, it works in conjunction with adrenaline and epinephrine to provide a boost to the body in stressful situations. It provides a burst of energy when a person is experiencing a fight/flight response. Its hormonal activity is also associated with decrease in appetite, and thus too much norepinephrine can create anorectic outcomes on the body. Its function as a neurotransmitter relates to both depression and mania. Inhibiting the reuptake of norepinephrine aids in alleviating depression, while elevated levels of this neurotransmitter can lead to mania.

Serotonin

Serotonin is referred to by some as the happiness transmitter. It too is monoamine but it belongs to the indolamine group. This neurochemical is responsible for reducing depression, alleviating anxiety, elevating mood, and increasing feelings of self-worth. It is closely associated with a new group of antidepressant drugs that includes Prozac, Paxil, Zoloft, Luvox, Lexapro, and Celexa. However, excessive amounts of serotonin can produce hallucinations.

Pharmacodynamics

Tolerance and withdrawal are two key components related to physical dependency that fall under the broader category of pharmacodynamics, which is an examination of what drugs do to the body.

Tolerance

Even though the DSM-V classified tolerance as simply another criteria to describe substance use disorders, it remains a significant contributing factor in the process of addiction development. After repeated use of a drug, the user may become more resistant to its effects. This loss of sensitivity is known as tolerance. Tolerance simply means that the body has adapted to the presence of the drug. With many chemical agents, the brain becomes used to the substance and the original effects of the drug diminish over time. Tolerant individuals may appear to walk and talk with no impairment but more complex and less observable behaviours, such as precise judgment or fine motor skills, will still be negatively affected. Tolerance may occur to both the desired effects of the drug of choice as well as to its adverse effects. Tolerance typically occurs after a period of chronic exposure, though for some drugs, like hallucinogens, it can occur after a single use.

Acute tolerance is evidenced in those persons who appear to become less intoxicated the more they drink. For these persons, there is a greater degree of impairment at the start of a drinking session than at its conclusion. With the chronic use of drugs such as alcohol, the liver also becomes slightly more efficient in breaking down the substance, requiring more to be taken to obtain the desired effect. The most common example of tolerance is the person who can "really hold his liquor." This is merely one indication of an individual who consumes alcohol on a regular basis.

Tolerance can be categorized as either dispositional—when the liver is able to process the drug more efficiently and excrete it faster from the body—or functional, also known as metabolic or pharmacodynamic tolerance. Functional tolerance occurs when actual physical changes take place in the body's receptors or when receptor sensitivity is altered. Drug sensitivity may also decrease over the course of a small number of administrations.

Functional tolerance development depends on a variety of factors, including:

- the pharmacological properties of the drug that is administered
- the effect being measured
- the selected dose, as generally the greater the dose, the faster the rate of tolerance development
- previous drug history, for if a person has been tolerant in the past, tolerance will develop much more quickly on subsequent drug exposures
- behavioural demands (If drug users are required to handle complex tasks during periods of intoxication, they will quickly develop tolerance to those drug effects that adversely affect their performance of that particular task.)
- behaviourally augmented tolerances
- the setting in which use takes place (If a person administers a drug in the same room each day, his or her body learns to expect the substance in that room. Conditioned compensatory changes occur in his or her brain that reduce the intensity of the experienced effect. If the same amount is consumed in a different environment, the person can overdose.) (Sproule, 2004)

In many instances, once an individual becomes tolerant to the effects of one drug, she or he will also show tolerance to other psychoactive drugs with similar effects on the central nervous system. This is called cross-tolerance. A phenomenon often referred to as reverse tolerance or sensitization has been noted with some drugs, notably hallucinogens, in which the desired effects may reportedly be achieved with smaller doses after the initial experience with the drug. Learning, environmental, and pharmacological mechanisms have been suggested to underlie this process. Finally, there is tachyphylaxis, a term derived from the Greek *tachys*, meaning "rapid," and *phylaxis*, meaning "protection," but which equates to nearly complete tolerance. This sudden decline in a drug effect could follow either one administration of that drug or multiple administrations of small doses. The underlying cause of this phenomenon might be a significant decrease of the neurotransmitter that mediates the drug effects or an acute downgrading of the available drug or neurotransmitter receptors. This downgrading could be due to the saturation of these receptors and commonly occurs with most hallucinogens, save cannabis, after only two or three days of consecutive use. It can also occur with psychotherapeutic agents, and if these are being used to help regulate a person's emotional state or behaviour, the consequences can be substantive.

Withdrawal

Withdrawal is the development of physical disturbances or physical illness when drug use is suddenly discontinued. It is the rebound effect that is a component of the process of physical dependence. When a drug ceases to be administered, the compensatory mechanisms cause a temporary overactivity of the cells; this overactivity, or rebounding, is the basis for withdrawal symptoms. The severity of the withdrawal reaction after stopping drug use is not necessarily related to the severity of dependence. Withdrawal from depressants generally results in symptoms of acute and toxic hyperactivation and physiological arousal, while the pattern following intense stimulant use usually involves sedation, depression, and extensive sleep to compensate for the artificially produced overarousal. Withdrawal symptoms can be prevented or promptly relieved by the use of the original drug, or one that is pharmacologically equivalent: the hair of the dog.

1.3 PHARMACOKINETICS
Routes of Administration
Distribution of Drugs throughout the Body
Breakdown and Elimination

Pharmacokinetics is the part of pharmacology that deals with how a drug gets from the external world into the body and to the specific site in the brain where it produces its effect. It involves the study of how a psychoactive drug is administered, absorbed, distributed, metabolized, and finally eliminated by the body. This is an extremely complex process, with a variety of factors being responsible for the effect, if any, that a psychoactive drug has. Three critical pharmacokinetics factors are

- how we get the drug into our body or the route of administration;
- distribution of the drug by the circulating blood to the various parts of the body; and
- the eventual breakdown of the drug into an inactive compound: metabolization and elimination.

Routes of Administration

Drugs can be administered in a variety of ways that determine both how quickly and how an individual's reaction to the drug will be:

- oral administration—through the mouth to the stomach and the intestines
- across mucous membranes—in the nose, gums, rectum, and vagina
- injection—directly into the vein, muscle, or under the skin
- inhalation—through the lungs
- transdermal—across the skin (see Table 1.1)

Oral Administration

In this commonly used process of drug administration, the substance is swallowed and is turned into a fluid in the stomach (if it is not already in that form). From the stomach, it moves to the small intestine, where it penetrates the lining. It then passes into the bloodstream, after being processed by the liver, and eventually reaches the central nervous system. How much of the drug is absorbed depends on its solubility—how efficiently it is turned into liquid in the stomach—and its permeability—how well it passes through the lining of the intestine, as well as by the presence or absence of food in the digestive tract. The more food that is present, the slower the entire process.

Alcohol is a pharmacological exception. Ethyl alcohol, that is, beverage alcohol, is absorbed directly through the stomach wall into the bloodstream and then moved to the central nervous system once it has been processed by the liver. This is faster than the route through the intestinal lining, especially on an empty stomach. However, when the stomach is full, the alcohol is absorbed by the food and is then processed by the intestine, slowing the rate of absorption.

Drugs administered orally in a liquid form are absorbed more rapidly than tablets or capsules. Sometimes drugs in tablet form, especially illicit ones, are poorly manufactured. They may not dissolve at all or may become encapsulated by food and will pass through both the stomach and the intestine and be excreted without ever being absorbed into the bloodstream. They thus never affect the central nervous system. There are several significant disadvantages with oral administration:

- losing the drug through vomiting
- stomach discomfort
- inability to accurately calculate the amount of the drug absorbed
- slowness of the process relative to other options

When administered orally, enzymes in the stomach and intestine can destroy some non-psychoactive drugs, such as insulin, before they can be absorbed. Likewise, cocaine, when administered orally, is metabolized in such a way that little if any psychoactive effect is produced in the central nervous system.

Across Mucous Membranes

Fewer layers of cells exist in mucous membrane areas than in other parts of the body, allowing for the quick absorption of psychoactive agents. Mucous membrane is found in the nose, lips, gums, vagina, and rectum. Drugs that can be sniffed, such as cocaine hydrochloride, stick to the nasal membranes and are transferred into the bloodstream and then to the central nervous system. Nicotine from chewing tobacco and pipe smoke crosses the mouth membrane into the blood and then moves to the CNS. Drugs administered in the form of suppositories are useful if a person is vomiting, unconscious, or unable to swallow. However, absorption is irregular and unpredictable across all mucous membranes, and many psychoactive drugs administered in this manner irritate the mucous membranes. More substantive long-term issues associated with this method of administration include the development of a deviated septum and oral cancers of the mouth and gums.

Injection

Natural biological barriers are bypassed by directly injecting a drug into the body. There are three ways in which to inject drugs:

- Intravenously: Injecting the drug directly into a vein is the fastest of the three injection options, with the initial effect generally perceived within 10 and 15 seconds.
- Subcutaneous: Injecting the drug just under the skin is also referred to as "skin popping." The effect takes place 5–10 minutes after the injection, depending on how quickly the drug penetrates the walls of the blood vessels and the rate of blood flow through the skin. Some users have been known to inject the drug between their toes to minimize the puncture marks that accumulate with multiple injections.
- Intramuscular: Injecting the drug into the skeletal muscle of the arms, legs, or buttocks is the slowest of the three injection methods, taking between 10 and 15 minutes to produce a psychoactive effect. However, this method of absorption is still quicker than when the drug is processed through the stomach. Absorption after an intramuscular injection is also dependent on the rate of blood flow to that muscle.

Advantages of injecting psychoactive drugs include the quickness and accuracy of dosage. The drawbacks include the lack of time to respond to an unexpected reaction or overdose, the painfulness of an injection, and the inability to recall the drug. The necessity of a sterile needle, especially in light of HIV risk, is a significant factor to consider, especially when injecting street drugs.

Inhalation

Gases such as nitrous oxide pass through the lung membranes and into the blood and to the CNS extremely quickly, in as little as 8–10 seconds. The almost immediate effect is a direct result of the large surface area of the lung. Nicotine in cigarettes and THC, the psychoactive agent found in marijuana smoke, act somewhat differently. These drugs are contained in small particles carried in the smoke, and although absorption is still quick, not all the drug particles get through. Thus, absorption is not as efficient as with other gases. Cocaine, which has anaesthetic properties, in the crack form is absorbed faster through the lungs than across the mucous membranes of the nose—even faster than when it is directly injected into a vein.

Transdermal

This is the least common method of administration, as few psychoactive substances are able to pass through the skin and reach the central nervous system via this organ. Also, as transdermal administration is a relatively slow means of producing an effect in the CNS, it is not a primary means of ingesting drugs. The primary psychoactive substances that can be used transdermally are opioids, used with individuals in chronic pain or who are terminally ill; nicotine in the form of a nicotine patch; and occasionally LSD, though the latter is primarily ingested orally.

TABLE 1.1: ROUTES OF ADMINISTRATION

Method	Example of Drug	Time Needed for Effect	Advantages of Route	Disadvantages of Route
oral	alcohol	30–60 minutes	convenient	slow, irregular
mucous membrane	cocaine	1–2 minutes	convenient	local tissue damage
intravenous injection	heroin	15 seconds	fast	overdose, infections
subcutaneous injection	heroin	5–10 minutes	safer and easier than intravenous	infection
intramuscular injection	morphine	10–15 minutes	controlled	painful
inhalation	nicotine	8 seconds	fast	lung damage
transdermal	nicotine	15–20 minutes	convenient	limited application

Distribution of Drugs throughout the Body

Substances are distributed throughout the body by the circulation of the blood. Once a psychoactive drug is absorbed into the blood, it is carried to most parts of the body, including the central nervous system, within a minute. However, psychoactive drugs create their effects by reaching specific cells found only in the CNS. To do so, the drug molecule must be small enough to pass through the pores in capillaries from the veins and then through the cell walls. Drug molecules must also be lipid (fat) soluble. The greater the lipid solubility of a drug, the easier the drug passes from the blood into the brain. The vast majority of psychoactive drugs are highly lipid soluble, meaning they pass easily into the brain to produce their effects. Ionization, which is the positive or negative charge a drug carries, is also a factor. Drugs with little ionization pass through lipid membranes more easily. The lower the ionization of a drug, either positive or negative, the more likely it will alter the CNS.

Breakdown and Elimination

The liver is the body's detoxification centre. For a drug to be removed from the bloodstream and to no longer affect the CNS, it must be metabolized by enzymes in the liver and eliminated from the body primarily in the form of urine or feces. Drugs must first be metabolized or changed so that they cannot pass from the kidney back into the blood. Anaesthetic gases and volatile drugs are eliminated through the lungs, as is approximately 5 percent of all beverage alcohol consumed. Other sites of elimination are the sweat glands, saliva, and breast milk.

After a drug is totally absorbed into the body, the concentration in the blood soon starts to fall. This drop is initially rapid because of the movement of the drug from the bloodstream into the body's tissues. The rate of decline slows as excretion begins. The rate of decline depends on both the type of drug and the concentration of the drug in the blood. The higher the drug concentration, the faster metabolism and excretion will proceed. This variability makes it difficult to compare the rate of metabolism of one drug to that of another. To address this difficulty, the concept of "half-life" was borrowed from nuclear physics. Half-life is a measure of the rate of metabolism of a drug. It indicates the length of time required for a drug's blood concentration to fall by one-half. By knowing the half-life of a drug, one can better assess the appropriate dosage, frequency, and amount required to treat a specific medical condition. In the later stages of metabolism and excretion, the half-life of a drug is constant, no matter how high the concentration actually is. The half-life of many drugs increases with the user's age. This may be due to increased amounts of body fat, which acts as a reservoir for highly lipid soluble drugs, or from impaired liver or kidney function. Ethyl alcohol, however, does not have a half-life, but rather is eliminated at a constant rate from the body (Sproule, 2004).

1.4 INCIDENCE OF DRUG USE AND ECONOMIC IMPLICATIONS
Global
Canada
Economic Implications

Global

It is estimated that, worldwide, half the adult population uses psychoactive drugs on a regular basis, excluding caffeine. Approximately 2 billion adults consume alcohol and 1 billion adults, one-quarter of the adult population of earth, smoke cigarettes (Anderson, 2006). In 2009, there were an estimated 149–271 million illicit drug users worldwide: 125–203 million cannabis users; 15–39 million problem users of opioids, amphetamines, or cocaine; and 11–21 million who injected drugs. While illicit drug use occurs among those individuals and nations of lower socio-economic status, it is greater in high-income countries and in nations neighbouring major drug production areas. Illicit opioid use is a major cause of mortality from overdose, HIV, hepatitis C and hepatitis B infections, and from unsafe injection practices. Adverse health outcomes such as mental health issues, traffic collisions, suicide, and violence are increased in illicit opioid, cocaine, and amphetamine users as compared to the non-using population (Degenhardt & Hall, 2012). While illicit drug use is a substantial global cause of premature mortality and morbidity, and globally, alcohol is used 10 times more than are illicit drugs, it is tobacco that contributes to disease burden more than any other psychoactive agent. Almost 6 million people die from tobacco use annually. At the current rate of consumption, tobacco is expected to kill 7.5 million people annually worldwide by 2020, accounting for 10 percent of all deaths. Smoking causes an estimated 71 percent of lung cancers, 42 percent of chronic respiratory disease, and almost 10 percent of cardiovascular disease. While illicit drug deaths combined account for less than 1 million deaths annually, and the concentration of illicit drug deaths occurs among younger people, tobacco deaths occur primarily among middle-aged and older adults (Degenhardt & Hall, 2012). North America has the highest mortality rate from illicit drugs in the world, at 155.8 per 1 million for those ages 15–64 (International Narcotics Control Board, 2014).

The consumer market for cannabis is more than 200 million people globally, though relative use remains low at 3–5 percent of the global population. Worldwide, the cannabis market continues to expand, with almost two-thirds of the nations who report drug use ranking cannabis as the primary illicit substance of abuse. Cannabis is being cultivated and seized in almost all countries in Africa. Nigeria remains the country with the largest seizures of cannabis, followed by Egypt. There was a tenfold increase in seizures of cannabis in Mozambique from 2010 to 2011, and a twofold increase in seizures in Burkina Faso from 2009 to 2011. Morocco, along with Afghanistan, remains the biggest source of cannabis resin in the world, although production in Morocco is decreasing. Spain remains the main entry point in Europe for cannabis resin originating in Morocco and the gateway to markets in Western and Central Europe. Cannabis originating in Afghanistan finds its way to Europe through Asian as well as North African smuggling routes. Egyptian authorities seized 3 tons of such cannabis on the shores of the Red Sea in a single operation in 2012. North America, Europe, and Africa are regions where cannabis use is greatest. It is estimated that in Africa, 7.5 percent of the population ages 15–64 use the drug, nearly double the global average. Paraguay is currently the largest cannabis producer in South America and accounts for 15 percent of the world's production. A total of 134 of the world's nations reported the cultivation of cannabis over the 1995–2005 period, with 146 countries reporting seizing cannabis plants over the same period (International Narcotics Control Board, 2014; United Nations Office on Drugs and Crime [UNODC], 2014).

Close to 25 million people in the world, or 0.6 percent of the population ages 15–64, consumed amphetamines in 2008. This is more than the number of adults who used either cocaine or heroin. This number has changed very little since the beginning of the new millennium. More than half of the world's amphetamines users live in Asia, with the majority being from East and Southeast Asia. The total number of amphetamines users in North America is estimated at 3.8 million people, and in Europe, at 2.8 million people, with North America accounting for about 15 percent and Europe 11 percent of the global total. The number of amphetamines users in Africa is estimated at 2.1 million, and in South America, including the Caribbean and Central America, at 1.9 million people, with each region accounting for approximately 8 percent of all adult users. The largest numbers of the world's estimated 14–21 million cocaine users are found in North America (6.4 million), followed by Western and Central Europe (3.9 million), South America (2.2 million), Africa (1.1 million), and Asia (0.3 million). Coca bush cultivation, which remains limited to a small portion of South America, namely Bolivia, Colombia and Peru, continued to decline with the net area under coca bush cultivation on December 31, 2012, totalling 133,700 hectares, a decline of 14 percent from the previous year's estimates and the lowest levels since the beginning of available estimates in 1990 (UNODC, 2008, 2014).

Global opioid abuse has stabilized at an estimated 15.6 million people, or 0.4 percent of the world's population ages 15–64. More than half of the world's illicit opioid users live in Asia, with the highest levels of abuse occurring along the main drug trafficking routes out of Afghanistan. Annual prevalence of opioids, including heroin, is high in the Islamic Republic of Iran, where the number of drug abusers is said to exceed 1.2 million or 2.8 percent of the general population ages 15–64. However, when licit use of opioids is factored in, a very different scenario emerges. Table 1.2 highlights nations with the lowest and highest total per capita opioid use rather than only illicit use. Nations with the least use are led by Nigeria, an African nation, followed by two countries in the heart of heroin production. Those at the top of the list are all developed nations, with Canada being the leader. After years of decline, the global area under illicit opium poppy cultivation in 2013 was 296,720 hectares, the highest level since 1998 when estimates became available. Thus, despite substantive successes in the reduction of cultivation and production in the Golden Triangle (Myanmar, Laos, Thailand), the overall global production of opium has increased by one-half since 1998, primarily in Afghanistan (UNODC, 2008, 2014).

TABLE 1.2: COMPARISON OF PER CAPITA OPIOID CONSUMPTION IN MORPHINE EQUIVALENCE AMONG LOWEST AND HIGHEST CONSUMPTION COUNTRIES, 2011

Lowest Consumption Countries	(mg per capita of morphine equivalence)	Highest Consumption Countries	(mg per capita of morphine equivalence)
Nigeria	0.0141	Canada	812.1855
Myanmar	0.0152	United States	749.7859
Pakistan	0.0184	Denmark	483.1678
		Australia	427.1240

Source: United Nations Office on Drugs and Crime (2014)

Worldwide consumption of alcohol in 2010 was equal to 6.2 L of pure alcohol consumed per person ages 15 years or older, which translates into 13.5 g of pure alcohol per day. Approximately 16.0 percent of drinkers ages 15 years or older engage in heavy episodic or binge drinking. Use of alcohol is a component cause of more than 200 disease and injury conditions, with direct alcohol-related deaths accounting for 3.8 percent of all deaths worldwide. More than half of these deaths occur from non-communicable diseases, including cancer, heart disease, and liver cirrhosis. However, when secondary factors such as drinking and driving deaths are added, the figure rises to 5.9 percent. Figure 1.2 illustrates per capita alcohol consumption in litres by nation. It is not surprising that the lowest consumption levels are found in nations with predominantly Muslim populations: Pakistan, Libya, and Kuwait. However, it is surprising that in nations where alcohol use is theoretically forbidden through religious edicts, individuals consume alcohol at all, let alone report it, especially when in some cases public use can lead to public caning or whipping. Likewise, few would be surprised that nations such as Russia, Lithuania, Moldova, and Belarus lead the world in average alcohol consumption. However, in general, the greater the economic wealth of a country, the more alcohol is consumed, and the fewer the number of abstainers. As a rule, high-income countries have the highest alcohol per capita consumption and the highest prevalence of binge drinking. However, people with lower socio-economic status appear to be more vulnerable to tangible problems and consequences of alcohol consumption, primarily because of a lack of resources to address their use once it becomes problematic (World Health Organization, 2011, 2014).

FIGURE 1.2: PER CAPITA ALCOHOL CONSUMPTION IN LITRES, 2010

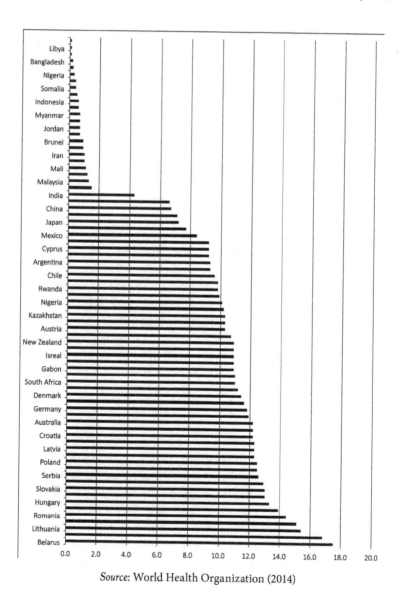

Source: World Health Organization (2014)

The demand for drug abuse treatment is another important indicator for assessing the world drug situation, as it reveals the drugs that place the largest burden on national health systems. Of the 25 million people (0.6 percent of the world's population ages 15–65) estimated to be heavily drug-dependent, about one out of six actually receives treatment, with an annual cost of $35 billion USD. In Africa, only 1 in 18 problem drug users receives treatment. In Latin America, the Caribbean, and Eastern and Southeastern Europe, approximately 1 in 11 problem drug users receives treatment, while in North America, an estimated one in three problem drug users receives treatment intervention of some type. If all dependent drug users had received treatment in 2010, the cost of such treatment would have been an estimated $200–$250 billion, or 0.3–0.4 percent of the global gross domestic product (GDP), which is still far less than the money earned through the illicit drug trade. Research findings clearly show that investment in treatment is cost-effective compared with the cost of untreated and continuing abuse. Research conducted in the United States reveals that every dollar invested in treatment yields a return of between $4 and $12 in reduced crime and health care costs.

In Asia and Europe, home to more than 70 percent of the world's total population, opioids account for the bulk of drug-related treatment demand, while in South America, cocaine continues to account for most of the drug abuse treatment (48 percent). High proportions of cocaine-related treatment demand are also encountered in North America (40 percent), while in Asia, cocaine-related treatment remains negligible. Most of the demand for drug-related treatment in Africa is related to cannabis abuse. Treatment demand for cannabis has increased globally over the past decade as THC content has risen. In the United States, between 2006 and 2010, there was a 59 percent increase in cannabis-related emergency department visits and a 14 percent increase in cannabis treatment admissions. This is in part because of increased use but also because tetrahydrocannabinol (THC) levels in seized or eradicated cannabis crops in the United States increased from 8.7 percent in 2007 to 11.9 percent in 2011 (UNODC, 2008, 2014).

Canada

Beer and liquor stores and agencies sold $21.4 billion worth of alcoholic beverages during the fiscal year ending March 31, 2013, up 2.2 percent from the previous year, which equates to a per capita use of $708.80. Beer remained the alcoholic drink of choice for Canadians, with $9.1 billion in sales, but the market share of wine continued to grow. The growth rate in wine sales (+4.9 percent) in 2013 outpaced that of spirits (+2.9 percent) and beer (-0.1 percent). The overall increase in alcoholic beverage sales slowed in 2013, with all three market segments (beer, wine, spirits) recording lower growth rates compared with a year earlier. New Brunswick had the lowest average per capita use at $646.60 per person, while those living in the Yukon spent the most on alcohol, more than double the amount spent in New Brunswick, at $1,319.60 per person (Statistics Canada, 2014). Health Canada's (2014a) national survey reported that 91.0 percent of Canadians 15 and older had in their lifetime consumed alcohol, with the average age of first drink being 16. In the past 12 months, the number of adult drinkers was 78.4 percent, of which 12.8 percent indicated they had exceeded the low-risk drinking guidelines once during the past year, whereas nearly one in five, or 18.6 percent, reported binge drinking on multiple occasions.

Approximately 4.6 million (16.1 percent of) Canadians smoked tobacco in 2013 (a dramatic decrease from 1965 when nearly half of Canadians did so), with 11.9 percent being regular smokers and more men (18.4 percent) than women (13.9 percent) presently using tobacco products. Smoking was most prevalent in Newfoundland/Labrador (19.7 percent) and Saskatchewan (18.5 percent) and least common in Prince Edward Island (15.2 percent) and Nova Scotia (15.6 percent). Daily smokers averaged 15 cigarettes per day. Surprisingly, use was highest among young adults ages 25–34 (21.8 percent) and 20–24 (20.3 percent). Canadians with a university degree were less likely to be smokers compared to those who had not attended a post-secondary institution (Reid, Hammond, Rynard, & Burkhalter, 2014).

Lifetime cannabis use was reported at 41.5 percent, while cannabis use in the past year was 20 percent among Canadians 24 years of age and younger and 8.4 percent of those 25 and older, with average age of first use being 16 for those under 25 and 19 for those over 25. British Columbia (13.8 percent) and Manitoba (13.2 percent) reported the highest percentage of cannabis users, with New Brunswick (8.5 percent) and Quebec (9.0 percent) reporting the lowest. Illicit drug use remained low among the general Canadian population, with 1.1 percent reporting cocaine or crack use, less than 1.0 percent methamphetamine/crystal meth use, 0.6 percent reporting ecstasy use, with other hallucinogen use being reported at 1.1 percent. As with cannabis, the majority of these users were under the age of 25. This pattern of illicit drug use has been consistent across time as less than 1.0 percent of Canadians reported the use of cocaine, heroin, or LSD in the 1990s as well (Single, Brewster, MacNeil, Hatcher, & Trainor, 1995).

Prescription opioid use was reported by 16.9 percent of those surveyed, with 10.2 percent reporting the use of benzodiazepines. The coroner's office in Nova Scotia identified just under 300 prescription deaths between 2007 and 2010, a rate of 7.8 per 100,000, which was over four times the number of deaths from illicit drugs. Between 1991 and 2004, opioid-related deaths doubled in Ontario and then doubled again between 2004 and 2012 when the highest single-year number was reported at 536. Likewise the number of opioid-specific treatment requests doubled between 2006 and 2012 (Health Canada, 2014a).

TABLE 1.3: STUDENT DRUG USE BY PROVINCE, GRADES 7–12

	Province								
	British Columbia	Alberta	Manitoba	Ontario	Quebec	New Brunswick	Prince Edward Island	Nova Scotia	New-foundland & Labrador
Depressants									
Alcohol	50.4%	48.5%	54.8%	61.8%	59.7%	50.3%	46.3%	51.7%	52.0%
Alcohol (binge drinking)	23.6%	19.3%	26.7%	26.9%	*	25.3%	26.1%	27.7%	29.7%
Inhalants	3.8%	5.3%	2.2%	8.7%	0.8%	2.6%	3.6%	4.4%	4.4%
Heroin	1.3%	0.8%	0.8%	1.1%	*	*	*	*	*
Stimulants									
Amphet-amines/ Metham-phetamine	2.2%	1.5%	2.8%	1.9%	7.3%	2.1%	1.2%	1.6%	2.4%
Cocaine	4.4%	3.3%	3.9%	4.2%	3.4%	2.9%	3.4%	4.3%	5.3%
Tobacco	3.0%	4.0%	5.0%	4.0%	5.0%	9.0%	7.0%	5.0%	6.0%
Hallucinogens									
Cannabis (past month use)	17.1%	9.3%	13.4%	16.8%	27.2%	11.3%	9.2%	13.7%	12.2%
Cannabis (daily)	3.6%	*	4.3%	2.6%	2.6%	4.0%	2.2%	5.3%	4.6%
LSD	*	*	*	*	*	4.3%	2.5%	3.7%	4.2%
MDMA (Ecstasy)	7.1%	5.7%	4.5%	4.4%	5.7%	5.2%	3.4%	6.9%	7.2%
Psyilocybin/ Mescaline	*	*	*	*	*	5.5%	4.9%	7.7%	4.2%

* data not collected

* *Note*: Saskatchewan does not collect information on student use of tobacco.

Sources: Propel Centre for Population Health Impact (2014); Young (2011)

Table 1.3 examines Canadian adolescent drug use by province. As with adults, the most common licit drug used after caffeine is alcohol, while cannabis is the most commonly used illicit drug. Overall use levels are lower than that of adults across all categories, with the inhalant category being the exception. The Centre for Addiction and Mental Health and its predecessor, the Addiction Research Foundation, have been tracking psychoactive drug use among teens in Ontario since the 1970s and have been able to develop trend data across 30 years (Table 1.4). In the past 30 years, the use of various drugs has dropped, increased, and plateaued at different times, and while there have been exceptions, such as methamphetamine use at the end of the 1990s and cocaine use at the beginning of the new millennium, the overall trend in use has been a downward one. Tobacco in particular is used by far fewer adolescents in Ontario, as is the case with alcohol, though, interestingly, cannabis levels remain at about the same rate. Also of note is that the study no longer tracks the amount of prescription psychoactive drugs authorized by physicians. This is an issue of ongoing concern, giving the medicalization of behavioural disorders such as anxiety and attention-deficit/hyperactivity and the increasing rate of prescription-related deaths among adults.

Economic Implications

Table 1.5 highlights the social and economic costs of alcohol abuse for a range of countries over nearly two decades. Economic costs range from $0.5 billion for Portugal (the first nation to adopt a decriminalization approach to drugs where drug trafficking is still prosecuted as a criminal offence, but drug possession for personal use is an administrative offence) to $193.5 billion in the United States, which has a far larger population but also far harsher penalties for illicit drug use. Lost productivity in the United States as a result of labour non-participation is a significant component of this cost. Studies in Australia and Canada identified losses of 0.3 percent of GDP and 0.4 percent of GDP, respectively. In those developed nations, the cost of lost productivity was estimated to be eight and three times higher, respectively, than health-related costs due to morbidity, ambulatory care, physician visits, and other related consequences. However, it is China that now consumes approximately 20 percent of the world's alcohol, with a value of nearly $60 billion, and that openly promotes the use of tobacco, which may have the greatest economic and health issues related to drug use. However, the Chinese government has yet to estimate what the economic and social costs of this level of consumption is or might become over time if use continues to increase (International Narcotics Control Board, 2014; Levy, Meek, & Rosenberg, 2014; Thavorncharoensap, Teerawattananon, Yothasamut, Lertpitakpong, & Chaikledkaew, 2009; World Health Organization, 2004).

TABLE 1.4: ONTARIO STUDENT PAST-YEAR DRUG USE (AT LEAST ONE USE)

Year	1977	1979	1981	1983	1985	1987	1989	1991	1993
Number	4,687	4,794	3,270	4,737	4,154	4,267	3,915	3,945	3,571
Depressants									
Alcohol	76.3%	76.9%	75.3%	71.7%	69.8%	68.1%	66.2%	58.7%	56.5%
Inhalants	9.1%	9.4%	5.3%	6.2%	3.8%	5.1%	4.2%	2.3%	3.4%
Medical Barbiturates	14.2%	12.8%	12.5%	11.0%	9.0%	7.8%	7.8%	4.4%	5.6%
Non-Medical Barbiturates	6.0%	6.8%	8.1%	6.0%	4.4%	3.3%	2.2%	2.2%	3.0%
Medical Sedative-Hypnotics	8.6%	6.9%	7.5%	6.5%	4.7%	4.9%	3.1%	2.9%	2.2%
Non-Medical Sedative-Hypnotics	4.9%	5.9%	4.9%	5.0%	3.3%	3.0%	2.4%	1.6%	1.1%
Opioids									
Heroin	2.0%	2.3%	1.5%	1.6%	1.5%	1.4%	1.2%	1.0%	1.2%
Non-Medical Opioids	*	*	*	*	*	*	*	*	*
Oxycontin/Oxyneo	*	*	*	*	*	*	*	*	*
Stimulants									
ADHD Drugs	*	*	*	*	*	*	*	*	*
Cocaine	3.8%	5.1%	4.8%	4.1%	4.5%	3.8%	2.7%	1.6%	1.5%
Crack	*	*	*	*	*	1.4%	1.0%	1.1%	1.0%
Medical Stimulants	6.6%	5.9%	6.1%	5.2%	4.3%	4.3%	3.3%	2.6%	4.0%
Non-Medical Stimulants	7.2%	10.6%	12.1%	15.4%	11.8%	7.9%	6.5%	4.0%	5.4%
Methamphetamine	2.7%	3.6%	3.0%	3.9%	3.1%	3.1%	2.5%	1.8%	2.0%
Tobacco	30.4%	34.7%	30.3%	29.1%	24.5%	24.0%	23.3%	21.7%	23.8%
Hallucinogens									
Cannabis	25.0%	31.7%	29.9%	23.7%	21.2%	15.9%	14.1%	11.7%	12.7%
Jimson Weed	*	*	*	*	*	*	*	*	*
Ketamine	*	*	*	*	*	*	*	*	*
LSD	6.1%	8.6%	10.2%	8.6%	7.4%	5.9%	5.9%	5.2%	6.9%
MDMA (Ecstasy)	*	*	*	*	*	*	*	*	0.6%
PCP	*	*	2.5%	2.0%	1.7%	1.3%	1.1%	0.5%	0.6%
Psyilocybin/Mescaline	4.3%	5.3%	4.7%	6.0%	4.8%	4.5%	4.3%	3.3%	3.1%
Salvia Divinorum	*	*	*	*	*	*	*	*	*

1995	1997	1999	2001	2003	2005	2007	2009	2011	2013
3,870	3,990	4,447	3,898	6,616	7,726	6,323	9,112	9,288	10,272
58.8%	59.6%	66.0%	63.9%	66.2%	62.0%	61.2%	58.2%	54.9%	49.5%
4.8%	3.5%	9.6%	7.6%	7.0%	6.0%	6.4%	6.0%	5.6%	3.4%
4.8%	6.0%	12.3%	11.8%	*	*	*	*	*	*
2.7%	2.5%	4.4%	4.0%	2.5%	1.7%	*	*	*	*
1.8%	2.1%	3.3%	3.2%	*	*	*	*	*	*
1.6%	1.7%	2.0%	2.2%	2.2%	1.6%	1.8%	1.6%	1.9%	2.4%
2.0%	1.8%	1.9%	1.1%	1.4%	0.9%	0.9%	0.7%	*	*
*	*	*	*	*	*	20.6%	17.8%	14.0%	12.4%
*	*	*	*	*	1.0%	1.8%	1.6%	1.2%	1.6%
*	*	*	*	*	*	1.0%	1.6%	1.0%	1.4%
2.4%	2.7%	3.4%	4.4%	4.8%	4.4%	3.4%	2.6%	2.1%	2.4%
1.7%	2.2%	2.5%	2.1%	2.7%	2.0%	1.0%	1.0%	0.7%	0.7%
4.1%	3.7%	6.8%	7.0%	*	*	*	*	*	*
6.3%	6.6%	7.3%	6.3%	5.8%	4.8%	5.7%	4.8%	4.1%	*
4.6%	3.6%	5.0%	3.9%	3.3%	2.2%	1.4%	1.6%	1.0%	1.0%
27.9%	27.6%	28.4%	23.1%	19.2%	14.4%	11.9%	11.7%	8.7%	8.5%
22.7%	24.9%	28.0%	28.6%	29.6%	26.5%	25.6%	25.6%	22.0%	23.0%
*	*	*	*	*	*	2.6%	2.3%	1.7%	1.3%
*	*	*	*	2.2%	1.3%	1.1%	1.6%	0.9%	*
9.2%	7.6%	6.8%	4.8%	2.9%	1.7%	1.6%	1.8%	1.2%	1.5%
1.8%	3.1%	4.0%	6.0%	4.1%	4.5%	3.5%	3.2%	3.3%	3.3%
1.7%	2.0%	3.0%	2.8%	2.2%	1.1%	0.7%	*	*	*
7.6%	10.1%	12.8%	11.1%	10.0%	6.7%	5.5%	5.0%	3.8%	3.7%
*	*	*	*	*	*	*	4.4%	3.7%	2.6%

* = data not collected

Note: Includes all data for Grades 7, 9, 11, and 13 until Grade 13 was eliminated, and then includes data for Grades 7, 9, 11, and 12.

Source: Boak, Hamilton, Adlaf, & Mann (2013)

TABLE 1.5: SOCIAL AND ECONOMIC COSTS OF ALCOHOL ABUSE BY NATION

Country	Year of Study	Population (millions)	Total Cost Estimate (billions of dollars)
Australia	1988	16.5	4.0
Australia	1998–1999	18.7	7.5
Canada	1992	28.3	7.5
Canada	2002	31.3	14.6
Chile	2000	15.2	3.0
Finland	1990	5.0	4.0
Germany	2002	82.5	27.4
Ireland	2000	3.8	2.4
Italy	2003	57.3	7.6
Japan	1987	122.1	5.7
Netherlands	2001	15.8	4.0
Portugal	1995	10.0	0.5
Scotland	2005–2006	5.1	2.25
South Korea	2000	47.0	0.15
Thailand	2006	65.9	4.75
United Kingdom	2000	59.4	23.6
United States	1998	283.2	184.6
United States	2011	311.6	193.5

Sources: Thavorncharoensap, Teerawattananon, Yothasamut, Lertpitakpong, & Chaikledkaew (2009); World Health Organization (2004, 2014)

In Canada the last complete estimate of the total cost of all substance abuse is more than a decade old, having been completed in 2002. At that time it was estimated that the total cost of substance abuse ran just under $40 billion, or approximately $1,267 per person per year. Of this, 80 percent was a result of the consumption of legal substances, primarily alcohol and tobacco, and only 20 percent a result of all illicit drug consumption (Rehm et al., 2006). A decade earlier the estimated cost had been $18.5 billion (Single, Robson, Xie, & Rehm, 1996). The highest contributor to total substance-attributable costs was productivity losses, which accounted for 61.0 percent ($24.3 billion) of the overall costs. This was followed by health care costs at 22.1 percent ($8.8 billion) and law enforcement costs at 13.6 percent ($5.4 billion). There were distinct regional variations across Canada, with the per capita costs of substance abuse being highest in Nunavut and the other territories, and lowest in Quebec and Prince Edward Island. Unfortunately, approximately 95 percent of all Canadian federal government expenditure addressing illicit drug use is spent on supply reduction, primarily through law enforcement initiatives, with only 5 percent spent on demand reduction, which includes both prevention and treatment (Haden, 2006). A 2006 study estimated that there were 4,258 deaths attributable to alcohol and 1,695 to illegal drugs, while 37,209 deaths were directly attributable to tobacco use. When combined, this represented 19.3 percent of the total mortality for 2002 in Canada. The number of days spent in acute care hospitals due to all forms of drug use was 17.8 percent of the total. In 2002, 761,638 criminal offences were attributable to alcohol, with 554,131 criminal offences attributable to illegal drugs, which constituted more than half of all the offences for that year. As well, just under 60 percent of all criminal charges were related to alcohol and illegal drug use.

In looking at ways to respond, Tragler, Caulkins, and Feichtinger (2001) stated that enforcement, while necessary, must be integrated with treatment. While they found that most nations needed to spend more on enforcement to control drug use, they countered that, of the drug control budget, even more should be proportionately spent on treatment. Regardless, crime committed under the influence of drugs is a major problem worldwide, even in small nations such as the Caribbean islands of Dominica, Saint Kitts and Nevis, Saint Lucia, and Saint Vincent and the Grenadines. There, 55 percent of convicted offenders reported that they were under the influence of drugs at the time of the offence, with only 19 percent of the offenders claiming that they would have committed the crime if they had not been under the influence of drugs. In the United States, 17 percent of state prisoners and 18 percent of federal inmates indicated that they had committed their current offence to obtain money for drugs. In the United Kingdom, it is estimated that economic-compulsive crime costs approximately $20 billion a year, the vast majority of those costs resulting from burglary, fraud, and robbery.

The other component of crime is the associated violence that comes not with drug use but with drug distribution. In the new millennium, murder rates have increased dramatically in the Caribbean and Latin America, particularly in Guatemala, where 6,290 drug deaths were recorded in 2008. In Jamaica, the murder rate reached 58 per 100,000 inhabitants, while in Mexico, approximately 20,000 individuals have been killed as a result of the drug war since 2006. Drug-related violence is an issue in every inhabited continent throughout the world. A study in Australia indicated costs of $3 billion a year associated with crime, while the result of fighting between the military and Colombian drug cartels in 1991 led to nearly 1 in 1,000 Colombians being murdered, 3 times the rate of Brazil and 10 times that of the United States. Systematic evidence-informed reviews suggest that, contrary to the conventional belief that increasing drug law enforcement will reduce violence, drug prohibition actually contributes to drug market violence and higher homicide rates. Well-intentioned policies and law enforcement strategies that aim to control drug markets and their associated violence have often had an opposite effect. Despite all the political and financial investment in repressive policies over the last 50 years, drugs are more available, and more widely used, than they have ever been (International Drug Policy Consortium, 2012; International Narcotics Control Board, 2014; Werb et al., 2010).

Brazil provides an example of this. In the 1980s, with the expansion of the cocaine trade, Brazil became part of a key drug route with an exponential growth in cocaine use within its own cities, especially in the slums of Rio de Janeiro. Young people living in poverty were openly courted by drug gangs, first through the provision of leisure activities, then through the exchange of money for favours, and then ultimately through their active recruitment as gang members. By the 1990s, heavy-calibre weapons could be found throughout Rio de Janeiro, and as the drug money increased, outsider groups, without links to the local communities, invaded and took control of some territories and their associated drug businesses. These outsider groups instigated an arms race with the local established groups and eventually with the police. By the end of the decade, police officers were given a productivity bonus—the "Western Bonus"—to actively execute traffickers. By this time, however, hundreds of Rio slums were under the territorial control of armed youth working in the drug business. Confrontation escalated further at the beginning of this century, with police using armoured vehicles and drug traffickers responding by buying weapons with increasingly destructive power. This rapidly escalated the arms race between the traffickers and the police, resulting in the official reported killings of 7,542 civilians and 220 police officers and leading to Rio de Janeiro having the highest death rate (46 per 100,000 inhabitants) from firearms in Brazil (International Drug Policy Consortium, 2010). Eventually the army was brought in to clear the slums in advance of the FIFA World Cup and the Summer Olympic Games. The similar preparation in Canada for the World's Fair and Winter Olympic Games contributed to Vancouver's Downtown Eastside becoming one of the most impoverished neighbourhoods in Canada, with high rates not only of drug use but also of poverty, sex trade, crime, and violence (Tayler, 2003).

Drug traffickers worldwide also corrupt officials at all levels of law enforcement and government in order to continue with their criminal activities. Non-involved citizens are thus indirectly and directly affected through the consequences of compromised law enforcement institutions. Drug trafficking is an issue in Kyrgyzstan, a nation in central Asia, in part because of the country's proximity to Afghanistan. As the major northern smuggling route passes through Kyrgyzstan, the country is a major transit area for transporting illicit shipments of unrefined opium, refined heroin, and cannabis from Afghanistan to Russia, its affiliated states, and Europe. The Kyrgyzstan–Tajikistan border consists of nearly 1000 km of mostly unregulated mountainous terrain. As well, cannabis plants grow wild on a total of at least about 10,000 hectares. Kyrgyzstan's drug control efforts are hampered by poverty in rural areas, unemployment in its urban centres, and uncontrolled labour migration. Thus, the income that can be derived from the sale and transportation of drugs has led to corruption at all levels in this nation of 6 million (International Narcotics Control Board, 2014).

However, corruption exists at much higher levels as well. Drug money worth $3.5 billion kept the global financial system afloat at the height of the 2008 economic crisis, according to Antonio Maria Costa, head of the United Nations Office on Drugs and Crime (Syal, 2009). He stated that there was evidence that the proceeds of organized crime were the only liquid investment capital available to some banks on the brink of collapse and that a majority of the drug profits were laundered and absorbed into the economic system as a result. The International Monetary Fund estimated that large American and European banks lost more than $1 trillion on toxic assets and bad loans from January 2007 to September 2009, and more than 200 mortgage lenders went bankrupt. During this period, a large portion of inter-bank loans were funded by money that originated from the illegal drug trade and related criminal activities as the system was basically paralyzed because of the unwillingness of banks to lend money to one another. Thus it may have been illicit drug profits that prevented the world from slipping into a global depression, as opposed to prudent central bank and government initiatives (Syal, 2009).

Table 1.6 further indicates why, despite legal restraints and prohibition, drug cultivation is a logical course of action, especially in developing nations. While a typical farmer in Afghanistan could make less than $1 a kilogram growing wheat or maize, he could earn more than $200 a kilogram for opium or from $12 to $95 a kilogram for cannabis. If a family's survival depends on farming, there is truly no decision to be made regarding which crop to cultivate. Economists Jeffrey Miron and Katherine Waldock (2010) completed a cost analysis on government savings of legalizing currently illicit drugs for the United States. They estimated that the various levels of government could save $41 billion per year in expenditures on the enforcement of current prohibitions, and while there would be different costs associated with increased use with regard to treatment and criminal offences, they would not be as great as the current costs.

TABLE 1.6: CHANGES IN AFGHANISTAN FARM-GATE PRICES OF SELECT LICIT AND ILLICIT CROPS, 2009–2013

Agricultural Product	Price (US dollars per kilogram)				
	2009	2010	2011	2012	2013
Fresh opium	48	128	180	163	143
Dry opium	64	169	241	196	172
Cannabis (prime grade)	35	86	95	68	n.a.
Cannabis (third grade)	12	39	39	26	n.a.
Rice	1.0	1.1	1.1	1.2	n.a.
Wheat	0.6	0.3	0.4	0.5	n.a.
Maize	0.4	0.3	0.3	0.3	n.a.

Source: International Narcotics Control Board (2014)

DISCUSSION QUESTIONS

1. Define
   (a) psychoactive drug
   (b) dependency
   (c) compulsive behaviour
   (d) addiction
2. What is the difference between a compulsive behaviour and an addiction? Why is it important for those in the helping professions to understand this?
3. Distinguish between the everyday, popular definition of addiction and the more precise definition provided in Chapter 1. What are the treatment, counselling, and policy implications for these two definitions?
4. What are the reasons a person becomes addicted to a psychoactive drug? How do those reasons align with the ideas from your discussion of question 1?
5. What distinguishes the different families of psychoactive drugs?
6. What factors contribute to how quickly a person becomes dependent on a psychoactive drug?
7. (a) What are the differences between drug use in Canada and drug use in different nations?
   (b) Was the incidence of drug use greater or lesser than you thought prior to completing the reading?
   (c) What factors influenced your thoughts on how many people in Canada and globally were using psychoactive drugs?
8. What are the economic implications of drug use?

NOTES

1. See Appendices A and B.
2. A more detailed discussion of the different drug groupings and individual psychoactive drugs is provided in Chapter 3.

Chapter 2
THEORIES ON ADDICTION

Why do people use psychoactive drugs? The opening chapter examined a variety of factors associated with drug use and abuse, but what are the actual reasons that lead to the continued use of drugs by a person? An entire spectrum of theories has been offered to explain the phenomenon of substance abuse. A theory is simply a collection of statements about how the world works. These statements are partially based on assumptions and beliefs combined with an empirical base. However, theory should be more than just a set of interrelated propositions or ideas pertaining to a possible explanation of a phenomenon. Theories should also provide us with a framework within which to further our studies and expand our understanding, and be relevant to planning and evaluating social interventions. However, it must also be recognized that theories raise moral questions and entail an examination of our values. In turn, our values shape our standpoint, and determine what we study and how we interpret information and what constitutes good evidence.

In studying addiction as a bio-psycho-social phenomenon, a good theory would be one that could explain drug use along five different dimensions, particularly if there was also substantial empirical support for the explanation. The five questions to consider are:

1. Why do people begin taking drugs (commencement)?
2. Why do people maintain their drug-taking behaviours (maintenance)?
3. How or why does drug-taking behaviour intensify (escalation)?
4. Why or how do people stop taking drugs (cessation)?
5. What accounts for the restarting of the drug-taking behaviour or cycle once it has stopped (recommencement or relapse)?

There is no shortage of theories and perspectives regarding addiction. However, of the dozens of theories that have been postulated to explain substance use and abuse, few can provide adequate responses to all five questions. Most theories also tend to be much easier to disprove than prove, which is one reason that they remain theory rather than becoming fact. However, these imperfect theories give credence to and shape the rise and development of different methods of intervention and treatment. If a treatment based on one theoretical model does not work, it indicates that the theory may be in some way flawed. Unfortunately, even if the treatment does work, it does not necessarily mean the theory behind it is complete. Following are descriptions of several perspectives that fall under one of four general areas: moral, biological, psychological, and sociological.

Before beginning your reading, complete Table 2.1, which provides you with a brief insight into how you view the causes of addiction. Record your scores, and once you have completed the chapter, re-do the assessment to determine if your perspective has changed.

2.1 THE MORAL MODEL

This model is based on the belief that using any drug is unacceptable, wrong, and even sinful. The moral model explains addiction as a consequence of personal choice and desire. Its formal origins can be traced back to the 17th century in Europe when alcohol was debated in religious circles as an example of how men must overcome temptation to exert control over themselves and their destinies (Valverde, 1998). Originally supported by zealous, religious grassroots groups in North America during the onset of the Industrial Revolution, the moral model still remains prominent worldwide today. It assumes that users are uniquely responsible for their own behaviour and are capable of making the choice not to use even once fully addicted to a psychoactive agent. Movements such as the Temperance Unions in Canada had their underpinnings in this doctrine. It is interesting to note that Temperance Unions were predominantly rural-based and arose in a larger effort to maintain the status quo and battle against urbanization in the 1800s and early 1900s in North America.

It is understandable in an era without medical or social science that lawmakers could only make sense of drug use as a moral problem or being due to a lack of moral fibre or decency, believing that if users had the proper character, they could just stop using or at least help themselves (Thombs, 2009). While the moral model has limited relevance in understanding why people use drugs, it still remains a prominent framework within which vices are judged and policy created. As recently as 1986, the Presbyterian Church in the United States stated that alcohol abuse was a sin because of the harm its use caused in oneself and to others. The Mormon faith and Islam are other examples of religions that have strict rules regarding abstinence from psychoactive substances, while the Buddha's Noble Eightfold Path encourages refraining from intoxicating substances as they dull the senses and lead to poor decision making. Every month, the day of the full moon in accordance with the Buddhist calendar, is a national holiday or "Poya day" on which alcohol is not served and cannot be purchased (Rahula, 2006).

TABLE 2.1: THEORETICAL ORIENTATION SELF-ASSESSMENT

		Strongly Agree	Agree	Neither Agree nor Disagree	Disagree	Strongly Disagree
1.	Poverty and poor environment are causes of substance abuse.	5	4	3	2	1
2.	The substance abuser is a victim of circumstance.	5	4	3	2	1
3.	If a substance abuser's environment is changed, use of drugs or alcohol will diminish.	5	4	3	2	1
4.	Substance abuse is a symptom of an underlying emotional disturbance.	5	4	3	2	1
5.	The main goal of drug abuse treatment is to gain insight about the reasons a person uses drugs.	5	4	3	2	1
6.	Drug or alcohol abuse results from an inability to cope with life's problems.	5	4	3	2	1
7.	What substance abusers need is advice to quit or cut down their use.	5	4	3	2	1
8.	Substance abuse is a moral issue.	5	4	3	2	1
9.	Jail sentences for possession of drugs are more effective in curbing drug abuse than drug diversion treatment programs.	5	4	3	2	1
10.	A substance abuser has a chronic progressive illness.	5	4	3	2	1
11.	Alcoholism has a biological basis.	5	4	3	2	1
12.	Addiction can't be cured.	5	4	3	2	1

Scoring: Use the following table to determine what your theoretical orientation is toward addiction.

Statement #	Score	Primary Theoretical Orientation
1–3	> 9	Social
4–6	> 9	Psychological
7–9	> 9	Moral
10–12	> 9	Biological

After reading the chapter, re-do Table 2.1 to determine if your views have changed.

Examples of initiatives spawned by the moral model perspective include prohibition, shifting attitudes toward public drunkenness, drunk tanks, anti-smoking lobbies, the criminalization of marijuana, random drug testing in the workplace, and the perpetual "War on Drugs." In the United States, the number of persons incarcerated since the beginning of the War on Drugs has dramatically increased (Figure 2.1) along class and racial lines, leading to severe overcrowding and to as many drug issues within the correctional system as outside (Kellen & Powers, 2010). During the beginning of the 21st century, on average an American was being jailed for a cannabis offence every 30 seconds, with a great disproportion being African-Americans (Brownsberger, 2000; Pettit, 2012).

The moral model perceives dependence on a drug as resulting from a weak moral character. The problem of addiction, from this perspective, can be remedied simply through building character, through personal willpower, by removing oneself from temptation, or through determination alone. This model offers no room for treatment and sees no need for extensive treatment networks, placing the responsibility and the blame solely on the user. Problems with this theory, other than the lack of research support, arise from a lack of consistency in its application. In North America, alcohol is often viewed as distinct from other drugs in this framework, and social class and economic status both significantly impinge on how the moral model is applied. Nevertheless, this view still plays a role in determining how drugs are classified and regulated under the law. An example is that alcohol remains classified as a food in Canada under the existing statutes, while cocaine, a stimulant, is categorized as a narcotic.

FIGURE 2.1: INCARCERATED AMERICANS AS A PERCENTAGE OF
POPULATION, 1920–2008

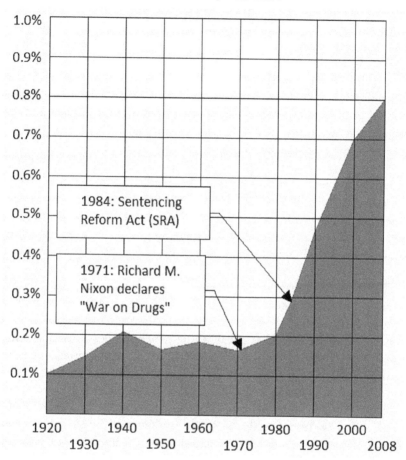

Source: Guerino, Harrison, & Sabol (2010)

The moral model remains a significant block in terms of adequate treatment funding and contributes to the oppression of substance users in North America. It is even a greater issue in many developing nations, where punitive and prohibitionist policies toward drugs are typically justified on both moral and utilitarian grounds. The ultimate form of the moral model is the application of the death penalty for drug use or drug trafficking. Typically, individuals involved in the drug trade are not accused of being guilty of individual, identifiable homicides, but rather as being purveyors of death whose crimes produce significant national harm. In this manner, the moral model presents drug offenders as threats to the life, values, and health of the state, against whom extraordinary penalties are therefore justified. It is also argued that drug trafficking corrupts a nation's youth, disrupts traditional values, is financed by and profits foreigners, and ultimately funds not only organized crime but also terrorist activity both inside and outside the nation (Edwards et al., 2009; Lines, 2007).

The death penalty has been abolished in law or practice in 135 nations. Of 63 stated retentionist countries that continue to use capital punishment, half have legislation applying the death penalty for drug-related offences, arguing that such offences fall under the umbrella of the most serious of crimes and thus are equal to treason and murder. Despite the international trend toward the abolition of capital punishment in the last quarter of the 20th century, the number of countries expanding the application of the death penalty to include drug offences actually increased from 22 nations in 1985 to 32 by the year 2010. The death penalty is applied for a wide variety of drug offences, including trafficking, cultivation, manufacturing, importing, exporting, and, under extraordinary circumstances, simple possession. Though the exact number of individuals executed annually for drug convictions is difficult to calculate, some data has been collected. China, Egypt, Gambia, Indonesia, Iran, Kuwait, Lao People's Democratic Republic, Malaysia, Saudi Arabia, Singapore, Sudan, Thailand, and Vietnam regularly execute individuals convicted of drug offences, with several prescribing the death penalty as a mandatory sentence for certain drug offences. In Gambia, if you are caught with more than one-quarter of a kilogram of either heroin or cocaine, the penalty is death. In Malaysia, between July 2004 and July 2005, 36 of 52 executions carried out were for drug trafficking, with a total of 229 people being executed for this offence between 1975 and 2005. Of the 50 executions carried out in Saudi Arabia in 2005, 26 were for drug-related crimes, while in 2006, another 33 individuals were put to death for drug offences. The government of Vietnam admitted in a 2003 submission to the United Nations Human Rights Committee that approximately 100 people per year are executed by firing squad primarily for drug-related offences. Amnesty International suggests that Singapore, with a population of just under 4.5 million, has the highest per capita execution rate in the world for drug offences, for in that nation the death penalty can be applied to anyone apprehended with more than 15 g of heroin, 30 g of cocaine, or 500 g of cannabis. In 2001 alone, over 50 people were convicted and publicly executed for drug crimes at mass rallies, at least one of which was broadcast on state television, while in 2002, there were 64 public executions (Edwards et al., 2009; International Drug Policy Consortium, 2012; Lines, 2007).

In Iran, a mandatory death sentence is imposed for possession of more than 30 g of heroin or 5 kg of opium. Under Iranian legislation, this quantity may be based on the amount seized during a single arrest, or it may be added together over a number of convictions. Both Sudan and Yemen have legislation that allows for the owner of an establishment where drugs are sold or even used, including hashish, to be subject to the death penalty. Egypt, Jordan, Oman, and Syria impose a mandatory death sentence if the offender of a major drug-related crime is a public official or government employee, while both Egypt and Iran call for a mandatory death sentence for anyone who, by whatever means, induces any other person to take any narcotic substance (Lines, 2007).

Harvard economist Jeffrey Miron (1999, 2005, 2008) has long been an advocate of eliminating drug prohibition fuelled by the moral model. He estimates that legalizing drugs in the United States would generate over $30 billion in revenue if cannabis, cocaine, and heroin were regulated and taxed in the same manner as alcohol and tobacco. To bolster his economic claims, he states that there are currently more people in the United States using illicit drugs than when the most recent War on Drugs began in earnest in the 1980s, and that the primary economic benefactors of prohibition are international organized crime and terrorist groups. Miron's views are supported by data released by the Colorado Department of Revenue (2015) on its first year of legal cannabis sales. The government generated over $50 million in revenue from taxes, licences, and fees, without even considering the additional income tax paid by employees working in this new field.

2.2 BIOLOGICAL THEORIES
Disease (Medical) Model
Neurobiology
Genetic Theory
Brain Dysfunction Theory
Biochemical Theories
Allergy Theory

This group of theories searches for a pre-existing or induced chemical, physiological, or structural abnormality as the cause for substance abuse. Much of the initial empirical work that serves as the foundation for these theories focused on alcohol, though most of the theories' premises can be readily extrapolated to other psychoactive drugs. While developed independently, the biological theories can also be viewed as interdependent, as brain function precedes chemistry and chemistry supports function. Trauma, regardless if the cause is autoimmune response or an environmental event, can initiate the disease process, while trauma experience can be passed on genetically. As well, stressful experiences early in life can modulate the genetic programming of specific brain circuits underlying emotional and cognitive aspects of behavioural adaptation to stressful experiences later in life.

Disease (Medical) Model

The most prominent biological theory revolves around the concept of substance dependency as a primary, chronic, fatal disease process (Miller, 1999; White & McLellan, 2008). It is currently the most prominent theory informing health professional education, research, policy, and drug abuse treatment and was the centrepiece of policy positions taken by the American National Council on Alcoholism and Drug Dependence and the American Society of Addiction Medicine through the latter half of the 20th century. Addiction, along with other mental health issues, has historically been presented as a medical disease in part to increase service use and overcome stigma and oppression (Pescosolido et al., 2010).

However, the initial conceptualization of repeated episodes of drunkenness as an illness rather than a vice arose in the late 18th century in the United States, when alcohol consumption was exploding and intemperance was described as a disease that was chronic and progressive. The following century saw new labels arise to describe the disease, such as dipsomania, chronic alcoholism, and inebriety, the latter of which acknowledged abuse of other drugs, such as opium, cocaine, and ether, an inhalant, for the first time. Nineteenth-century addiction medical journals consistently characterized alcohol and other drug addiction as a chronic, relapsing disease. The disease concept fell out of favour in the early decades of the 20th century with the rise of the Prohibition movement and the re-emergence of the moral model as the dominant addiction standpoint. However, a reformulated disease concept emerged following the repeal of Prohibition. In 1938, the Scientific Committee of the Research Council on Problems of Alcohol stated that an alcoholic should be regarded as a sick person, just as is one who is suffering from tuberculosis, cancer, heart disease, or another serious chronic disorder (White, Boyle, & Loveland, 2002).

Ludwig (1975) stated that sufficient deviation from the normal represents disease; that it is due to known or unknown natural causes; and that elimination of these causes will result in cure or improvement in individual patients. Proponents of the disease theory believe that substance dependency is an involuntary biological trait to which certain people are susceptible, and thus drug users are not responsible for their compulsive drug consumption. Drug use in this theory is thought to be an inherited characteristic that worsens over time with increased consumption, leading to a loss of control over use. In this model the emphasis focuses exclusively on the person, with individuals no longer being scorned or shunned for their illness; rather, they are now considered and labelled sick. Initially, labelling alcoholism as a disease helped remove some of the social disgrace and disapproval of having a problem with alcohol. This change of attitude subsequently resulted in more persons receiving treatment, even while the majority of society still felt that those with an addiction could simply will themselves to stop using drugs without any formal support or treatment.

While addicted persons are still held responsible for their affliction and uncontrollable cravings in this model, they are now viewed as requiring care, including hospitalization, like any other ill individual (Miller & Gold, 1990). This theory views substance abuse as a progressive disorder that continues to worsen until treated, as illustrated by Glatt's (1958) proposal of the decline of an alcohol-dependent person until he has reached bottom, followed by a slow, staged recovery process (Figure 2.2). Glatt's model was influenced by Jellinek's (1952) seminal work on the increasing progressive stages of dependence on alcohol. Glatt drew on Jellinek's research to create a model with an inverted bell curve: the downward half of the curve describes the nature of alcoholism, and the upward half of the curve, the subsequent potential progression of recovery. Jellinek examined the drinking histories of over 2,000 individuals, mostly men, and from those devised a four-step progression model. The model begins as a person moves from the pre-alcoholic phase of social or integrated drinking, to the blackout stage with its increasing preoccupation with alcohol, to the stage of loss of control over alcohol consumption, and finally to the chronic phase of prolonged intoxications where drinking takes on its obsessive nature. Jellinek stated that two options arose for an individual at this point—either continue the path of deterioration to death, or find a pathway out of alcoholism through a new understanding of life, which many equate with the Alcoholics Anonymous (AA) stage of experiencing a spiritual awakening. Likewise, the low point of Jellinek's model, when the alcohol-dependent person admits to being defeated by his or her use of alcohol, aligns with AA's point of hitting rock bottom. Glatt enhanced Jellinek's idea by adding the ascending component that highlights the process of recovery, beginning with an honest desire for help, followed by steps to stop consuming alcohol and becoming open to a new abstinent way of life, and finally to obtaining a state of grace.

In 1956, the American Medical Association declared that alcoholism was a disease at its annual conference, though it would be another decade before they formally ratified this position. The acceptance of the disease concept by the medical profession led to a paradigm shift for the addiction field, and part of its historical significance is the fact that it was the antecedent event that led to the enormous humanitarian move away from the moral model that transpired throughout the latter half of the 20th century. The disease model allowed drug-dependent persons to receive formal and proper medical care. In Canada, the majority of treatment costs were—and to a large extent remain—directly or indirectly covered under provincial medical plans or through subsidized social service initiatives. In the United States, many private medical plans provide coverage for substance abusers, though with the move to managed care and third-party benefit providers, this is beginning to return to a more moralistic perspective. However, even Jellinek (1960) later stated that alcoholism was labelled as a disease primarily because the medical professional considered it a disease, even if this was not a unanimous belief. This sentiment was subsequently echoed by others (Berridge & Edwards, 1981; Conrad, 2007; Conrad & Barker, 2010; Fingarette, 1988, 1989; Peele & Brodsky, 1992).

By diseasing drug-using behaviour, this theory allowed for the medical community to take the lead in the care of drug abusers. This subsequently also led to the diseasing of many other behaviours that did not have the same biological basis as addiction (as witnessed in the Canadian Society of Addiction Medicine's [2008] definition, which states that addiction is a primary chronic disease characterized by impaired control over psychoactive drugs and also behaviours). The development and expansion of the disease model in Canada and the United States was also in part a response to the large-scale experimentation and drug use in the 1960s and 1970s by white middle-class youth, along with the lengthy prison sentences imposed for the possession of minor amounts of marijuana on the children and youth of affluent middle-class families during that era (Acker, 2002).

The disease model, like most theories, has its limitations. There is a major dearth of empirical research to substantiate the fact that alcoholism, or any other substance-related problem, is the result of a medical disorder. There is no uniformity of the disease nature of the drug action, nor any standard way to diagnose this disease, nor any reliable or consistent medical method to care for the sick, nor a need for medical care in much of the recovery process. The progressive nature of the disorder has been challenged for 30 years, and there are many aspects of the disease process that remain deficient. In reality, alcoholism is not an inevitable progression of symptoms and stages, nor a consistent loss of control (Fingarette, 1989; Fisher & Harrison, 1977; Pattison, Sobell, & Sobell, 1977). As well, through labelling alcoholism and drug dependency a disease, some individuals feel just as stigmatized as under the moral model. Recent empirical reviews have found that despite the fact that addiction in the medical model is described as a chronic, relapsing disease, population-wide surveys suggest that this is not the case. Approximately 80 percent of individuals formerly dependent on an illegal drug, or on a medicine used for non-medical purposes, have been in remission for at least a year. These remission rates are much higher than for other chronic mental health disorders, with the likelihood of relapse unrelated to the cumulative amount of drugs consumed (Berghmans, de Jong, Tibben, & de Wert, 2009).

Under the disease model, abstinence alone is considered the cure for alcoholism and drug dependency. However, this can be equated to treating a broken leg by amputating it. Neither solves the true problem, though both are remedies. As well, once a person stops drinking or drugging they are not recovered but in recovery, a state that stays with them until their death. The disease becomes an inescapable component of their persona in perpetuity. The person must become even more vigilant about their recognized disease, entailing a moral obligation to engage in the recovery process (May, 2001). Psychologist Stanton Peele (1983, 1989) has claimed that while the disease concept of alcoholism is deeply entrenched in the United States, in many other countries, such as England, it is less of an economic utility as reimbursement for doctors is not dependent on what is defined as a disease. In the United States, however, the reward structure is built on fitting as many things as possible into the doctor's bag. This has led to quite distinct vested interests between Canada and the United States in labelling drug use a disease (Alexander, 1988; Fingarette, 1988). As well, there are huge economic benefits for pharmaceutical companies that develop lifelong drug treatments for this disease. Many psychoactive drugs, from barbiturates, to benzodiazepines, to amphetamines, to all the current psychotherapeutic agents, have been developed since the beginning of the 20th century to treat illnesses. Others for which no profitable therapeutic use can be found, such as LSD and MDMA (ecstasy), became prohibited substances (Singer, 2006), though renewed interest re-emerges even in these as treatment alternatives as new syndromes such as post-traumatic stress disorder (PTSD) are categorized.

Despite its shortcomings, the disease model remains extremely popular for several reasons:

- It is a simple solution to a complex problem.
- The medical profession, especially in the United States, benefits economically and socially from maintaining ownership of the issue.
- It provides a foundation for the most popular model of addiction recovery, Alcoholics Anonymous.
- Tradition and history create biases that are difficult to change.
- Politically, if drug use is a disease and each individual is personally responsible for his/her condition, then there is no reason to make social reforms that might prevent the problem.
- There is money to be made in the field and in related adjunct industries.

However, outside of assisting with detoxification using a few specific drugs, there is limited need for medical practitioners to be directly involved in the treatment of clients with addiction problems. Despite this, support for this perspective continues. In 2012, Gil Kerlikowske, director of the White House Office of National Drug Control Policy, clearly stated when speaking at the Betty Ford Center in California that the American government's view is that "addiction is a disease, not a moral failure" (Join Together, 2012).

Alcoholism as a disease has become a great model for treating all kinds of problems as disease. It is self-sustaining, it fits into the American culture, it is economically rewarding, and basically nobody really cares if it has any effect or not: it relieves everybody of guilt. So, calling it a disease essentially means we ignore it as a social condition. (McConnell, 1989, p. 16)

FIGURE 2.2: MEDICAL MODEL PROCESS OF ALCOHOL ABUSE AND RECOVERY

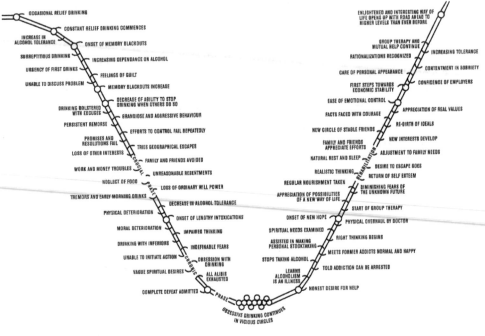

Source: Glatt (1958)

Neurobiology

In 1997, Dr. Alan Leshner, the director of the National Institute on Drug Abuse (NIDA), published a seminal article, "Addiction Is a Brain Disease, and It Matters." The article would focus research initiatives drawing from more established theories, including brain dysfunction and biochemical, into a more evidence-informed examination of how psychoactive drugs compromise the brain. During the past two decades, molecular neurobiological studies of addiction have undergone tremendous development. They have yielded enormous amounts of valuable information about neuronal response mechanisms and their adaptive changes through an array of techniques, ranging from in vitro molecular methods to brain imaging procedures in conscious subjects actively performing a range of behavioural tasks. This research has demonstrated that brain structures do change over time due to exposure to psychoactive drugs until they reach a threshold. At this threshold point, the primary symptom of dependence occurs, making it difficult to stop excessive drug use without professional help (Erickson & White, 2009).

The brain continually attempts to keep the body at or return it to a point of balance or homeostasis, and in so doing, it will adapt to the prolonged or excessive presence of drugs by making changes in brain cells and neural pathways. When people administer a psychoactive drug, it activates the same reinforcement system in the brain that is normally activated by food, water, and sex, sometimes to a lesser extent but sometimes to a far greater one. Some theories have viewed the role of the limbic system (Nestler, 2005), particularly the amygdala, the part of the brain responsible for emotions such as fear and anxiety (Chambers et al., 2007), as crucial to this process. Others have looked at the effect of reinforcement of dopamine receptors in the mesolimbic system, which originate in the ventral tegmental area (VTA) and terminate in nucleus accumbens (Koob & Roberts, 1999; Saal, Dong, Bonci, & Malenka, 2003). All of these reinforcers share one physiological effect—increased amounts of dopamine being released in the brain either directly or indirectly through the activation of other neurotransmitters. During this process, prominent physical changes occur in areas of the brain that are critical to judgment, decision making, learning and memory, and behavioural control (Anton, 1999; Chandler, 2003; Naqvi, Rudrauf, Damasio, & Antoine Bechara, 2007; National Institute on Drug Abuse, 2007).

The popular term "the highjacked brain" has underscored neurobiological research in three new areas:

1. drug actions on intracellular signalling systems that mediate cell responses;
2. synaptic plasticity in the course of chronic drug exposure;
3. the role of dopaminergic and other components of the human reward system; along with a fourth long-established area:
4. genetic factors that will be examined as a distinct theoretical construct.

Intracellular Signalling

Nerve cells are the dynamic component of the CNS that have the ability to adapt to changes produced by external influences, such as psychoactive drugs. This adaption follows basic physics and occurs in an equal and opposite direction to the initial effect, working to return the body to the initial state of homeostasis. This is the foundation for the development of tolerance. When a person no longer uses the drug, the adaption becomes apparent through the pain of withdrawal. The process occurs through membrane receptors, ion channels, and enzymes, as well as in alterations in cellular metabolism, ion movement, and activation of genes that direct the synthesis of proteins. This process has been demonstrated with CNS depressants, stimulants, and cannabis, and thus chronic exposure to any of these drugs leads to increases or decreases in the cells' internal signalling mechanisms. However, this adaption is not unique to psychoactive drugs but occurs with a range of sensory stimuli. Thus, signalling pathways are the foundation of all human biological adaption to any stressor and not only to psychoactive drugs (Kallant, 2009).

Synaptic Plasticity

The process of addiction shares many similarities with neural plasticity, which is the biological means through which learning and memory is shaped. Environmental stimuli repeatedly linked to psychoactive drugs become learned associations, and those stimuli then elicit memories or sensations that motivate continued drug use. Dopamine and glutamate are widely distributed throughout the brain, but it is specific concentrations in the limbic system and basal ganglia, that appear to play a key, integrative role in motivation, learning, and memory. It is currently believed that coordinated molecular signalling of dopamine and glutamate systems are critical events in the induction of intracellular messaging and neuron cascades that lead to adaptive changes in gene expression and synaptic plasticity, which can reconfigure neural networks and ultimately behaviour (Kelly, 2004; Tang & Dani, 2009).

Adaptive responses occur not only within single neurons but also at synapses between neurons. This synaptic adaptive response has two opposite components: long-term potentiation (LTP) and long-term depression (LTD). LTP involves the long-lasting impulse transmission from one neuron to another, where the synapse between them is used repeatedly to convey the chemical message. LTD involves the opposite, a long-lasting decrease in impulse transmission. Both arise due to changes in different neurotransmitter receptors, and as with intracelluar signalling, they are core human adaptive processes triggered by a range of stimuli and not only psychoactive drugs. Thus, when examining addiction, synaptic changes explain how the physical aspect of addiction arises but not, unfortunately, why (Cruz, Rubio, & Hope, 2014; Kallant, 2009).

Dopamine and the Reward System

The more a psychoactive drug produces physical dependency, the greater the release of dopamine at the axon terminals of the neurons. This creates the euphoria, or the pleasure response, in the substance user. The core reward circuitry consists of the ventral tegmental area (VTA), nucleus accumbens, and ventral pallidum via the medial forebrain bundle. This system does more than just produce pleasure, however; it is now believed that it is also responsible for more complex cognitive functions, such as attention, reward anticipation, negating reward expectation, and incentive motivation. Drugs that alter endocannabinoids, endorphins, GABA, glutamate, and serotonin indirectly enhance the dopamine reward synaptic function in the nucleus accumbens, as do all psychoactive drugs that directly affect dopamine. Drug self-administration is regulated by dopamine levels in the nucleus accumbens. Likewise, chronic alcohol intake seems to render mesolimbic circuits hypersensitive to alcohol and alter the motivational reward system, including dopamine neurotransmission (Hagele, Friedel, Kienast, & Kiefer, 2014).

However, for some substances, tolerance develops with chronic use. When this occurs, users no longer self-administer to feel euphoria but simply to restore a homeostatic level. A greater amount of the drug is now required to be present in the brain for the body to be able to function normally (Gardner, 2011). While different drug groups work through different biological reactions, the outcome is similar—an increase in dopamine activity in the nucleus accumbens and prefrontal cortex. However, what is not yet understood is why only a minority of people become addicted when all psychoactive drugs act the same way in the VTA and the majority of people use some type of psychoactive drug (Kallant, 2009).

Despite intense research and increasing empirical support, neurobiological theory still has distinct limits. Its contribution to understanding addiction is the knowledge that almost every cell function appears to be involved. Thus we are aware that neurons adapt to psychoactive drugs, but they likewise adapt to all types of functional disturbances. This reductionist approach is unable to explain what causes these mechanisms to be brought into play with some individuals but not others, and why this occurs only through self-administration and not passive exposure (Kallant, 2009).

Sociologists in particular have criticized the reductive tendencies of the neurobiological approach that claims a causal link between addiction and physiological processes. It simply cannot fully account for the complexity of human behaviour (Oksanen, 2013). Even more problematic may be the concern that the neurobiological discussion of addiction as a brain disease is simply presenting a revised form of the disease model in an attempt to decrease the oppression faced by those with an addiction and to continue to counter and rebut the still dominant view of addiction as a moral issue. Inherent limits found in the disease model are also present here. While presenting addiction as a neurobiological condition does allow for the same medical care as that for individuals living with other diseases, and while it helps to promote enlightened social and legal policies, such claims may still unintentionally foster the discrimination commonly associated with any pathology. Specifically, the language of neuroscience can reduce blame and responsibility while inadvertently identifying addicted persons as neurobiological "others" and increasing the social isolation of this vulnerable group (Buchman, Illes, & Reine, 2010).

Genetic Theory

Despite the vast numbers of individuals who experiment with psychoactive drugs, the majority do not become addicted. However, there is a proportion of every human culture who do, and they also tend to differ from the general population in having pre-existing co-morbid traits, including novelty seeking and antisocial behaviour. This has become part of the argument for a genetic basis for the susceptibility to dependence (Hiroi & Agatsuma, 2005). Genetic theory was for a short time out of favour in the 20th century, but it has had a dramatic rebound in prominence with advances in human genome research. Humans have only approximately 20,000 genes, about the same as the nematode worm that grows to only 2.5 mm in length. Human genes must therefore perform multiple tasks, leaving them open to a range of potential coding errors as they produce the range of enzymes, hormones, proteins, neurotransmitters, and all other biological material.

Genetic theory proposes that alcohol dependency and other forms of substance abuse are an inherited disorder, though the majority of research in this area remains alcohol-specific. It has been documented that, historically, certain Asian and related populations have a lower mortality from alcoholism than Europeans. These Asian groups lack a gene that allows for the efficient processing of alcohol. Thus, when alcohol is consumed, an unpleasant physical response and flushing of the face occurs at much lower dose amounts than for Europeans. This, in turn, historically led these groups to avoid using large amounts of alcohol, and fewer individuals fell into an alcohol-dependency cycle (Maisto, Galizio, & Connors, 1995; Stohl, 1988). Genetic studies conducted in various ethnic groups have confirmed that certain genetic allele variations of the enzymes ADH and ALDH are linked either in development of or in protection from alcohol addiction, though the exact mechanism has still not been determined (Moussas, Christodoulou, & Douzenis, 2009). Likewise, some people have a gene that leads to caffeine being metabolized slowly, while others have a gene that allows for far faster metabolism. Those who are fast metabolizers can literally consume coffee after coffee, whereas those who are slow metabolizers are at four times greater risk of having a heart attack by the age of 50 if they drink as little as four cups a day (Cornelis & El-Sohemy, 2007).

Alcoholism has been documented to be strongly familial, running through several generations. The increase in risk for developing alcoholism is from four- to sevenfold among the first-degree relatives of persons with an alcohol dependence compared to the general population, regardless of nationality (Hesselbrock, Hesselbrock, & Chartier, 2013). Inherited personality traits may also influence susceptibility to alcoholism, and neurological disorders that lead to alcohol and substance abuse, such as attention-deficit/hyperactivity disorder, may be transferred from generation to generation. As well, there may be actual cell differences in alcohol-dependent persons that are inherited (Reich, 1988). Fraternal and paternal twin studies, conducted with families where a child was adopted at a young age, have also indicated a genetic component to the development of substance abuse (Bierut, 2011). Approximately one-quarter of the fathers and brothers of those with an alcohol dependency are themselves alcohol-dependent. This compares with an overall rate among men of 3–5 percent while 5 percent of daughters and sisters develop alcoholism (Shuckit, 1999). When adopted offspring of persons with a dependency to alcohol were compared to adopted children of biological parents who were not alcohol-dependent, an alcoholism rate three to four times greater than for those whose biological parents were dependent was observed (Goodwin, Schulsinger, Hermansen, Guze, & Winokur, 1973). In the Minnesota Twin Family Study, which examined 1,080 twins, there was also evidence for the existence of a highly heritable factor that underlies the association among multiple forms of psychopathology (McGue, Iacono, & Krueger, 2006). Research has also found a degree of heritability to acute adverse and affective responses to opioids (Angst et al., 2012).

Jung (1994) compared brothers who were adopted from families where alcoholism was prevalent to those who remained with their natural parents and found rates of abuse to be similar. Heath, Jardine, and Martin (1989), in one of the first studies to examine female twins, found greater levels of alcohol dependency between identical twins than between fraternal twins, a similar finding to that of Kendler, Heath, Neale, Kessler, and Eaves (1992). Individuals with a family history of alcohol dependency tend to develop tolerance to alcohol quicker than those without (Morzorati, Ramchandani, Li, Fleury, & O'Connor, 2002). Van den Bree, Johnson, and Neale (1998) examined 54 identical and 65 fraternal twins in public and private alcohol and drug abuse treatment programs in Minnesota during the 1980s and found evidence to suggest genetic influences in persons prone to developing an addiction to alcohol.

Good laboratory and field studies exist supporting the genetic theory (Zubieta et al., 2003), with the heritability of drug dependency estimated at 50 percent (Buscemi & Turchi, 2011; Enoch, 2012; National Institute on Alcohol Abuse and Alcoholism, 2000; Sartor et al., 2009), yet evidence for a specific genetic factor has still not been discovered. Some researchers have begun to examine specific genes that they believe play a role in the development of substance dependency, specifically with regard to dopamine. However, a single gene cannot explain the majority of cases due to the great heterogeneity of those who develop an addiction. Thus, any genetic link to substance dependency will be polygenic to account for these differences among substance-dependent persons (Plomin, Haworth, & Davis, 2009).

Genome studies have implicated several regions and genes that may be related to the addiction to various substances, with specific attention now being focused on 11 distinct chromosome regions (Li & Burmeister, 2009). DNA analysis has indicated that genes contributing to the susceptibility for alcohol dependence may be located on chromosomes 1, 2, 4, and 7. Two specific neurotransmitter genes, $GABRA_2$, a GABA gene, and $CHRM_2$, a gene involved in neuronal excitability and feedback regulation of another neurotransmitter, acetylcholine, have been shown to be linked to the vulnerability for alcohol dependence (Hesselbrock, Hesselbrock, & Chartier, 2013), as has the alcohol-metabolizing enzyme alcohol dehydrogenase (Kimura & Higuchi, 2011). Genetic variations in the μ-opioid receptor sites in the brain's reward system seem to influence the release of the neurotransmitter dopamine and the degree of pleasure that individuals derive from drinking. Individuals who possess this receptor variant may experience enhanced pleasurable effects from alcohol that could increase their risk for developing alcohol abuse and dependence (Ramchandani et al., 2011). Other genes, such as CYP_2E_1, located on chromosome 10, provide instructions for making an enzyme that breaks down alcohol. If these can be activated, they may be able to provide protection against alcohol abuse and decrease the risk of developing a dependency (Schuckit et al., 2005; Webb et al., 2011).

Consistent but indirect evidence has implicated genetic factors for smoking behaviour at chromosomes 9, 10, 11, and 15 (Tobacco and Genetics Consortium, 2010). Distinct genetic influences have been found indicating the likelihood of a person becoming physically dependent on smoking cigarettes (Munafo & Johnstone, 2008) or developing lung cancer from doing so (Amos et al., 2010), though environmental interactions were also found to be a factor. In a study involving twins from Finland, 76 percent of the total variance in abstinence or choosing to begin to drink alcohol was explained by common environmental effects (Rose, Dick, Viken, Pulkkinen, & Kaprio, 2001). While a more recent Swedish twin study found that drug abuse is influenced by a diverse set of genetic risks, with a specific liability relating to the neurotransmitter dopamine, vulnerability was also created by environmental factors, especially family instability (Kendler et al., 2012). Environmental factors are also important in determining whether teens experiment with alcohol or other drugs, but it is genetics that is more important than the environment in determining if they will become addicted or not once they do start using (Fowler et al., 2007).

While an important contributing factor, genetics cannot at this time explain the majority of cases of substance abuse. As well, heritable should never be confused with unchangeable. What this theory does indicate, however, is that some persons may be born with a greater predisposition or inherited risk to develop a substance abuse problem. Thus, genetics may influence the extent of use once an individual has already begun to use. In this regard genetic factors may be as potent as psychological, physiological, or other biological factors that are necessary for a substance abuse problem to develop and escalate. Nevertheless, genes and chromosomes are not omnipotent, and consideration must be also given to social, cultural, economic, historical, and other environmental factors that are involved in the process of substance-dependency development.

Brain Dysfunction Theory

Chronic drug abuse can severely damage the nervous system, particularly cognitive functions, cerebral metabolism, and brain morphology. This damage can lead to memory loss, concentration deficits, and increased impulsivity. Under the early biological theory of brain dysfunction, addiction was conceptualized as a chronic relapsing brain disorder that affected circuits that regulate reward, motivation, memory, and decision making. It is now consistently argued that drug-induced changes in the brain create behaviours that continue despite adverse bio-psycho-social consequences (Cadet, Bisagno, & Milroy, 2014). In its definition of addiction, the American National Institute on Drug Abuse states that it is, in part, a result of prolonged drug use on brain functioning.

That brain damage occurs as a consequence of heavy alcohol intake is a well-established argument found in the alcohol literature of the past 200 years. Jellinek (1960) equated this disorder to what he termed "gamma alcoholism." Brain dysfunction theories postulate that continued consumption of large amounts of alcohol and other drugs leads to damage of brain cells responsible for willpower and judgment. Once a specific level of damage is reached, a single incidence of drug use can paralyze the remaining cells and lead to uncontrolled and excessive drug use as occurs in bingeing. The theory hypothesizes that drug-dependent persons are biologically different, and ongoing research has demonstrated that the brains of dependent and non-dependent individuals are in fact different. Early electroencephalograph studies have indicated that there may be a cerebral condition predisposing individuals to alcohol dependency. Regardless, no evidence exists that there are any specific brain cells responsible for willpower or judgment that can be differentially affected by drugs (Chaudron & Wilkinson, 1988).

Brain damage from alcohol due to nutritional deficiencies can partially explain the pathology of alcoholism, namely, the permanent loss of control over drinking. It has historically been believed that if a biological problem does arise, it is the result of heavy and/or excessive consumption, not an initial breakdown of a select group of cells. Chronic exposure to drugs does create many modifications to the physiology of the brain, such as impairment of the brain's synapses. By limiting synapse plasticity, new learning can also be impaired. This could allow drug-using behaviour to become more established and lead to even more compulsive use (Ksaanetz et al., 2010). Studies with animals have also shown that heavy alcohol use actually rewires brain circuitry, making it harder to recover psychologically from a traumatic experience. A history of heavy alcohol abuse could impair a critical mechanism for recovering from trauma, placing people at greater risk for PTSD (Holmes et al., 2012). While alcohol can produce irreversible neuron death, it also degrades the cerebrospinal fluid, which acts as a buffer for the brain. With abstinence, this can be reversed. Individuals can experience brain volume recovery often within the first two weeks of abstinence, though this varies between brain regions. While motor skills appear to return quickly, higher cognitive functions such as divided attention, which are processed in specific cortical areas, take a longer time to recover (Ejik et al., 2012).

Psychoactive drugs from different families as distinct as cocaine, alcohol, and morphine all affect neurons in the same part of the brain (Saal, Dong, Bonci, & Malenka, 2003). Chronic drug use does change brain function, and some of these changes persist after cessation. Wilkinson (1998) contends that addiction is tied to changes in brain structure and function. At its core, addiction is the product of changes in the brain, and thus treatment must focus on reversing or compensating for those brain changes. It has long been argued that the same process that leads excessive alcohol consumption to produce liver damage can create brain damage (Pratt, Rooprai, Shaw, & Thomson, 1990). Li and Wolf (2015) found that cocaine influences brain-derived neurotrophic factor (BDNF) levels in the VTA, along with the amygdala, hippocampus, and frontal cortex. BDNF is a protein that regulates cell growth, survival, and differentiation during central and peripheral nervous system development. Differences in the brains of dependent and non-dependent persons have also been identified, some of which are permanent and others that disappear after cessation of use (Chandler, 2003). Brain dysfunction theory was among the earliest addiction theories proposed, and much of what was earlier argued and the ongoing supporting arguments have been incorporated into the broader domain of neurobiological theory.

Biochemical Theories

This broad grouping of theories comprises a variety of related physiological hypotheses. Various metabolic disturbances and sensitivities, and vitamin and other dietary deficiencies, including hypoglycemia, leading to abnormal cravings, endocrine gland deficiencies, and malfunctioning control centres in the brain, are among the perspectives included. Biochemical theories propose that chemical imbalances exist in the body or are created by the use and then withdrawal process (May, 2001; Rose et al., 2007), or that alcohol is metabolized in some abnormal way that contributes to increased consumption (Fingarette, 1988) or decreased intoxication (Blednov, Cravatt, Boehm, Walker, & Harris, 2007).

For example, if the cause is diet-related, an individual experiences a "pick up" for a short period after ingesting his or her food of choice. Once the food has been processed, the person begins to suffer from withdrawal. In the case of alcoholism, individuals may become physically dependent on food elements in alcoholic beverages, such as malt or corn. Alcohol promotes a rapid absorption of these substances, thus increasing their "pick up" effects and helping to relieve withdrawal effects. It has also long been argued that there may be a reciprocal relationship between hypoglycemia and alcoholic tendencies (Tintera, 1966). As well, monoamine oxidase (MAO), a genetically controlled enzyme involved in regulating the neurotransmitters dopamine and norepinephrine, may be a causative factor, as members of families with a history of alcoholism generally have lower MAO levels than members of families with no such history (Pandey, Fawcett, Gibbons, Clark, & Davis, 1988). Researchers at Johns Hopkins University have also hypothesized that children of alcoholics have altered brain chemistry that makes them most susceptible to becoming alcohol-dependent themselves (Wand, Mangold, El Deiry, McCaul, & Hoover, 1998). Goldstein (1976) and Snyder (1977) earlier hypothesized that some individuals might have lowered levels of endorphins that leave them unusually sensitive to pain and thus with a far greater reinforcing response to opioids. Similarly, stress hormones such as corticotropin have been shown to play a critical role in the development and continuation of alcohol dependence in lab animals. Thus, if this chemical could be blocked, alcohol dependence could be alleviated (Roberto et al., 2010).

Research has also indicated that exposure to the heavy metals, such as lead and cadmium, may also make people more susceptible to alcohol and drug addiction by requiring greater amounts of the drug of choice to be ingested to obtain a significant feeling of euphoria (Nation, Cardon, Heard, Valles, & Bratton, 2003; Nation, Livermore, & Bratton, 1995; Overstreet, Miller, Janowksy, & Russell, 1996). Cadmium, a component of cigarettes, enters the body when a person smokes and can be retained for years. It also crosses the placenta of a smoking mother to the fetus. In experiments in which laboratory rats were exposed to lead, they became supersensitive. Supersensitivity has also been linked with drug use among persons with concurrent disorders. Individuals with existing mental health problems, such as schizophrenia, might be supersensitive due to their other chemical imbalances. When they consume alcohol, nicotine, or another psychoactive substance, their system reacts much more dramatically or quickly, thus explaining the higher incidence of substance abuse among some groups with other mental health problems. Despite these interesting hypotheses, the actual cause-effect relationships still require additional research, and ideas from this theory have been minimized by or incorporated into the broader ideas represented in neurobiological theory.

Allergy Theory

It has been argued that for some persons an initial contact with a drug leads to an allergic reaction, which produces the subsequent loss of control over consumption. Early support was given to the belief that alcoholism and certain types of drug dependency were the result of an allergic reaction to the substance. This support was crystallized by the physician who treated founding members of Alcoholics Anonymous, Dr. William Silkworth. Silkworth stated that alcoholism was a physical allergy combined with a mental obsession. At the request of the co-founders of Alcoholics Anonymous, Bill Wilson and Dr. Bob Smith, Silkworth included his views in the book *Alcoholics Anonymous*, which gave great prominence to the view in the early days of the addiction recovery movement. Silkworth wrote:

> We believe, and so suggested a few years ago, that the action of al-
> cohol on these chronic alcoholics is the manifestation of an allergy;
> that the phenomenon of craving is limited to this class and never
> occurs in the average temperate drinker. These allergic types can
> never safely use alcohol in any form at all; and once having formed
> the habit and found they cannot break it, once having lost their self-
> confidence, their reliance upon things human, their problems pile
> up on them and they become astonishing difficult to solve. (*Alcoholics
> Anonymous*, 1976, p. xxviii)

Supporters and members of Alcoholics Anonymous and related 12-step groups, such as Narcotics Anonymous (NA), have championed this view and continue to do so, though early references in the AA literature use allergy more as a metaphor than an actuality.

Randolph (1956) supported the position that alcoholism was a masked food allergy, and that certain food allergens whose manifestations must be counteracted through specific alcoholic beverages create a craving for alco-hol. However, subsequent research failed to confirm that alcohol stimulated production of any type of anti-alcohol antibody (Jellinek, 1960). As with the disease model, no specific mechanism, pathway, or system has ever been pro-posed to support this view, nor has an allergic reaction been linked to a single use of any drug. While certain individuals may become dependent on a drug after a single usage, the proportion is statistically insignificant and usually better attributable to other factors. Nonetheless, Ohlendorf-Moffat (1993) argued that if food allergies can cause migraines, why not a dependency to alcohol?

While this theory is largely out of favour, there may still be some value to examining the allergy link to addiction. Speaking at the 2011 annual meet-ing of the American Academy of Allergy, Asthma and Immunology, former president Dr. Sami Bahna stated that alcoholic beverages can trigger allergic reactions or exacerbate existing allergies (Rabasseda, 2011). While rare, some individuals have allergies to the alcohol itself, while others are allergic to various substances in alcoholic beverages such as beer and wine. Symptoms may include red, itchy eyes, nasal congestion, upset stomach, and difficulty breathing. Allergic reactions to an alcoholic beverage can range in severity from a minor rash to a life-threatening asthma attack and anaphylaxis. Re-searchers have pointed out that alcohol could also aggravate existing allergies (Dallas, 2011).

2.3 PSYCHOLOGICAL THEORIES
Learning Theory
Personality Theory
Psychodynamic Theory
Humanistic Theory
Attachment Theory
Rational Theory

Psychological theories examine the experience of drug dependency from within the context of an individual's behaviour. They have been advanced as an alternative to the notion that drug dependency is a unitary disease with a specific cause. This viewpoint also focuses on observable behaviours of drug use, how the behaviour is learned, modified, and reinforced, and that there may be some psychological component that exists that predisposes an individual to an accelerated pattern of use.

Learning Theory
Among the earliest investigations into why people became addicted were theories that looked at stimuli that give pleasure, relief, or excitement, and how reliably and quickly they could be produced. Learning is a change in behaviour brought on by a negative or positive experience: reinforcement. If the potential of an action or behaviour reoccurring is increased when another event—the stimulus—occurs, then learning can take place. If the occurrence of the stimulus increases the likelihood of the behaviour, this is positive reinforcement. Negative reinforcement is the process of decreasing the likelihood of a particular action occurring through a process of punishment, which can be physical (such as a shock) or psychological (such as a verbal rebuke) (Wilson, 1988).

Drug abuse researchers have identified Pavlovian sign-tracking as a major contributor to the transition from voluntary drug use to poorly controlled drug abuse. Sign-tracking is the conditioning of directed motor action that arises from the pairing of an object with a reward. In Pavlovian sign-tracking procedures, a small object (conditioned stimulus [CS]) is paired with a reward (unconditioned stimulus [US]), producing a conditioned response (CR). The response typically consists of approaching the CS, interacting with it, and eventually consuming it. When sign-tracking behaviour is poorly controlled, it resembles the process of relapse among drug users. Sign-tracking itself resembles psychomotor activation, a behavioural response produced by physical dependency–producing drugs. The effects of sign-tracking on corticosterone levels and dopamine pathways resemble the neurobiological effects of drug use, which supports the classical conditioning explanation for drug abuse (Tomie, Grimes, & Pohorecky, 2008).

Social learning theory also provides a very plausible explanation for drug abuse (Bandura, 1986). It states that people will repeat any behaviour that brings them some kind of pleasure or reward and will discontinue any behaviour that brings them discomfort or punishment. If a drug brings pleasure or relief in a stressful situation, reduces anxiety or fear, or provides status or popularity in an insecure or lonely situation, its use will become a repeated behaviour. Psychoactive drugs also have a negative reinforcement component—withdrawal—which further maintains and facilitates usage. If a person lacks alternative coping strategies, if external stressors are too great to deal with, or if there appear to be no apparent avenues of problem resolution, escape through drug use can be a powerful and extremely easily learned behaviour. Many researchers agree that reinforcement is a critical issue in understanding substance dependency (Donegan, Rodin, O'Brien, & Solomon, 1983; Gifford & Humphreys, 2007; Lewis & Lockmuller, 1990; Peralta & Steele, 2010; Woods & Schuster, 1971).

Tolerance is also an important process within this theory and is associated with habituation. Habituation is seen through reduced responses to a drug either because of prior exposure to the substance or because of the presentation of environmental stimuli that in the past have reliably predicted the presence of the drug. Opioid-dependent persons, under specific circumstances, have been observed to respond to the mere anticipation of drug effects, to an injection of saline or to an opioid injected while an antagonist is present, as if they had actually received an opioid drug (Mirin, 1984).

The final process to consider in learning theory is extinction. Extinction is the process whereby the link between previously established behaviour is weakened until a point is reached when the behaviour no longer has any reinforcing benefit or purpose. This is what the treatment process attempts to accomplish in terminating an individual's misuse or abuse of a substance. Learning theory holds much promise and insight into understanding how drug abuse develops and why drug use continues, and it has been incorporated into both treatment and prevention initiatives.

Personality Theory

Traditional personality theory has categorized personality traits into five categories:

- extraversion—talkative, lively, impulsive, risk taking, outgoing versus shy, quiet, conforming, passive
- agreeableness—sympathetic, kind, warm, cooperative, sincere, compassionate versus harsh, rude, rough, antagonistic, callous, cold
- conscientiousness—organized, systemic, efficient, precise, thorough, practical versus careless, sloppy, absent-minded, disorderly, unreliable

- emotional stability—relaxed, unemotional, easygoing, unexcitable versus moody, jealous, possessive, anxious, high-strung
- openness to experience—intellectual, complex, philosophical, innovative, unconventional versus simple, conventional, uninquisitive, shallow (Hofstee, De Raad, & Goldberg, 1992; Saucier & Goldberg, 1996)

Of these five categories, extraversion has been most closely associated with excessive substance use, particularly the attribute of impulsivity. However, the idea of an alcoholic personality was extremely popular well before the development of the five personality dimensions and contributed to the rise in popularity of personality tests for those with addiction issues in the mid-20th century (Cox & Klinger, 1988).

The most popular personality theory of substance abuse views the problem as an expression of abnormal personality traits. The characteristics commonly attributed to a drug abuser include:

- highly emotional with a low frustration tolerance
- nonconformity, impulsivity, and reward seeking
- negative affect and low self-esteem
- immature in personal relationships
- inability to express anger adequately
- ambivalence to authority
- excessive anxiety
- perfectionism and compulsiveness
- rigidity
- feelings of isolation
- sex-role confusion (Barnes, 1979; Cox, 1979; Cox & Klinger, 1988; Dolan, Bechara, & Nathan, 2007; Dom, D'Haene, Hulstiin, & Sabbe, 2006; Linn, 1975)

This broad list supports Miller's (1983a, 1995) point that alcohol-dependent persons have as broad a range of personality characteristics as those who are non-alcohol-dependent, and that no consistent personality pattern has been established with one drug, let alone across the range of psychoactive substances.

Bill Wilson, co-founder of Alcoholics Anonymous, observed that many alcohol dependent men had a craving for attention and power, just as many ardent prohibitionists of the time did (Alcoholics Anonymous, 1976). Contrarily, persons with alcoholic personalities have also been characterized as passive and dependent, as reflected by their fixation on an external locus of control (the belief that people and agents other than themselves control behaviours and reinforcements). These individuals tend to have low self-worth, be self-derogatory, and are more likely to be depressed, anxious, and impulsive (Cox, 1988).

A difference between alcoholic and pre-alcoholic personalities is believed to exist, with distinctive personality characteristics predating the drug dependency, though empirical support is difficult to obtain for this assumption. Impulsivity, independence, and rejection of conventional values have characterized the personalities of persons who later in life developed problems with alcohol and other psychoactive drugs. These people impulsively find gratification through drug use, but they have difficulty working toward long-range goals that will bring enduring satisfaction. It is also claimed that the same personality characteristics that existed among pre-alcoholics are also apparent among those in treatment for alcoholism. However, unlike pre-alcoholics, persons assessed as being addicted to alcohol have low self-esteem and show strong negative affect, particularly depression and anxiety. Although the cognitive-perceptual style of those with alcoholism is characteristically different from those who are not dependent on alcohol, it is unclear whether this distinctive style is a precursor to or a consequence of the use of the drug (Cox, 1988).

Another view suggests that substance abuse does not constitute a specific entity. Rather it is the symptom of some underlying psychiatric disturbance. Substance abusers do not differ significantly, diagnostically, from other mental health patients, according to proponents of this theory. Albert Ellis (1995), originator of Rational Emotive Behavior Therapy (REBT), states that most destructive persons with an addiction suffer from one or more severe personality disorders and that there is an underlying biological tendency to easily overreact or underreact to the stresses and strains of living. As well, most persons with a severe personality disorder come from households where their close relatives were also innately highly disruptive, leading them to experience above-average daily life stressors. According to Ellis, extensive therapy is required for these individuals to deal with their underlying behavioural issues.

Another theory relating to personality was postulated by Robert Cloninger (1987), who attempted to establish a relationship between neurotransmitter levels and personality dimensions, thus linking the biological and psychological dimensions of addiction. As dopamine facilitates the perception of pleasure or excitement, Cloninger states that those who exhibit personality traits of exploration, excitability, impulsiveness, extravagance, and disorderliness have active dopamine systems. Those with lower dopamine activity would register lower in novelty-seeking traits. Likewise, those with inactive serotonin systems would exhibit harm-avoidance behaviours in actions that seek to avoid pain and anxiety. Cloninger believed that individuals with inactive norepinephrine systems would develop strong sentimental attachments, as this neurotransmitter inhibits signals associated with reward.

Despite these varied perspectives on personality theory, the literature generally tends to side with the view that personality does not predict illness. Research continues to attempt to determine if those with certain personality characteristics become drug abusers, or if drug use creates a specific type of personality. Thus, the question remains whether the characteristics precede alcoholism and contribute to its development, or whether the traits are a result of alcohol use, misuse, and abuse. One study investigating this began by following 12,600 children from birth until the age of 16, though by that time only 4,600 participants remained. Parents were asked about their children's personalities in the first five years of life, after which the researchers interviewed both the children and their parents. The research team found that the personality traits in toddlers most closely associated with teen alcohol use fell into two categories: (1) emotional instability and relatively low sociability, and (2) high sociability, which may lead to sensation-seeking later in adolescence. Childhood temperament prior to age five was a predictor of adolescent alcohol use problems by age 16, after controlling for both socio-demographic factors and parental alcohol problems. Thus, the heterogeneity of drug users was again demonstrated as the researchers found not one high risk group but two. However, in both groups not all of the children were using drugs problematically, with many remaining abstinent (Dick et al., 2013). It is both interesting and important to note that while some would like to label those with addiction issues as having an addictive personality, we do not label those with diabetes as having a diabetic personality.

Psychodynamic Theory

This perspective arises from Freudian and post-Freudian thought, though Freud himself did not devote much attention to addiction in his extensive writings, despite his own drug dependency on tobacco and cocaine. Freud's work launched the fields of counselling and psychotherapy, yet given the growing interest in neurobiology, it is not without irony that Freud himself was trained as a neurologist. He initially turned to hypnosis to aid his patients in talking about their difficult problems before abandoning this option for psychotherapy. Sigmund Freud was the first to provide a systemic explanation of mental health issues, and his views remain influential. In Freud's perspective, there were three potential explanations for all maladaptive behaviour:

1. seeking sensuous satisfaction
2. conflicts among the components of oneself
3. fixation in the infantile past (Kottler & Montgomery, 2010)

Freud (1905) did state that alcoholism may be due to the inability to successfully resolve issues among the three components of oneself: (1) the id or instinctual striving for pleasure and/or relief, (2) the superego or conscience, and (3) the ego or coping component of the person. Failure of the ego to resolve issues between conscience and basic instincts can lead to maladaptive coping responses, including use of psychoactive drugs. In Freud's few writings directly pertaining to alcohol abuse, he commented that drug abuse could pertain to a fixation at the oral stage of psychosexual development, thus representing the need for the person to obtain immediate oral gratification and pleasure. Early followers of Freud also proposed that all addiction-related behaviours were displacements and re-enactments of early childhood sexual behaviour. This theory evolved to linking addiction to symbolic gratification and Oedipal wishes (Bonaparte, Freud, & Kris, 1954). Much later in his career, Freud also wrote simply that alcohol was misused by those exhibiting psychopathology to ward off unpleasant feelings (Barry, 1988).

Psychodynamic theory incorporated ideas that were very popular in the mid-20th century, such as denial, justification, rationalization, and intellectualization. This theory views the development of addiction as a futile attempt to repair development deficiencies of the self. As a result of these deficiencies, the capacities for regulating tension, for self-soothing, for affect recognition, and for affect consistency are all impaired (Sachs, 2009). Despite the substantive shortcomings of this view, sensuous satisfaction can apply to any behaviour that brings relief to anxiety, and psychoactive drugs fit very well into this more generalized understanding of sensuality and sexuality. Thus, addiction became generalized with the idea that the voluntary consumption of drugs is initially motivated by the desire for its pleasurable effects. Those who experience unusually strong pleasurable effects from drugs will use them excessively, even to the displacement of normative sexual behaviour, and even when the effects become destructive. The pleasurable effect is usually attributed to relief from anxieties and conflicts or as a substitute for a lack of sexual fulfillment, rather than necessarily a direct sensuous satisfaction (Salmon & Salmon, 1977).

Another psychodynamic orientation proposes that a block in emotional development of the child may result in chronic immaturity and a desire to escape from reality, or, alternatively, conflicts among components of the self may lead to substance dependency. This theory emphasizes the importance of parents in shaping an individual's life and meeting his or her needs. If a child's early needs are not met, a deficit may occur that finds resolution later in life through drug use. Psychodynamic theory states that people vulnerable to substance abuse have powerful dependency needs that can be traced to their early years. If an individual's needs are unmet at a young age, they may turn, as they mature, to substances to fulfill them. Although Freud's view is generally centred on sexual fulfillment, it can be applied to addiction as well, as an individual may turn to drugs to fulfill a need that he or she is unable to fulfill consciously (Barry, 1988). Several studies report that psychodynamic factors create internal conflicts within an individual's psychic structure, which predisposes them to the development, maintenance, and relapse of drug use (Khantzian, 2003). Studies also assert that psychotherapeutic techniques addressing these internal conflicts can be successful in the cessation of substance use (Woody, 2003).

McClelland, Davis, Kalin, and Wanner (1972) countered that addiction could also be viewed as being power-based. They interpreted the independence and aggressiveness of many male drinkers as a direct manifestation of a drive for power rather than passivity. They believed that drinking and drug use allowed men to engage in fantasies and feelings of power, and thus it was powerlessness that led to substance abuse. For women, drinking served to reduce rather than enhance fantasies of power, as women who abused substances were more anxious about their femininity (Wilsnack, 1973, 1974).

Neo-Freudian theorists and practitioners have also argued that the use of drugs allows expression of otherwise repressed tendencies, such as the need for ongoing overt oral gratification or some form of societally suppressed sexuality. The underlying premise remains that drug use relieves unconscious conflicts that individuals cannot deal with at the conscious level. Oral passivity and regression, a lack of security, a replacement for masturbation, internalized conflicts and ego deficits, guilt and unacceptable aggression, leading to desires for self-punishment and sexual denial, have all been proposed by various neo-Freudians to explain drug-dependent behaviour during the first half of the 20th century (Bonaparte, Freud, & Kris, 1954; Glover, 1928; Schilder, 1941). However, rather limited empirical research was done then to support these views as the ideas are difficult to conceptualize, and there are ethical implications for studying the concepts, especially as the events that often lead to the misuse of drugs occur many years before the onset of addiction.

The evidence in this is sparse, yet therapists remain who are willing to engage clients in extensive, long-term psychotherapy to help resolve underlying problems that manifest themselves in drug-using behaviour. Freudian theory was most popular in the early to mid-20th century when science was gaining prominence in Western civilization and faith in traditional religious teachings was waning. Freudian teaching remained a prominent component of many university counselling programs up until the 1970s, including the departments of psychiatry at Harvard, Columbia, and Johns Hopkins universities. Some of the past and present appeal of Freud's theories, much like Marx's views, was and is a result of the spiritual void they fill. As such, psychodynamic theory also has a direct evolutionary link to the peer-based methods of helping in the addiction field that arose in the 20th century (Paris, 2005).

Humanistic Theory

Humanistic theory is in part an outgrowth of and response to Freudian-based theories. This theory, however, examines mental health rather than mental illness. This theoretical perspective, developed by Abraham Maslow (1970), has a much more positive perspective on human motivation and activities. Maslow, who initially trained as an anthropologist, came to believe that all humans strove for critical understanding and empowerment, and a desire for autonomy and independence. His initial model consisted of five distinct stages of human needs that attempt to explain behaviour: physiological, safety, belongingness, self-esteem, and self-actualization. Over the course of his career, he added three additional stages: cognitive needs, aesthetic needs, and transcendence (see Figure 2.3).

These eight stages can all be directly applied to why drug use begins, is maintained, escalates, stops, and recommences. Stage one in the hierarchy comprises basic human physiological needs, which incorporates all the necessities to maintain life: air, drink, food, sex, and sleep. Physiological needs are the most basic of life's needs, and without the ability to satisfy these core needs, there can be neither personal nor societal advancement. Stage two in the hierarchy includes safety needs, such as the need for health, personal and financial security, and the need for familiarity. This second level of need entails the search for a safe, ordered, and secure world with protection from both physically and socially harmful elements. Stage three relates to the need of belonging or, in other words, social and love needs. This includes the need to be able to relate to others, the need for friends and family, and the capacity to develop affectionate, close, personal relationships, including romantic relationships. This category involves not only receiving love but also giving love.

Stage four of Maslow's hierarchy relates to esteem needs, which include the needs required for a stable, positive regard for oneself. This involves not only self-respect, but also respect from others. Esteem needs also consist of the desire for acknowledgement, freedom, importance, independence, prestige, reputation, responsibility, and status. Those searching for esteem needs are seeking feelings of self-confidence and worth. Following this is the first of the additions to the original model, that of cognitive needs. As Maslow applied his theory, he observed that people also had a need to increase their knowledge. Cognitive needs include the human need to discover, explore, and learn more about oneself and one's environment. Another addition was that of aesthetic needs, the search for beauty both in nature and in personal artistic expression.

FIGURE 2.3: MASLOW'S ENHANCED HIERARCHY OF NEEDS MODEL

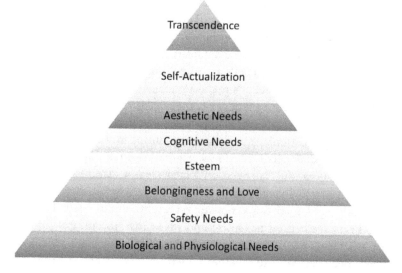

Sources: Koltko-Rivera (2006); Maslow (1970)

The initial peak of Maslow's final level in the hierarchy was self-actualization; realizing one's personal potential and obtaining a state of self-fulfillment. This was attained through seeking personal growth and achieving peak experiences, though for most people, it is the search rather than the actual accomplishment of this step that is critical. Self-actualization involves becoming what one has the capability of being. It is the need and the desire for self-fulfillment, using one's skills, talents, and experience to maximum benefit both for oneself and others. However, Maslow also added one additional level beyond self-actualization: transcendence. The level of self-actualization initially had a spiritual component. With continued research, however, Maslow noted that humans across cultures strove to aid others to reach their maximum potential. They reached out to help others in need, thereby securing a larger sense of purpose and meaning. After reaching a level of self-actualization, Maslow states that further striving leads people to connect with a greater whole or a higher truth. This provides a broader understanding of the motivational roots of social progress and human behaviour, such as altruism, and underscores the spiritual dimension of humanity (Koltko-Rivera, 2006).

The humanistic perspective views the causes of drug dependency as boredom, frustration, and the inability to reach one's potential because of blockages in Maslow's hierarchy of need fulfillment. When people are denied either access to or the opportunity to meet their next level of need, they turn to drugs to compensate for or escape from their plight. And while drugs can provide an artificial sense of security, in actuality they create greater vulnerability. Individual or group therapy is again the primary method to remedy the drug-dependence problem. Individuals are viewed as much more functional than in psychodynamic theory, with greater ability to change and adapt in a positive manner. In the application of this theoretical model, the counsellor focuses on what blocks are impeding a person from realizing her or his potential. The counsellor's role is to determine what needs are not being met and how drug use satisfies or counterbalances the blockage.

Humanistic theory has been critiqued for being very weak theoretically, for being overly reductionist, and for not accounting for the origin and nature of the self and human needs. Maslow's original research that examined what makes people successful has been criticized for not being rigorous. Critics also note that Maslow's conclusions did not directly relate to his field of research, resulting in a far too simplistic representation of need. This theory has also been deemed ethnocentric and insensitive to cultural differences (Geller, 1982; Hofstede, 1984; Neher, 1991; Smith & Feigenbaum, 2012). Questions have been raised as to whether a hierarchy exists and if fundamental human needs are hierarchical in nature (Cianci & Gambrel, 2003; Wahba & Bridgewell, 1976).

Attachment Theory

Attachment theory examines the relationships between people with a focus on long-term emotional bonds, which begin with early parent-child interaction. Prominent theorists in this area are John Bowlby (1958, 1969), who describes attachment as the lasting psychological connectedness between people, and Mary Ainsworth (1973), who observed what occurred when children ages 12–18 months were separated from and then reunited with their mothers. Her work led to the categorization of three major styles of attachment:

1. Secure attachment, where children express distress when separated from their caregivers and joy upon their return. Children with secure attachment know their primary caregivers will provide comfort and reassurance, so they are comfortable seeking them out in times of need.
2. Ambivalent-insecure attachment, where children become extremely and inconsolably distressed when their caregivers leave. This typically occurs in instances where the caregivers are not regularly available and the child cannot depend upon them to return when the child needs them.
3. Avoidant-insecure attachment, where children avoid the primary caregivers and, when given a choice, do not select the parent over a stranger. This is most commonly the result of neglectful or abusive caregiving (Ainsworth, Blehar, Waters, & Wall, 1978).

To these three stages, Main and Solomon (1986) added a fourth, that of disorganized-insecure attachment. Children who appear disorientated, confused, and even dazed, and who avoid and even resist their caregivers, are placed in this category. This behaviour is typically the result of inconsistent parenting, where caregivers do provide comfort but also invoke fear. This leads the child to display inconsistent attachment patterns, which persist into adulthood.

The core idea behind attachment theory is that primary caregivers who are available and responsive to children's needs allow them to develop a sense of security, which some label as love. This then allows the children to explore their environment in a confident manner, knowing they are protected. Children who are securely attached as infants tend to develop stronger self-esteem, and are more sociable and self-reliant as they grow older. They generally become independent and exhibit good school performance. All of these qualities establish a foundation for successful adulthood interactions. Individuals who are more securely attached in childhood tend to have good self-esteem, positive romantic relationships, and the ability to self-disclose to others (Hazan & Shaver, 1987). Failure to form secure attachments early in life can produce a range of mental health issues, including the greater likelihood of turning to psychoactive drugs to achieve a sense of comfort (Ainsworth, 1991; Prior & Glaser, 2006).

Attachment theory views addiction as an attempt to fill the void resulting from the lack of a secure attachment during childhood, including painful, rejecting, or shaming relationships. As a result, excessive drug use is viewed as an individual's attempt to self-repair psychological deficits and fill the emptiness from childhood. The vulnerability caused by developmental failures and early environmental deprivation leads to an ineffective attachment style as an adolescent and/or adult. Inappropriate attachment behaviours tend to be intensified through the excessive use of psychoactive drugs as observed through problematic regulation of appropriate affect, behaviour, and self-care (Flores, 2001, 2006). In a study of attachment, fear of intimacy, and differentiation of self, 158 volunteers, 99 of whom were enrolled in an addiction treatment program, reported higher levels of insecure attachment and fear of intimacy, and lower levels of secure attachment and differentiation of self when compared to a control group (Thorberg & Lyvers, 2006). Similar results were also found in a study of substance-dependent German adolescents (Schindler et al., 2005).

Rational Theory

The last of the psychological theories to be discussed proposes that some, if not most, people drink or use other psychoactive drugs without realizing the potential dangers. They are aware of or care about only the positive, short-term effects produced by the substance and generally do not believe they will experience any long-term harm. The theory states that as persons become more knowledgeable and informed about psychoactive drugs, their use of drugs should correspondingly decrease. This theory is based on sound theoretical arguments and empirical outcomes, and the belief that a rational human being will strive toward health and longevity (Allott, Paxton, & Leonard, 1999; Brown, 2001). Health promotion and drug awareness campaigns have been correlated with decreases in drug use. For example, since 1964, smoking rates have dropped by more than half in North America as a direct result of successful education, legislative, and smoking cessation efforts. Education is an essential component in drug use prevention and should be a core component of any treatment practice. School systems now recognize the importance of primary prevention and early intervention, and many school boards now begin their drug education programming in the junior grades (United Nations Office on Drug and Crime, 2004). In 2002, Caulkins, Pacula, Paddock, and Chiesa reported that well-developed and -delivered school-based substance abuse–prevention programs consistently reduce drug use among adolescents. Likewise, educated health care practitioners can also lead to a decrease in the prescription of psychotherapeutic agents (Ray et al., 1993).

However, the rational model approach does not always work, or, in a worst-case scenario, is subverted. In 2011, a warning was issued in Vancouver regarding high-potency heroin and a subsequent increase in fatal overdoses. After the education campaign, semi-structured qualitative interviews were conducted with 18 active heroin injectors to ascertain why, despite being aware of the danger, they did not stop their heroin use. Researchers were surprised to learn that, rather than responding with caution, many users actively sought out the higher potency heroin. The education campaign was negated by the sales tactics of dealers, the pain and fear of withdrawal, entrenched injecting routines, and the desire for intense intoxication. While the campaign provided accurate information, it did not address the underlying issues pertaining to drug use (Kerr, Small, Hyshkal, Maher, & Shannon, 2013).

Even more concerning is that the rational approach is actively used by pharmaceutical companies to misinform or at least distract physicians. Pharmaceutical companies covertly influence the publication of research papers (Angell, 2008; Spielmans & Parry, 2010), and many journals now require conflict-of-interest statements from authors along with a disclosure as to who funded their research. Further, the majority of contributors to the last two editions of the *Diagnostic and Statistical Manual of Mental Disorders* have held consulting contracts with pharmaceutical companies (Cosgrove & Krimsky, 2012; Cosgrove, Krimsky, Vijayaraghavan, & Schneider, 2006). In addition are the findings of a content analysis of 11 prominent medical journals used by German physicians to keep abreast of new developments in their field. Researchers identified 313 journal issues containing drug advertisements and 412 articles where specific drug recommendations were made by the authors. Free journals almost exclusively recommended the use of the specified drugs.

In contrast, journals financed entirely by subscription fees tended to recommend against the use of the very same drugs. Thus, a distinct bias was found in medical journals that focus on continuing physician education based on whether the journal was funded by the reader or the advertiser (Becker et al., 2011). Unfortunately, this is not a new trend. The promotional influence of pharmaceutical manufacturers on the prescribing behaviour of physicians has been noted for nearly half a century. Studies have found that physicians' knowledge of drug properties is more consistent with sales information than with the evidence published in the medical literature. Direct-to-physician promotion of pharmaceuticals has led to the widespread inappropriate use of psychoactive drugs, which in turn has resulted in increased morbidity and mortality for patients. Commercial sources of information for many drugs have consistently overstated their benefits and underestimated their risks, thus demonstrating the utility of the rational model, though not in a positive manner (Kesselheim, 2011).

2.4 SOCIOLOGICAL THEORIES
Cultural Theories
Subcultural Theories
Deviant Behaviour Theory
Marxist Theory
Availability-Control Theory
Environmental Stress

The classification of drugs as licit or illicit is not typically a result of the biological attributes of the substance but rather a social construct. Sociological models not only examine drug use in the context of the entire society, but also how addiction is produced through social practices. They hypothesize that larger socio-cultural events influence trends in drug use and that drug abuse does not occur in isolation. Events in the broader environment such as ceremonies, cultural norms, politics, the political economy, rituals, and the media, also need to be considered, as well as the manner in which drugs are regarded and regulated by society.

Cultural Theories

Perhaps in order to understand Japanese alcohol use from a Japanese perspective, it is important to understand that for many Japanese drinking is their sole hobby, and when asked what their hobby is they will openly say "drinking." At company parties it is custom to keep drinking until your boss stops. Not to drink can be insulting to your colleagues, though I do know some Japanese non-drinkers and I am not sure how they get around the drinking party custom. It doesn't matter what happens while drunk, it is never discussed the next day. Furthermore, drinking alcohol is acceptable in the park, and even on the train. (Heather Dorion, personal communication, 2007)

Culture is a set of thoughts shared by members of a social unit that include common understandings, patterns of beliefs, and expectations. Cultural guidelines are generally unwritten rules of conduct and direction for acceptable behaviour and actions reflecting the morals and values of a specific group. Cultural theory begins with this premise in attempting to describe and explain the process of drug use in relation to societal norms. This perspective moves significantly beyond the simpler disease and related biological models and its predecessor, the moral model, in understanding the process of addiction. Regardless of how potent a psychoactive substance may be, its effects are moderated by the practices, norms, and environmental context of the user (Waldorf, Reinarman, & Murphy, 1991).

Socio-cultural theorists support the demystification of substance use and the study of drugs within an integrated life model. As early as 1943, Horton asserted that the primary function of alcohol in a culture was to reduce anxiety. Thus, substance abuse would be more prevalent in societies where anxiety abounded and where few alternatives to drinking alcohol and using drugs as tension-releasers existed. These societies would also exhibit the highest rates of intoxication. Bales (1946) built and expanded on Horton's premise using cultural and cross-cultural studies. He stated that cultures influence alcohol use in three distinct ways:

1. by the degree to which they operate to bring about acute needs for adjustment of inner tensions such as guilt, suppression, aggression, conflict, and sexual tension in their members
2. by the attitudes toward drinking that they produce in the members, seen in the information exchange, including advertising
3. by the degree to which the culture provides substitute means of satisfaction beyond substance use in the form of positive alternative lifestyle options

Four distinct cultural patterns of drug use have been identified (Schutten & Eijnden, 2003). The first are abstinent cultures, where the overall attitude toward drugs, including alcohol, is negative and all alcoholic beverages are forbidden. Middle Eastern nations, such as Saudi Arabia, typify this pattern. The second are ambivalent cultures, where the attitude toward alcohol use is positive in social settings but negative in others. The African nation of Morocco is an example of this cultural pattern. Morocco is a democratic Islamic nation that has a parliament, but where the hereditary king's decisions supersede parliament. Islam forbids the drinking of alcohol, but it is widely available throughout the nation. Along with the availability of alcohol in hotels and upscale restaurants in the larger urban centres, wine and beer can be bought from liquor stores and supermarkets and even in small communities in the Atlas Mountains. Likewise, while marijuana is an illicit drug, it is openly cultivated and is a major economic vehicle in the north of the nation, where other cash crops are difficult to grow.

Permissive cultures are ones where the use of alcoholic beverages is acceptable, though a negative attitude toward drunkenness remains, such as Canada. Finally, ultra-permissive cultures are those where the attitude is permissive toward both drinking and alcohol-related problems. This last model is most likely to be observed in a culture that is experiencing a rapid social change, especially where there is a heavy economic interest in alcohol production and distribution. The most recent example of this is what has occurred in Russia since its attempted transition to a free market economy and its retrenchment under the protracted leadership of Putin.

Cultures tend to have lower rates of alcohol problems when the rules governing the use of substances are clear, uniform, and prohibitive with specific social sanctions associated with use; when members of the culture are exposed to alcohol at an early age and observe adults using alcohol in moderate amounts in settings that discourage the use of the drug as an intoxicant, such as at meals or during religious ceremonies; and when the excessive use of alcohol, including drunkenness, is uniformly discouraged and proscribed (Whitehead & Harvey, 1974). Examples of this pattern of drug use are the traditional Chinese and Jewish populations.

Boyd (1983) contrasted the difficulties Chinese policy-makers of the early 20th century had in attempting to curb opium use with those of a neighbouring nation, India, which had far fewer problems with opium despite an even longer history of use. The difference according to Boyd was that in India, opium had been employed for centuries for medicinal and ceremonial purposes, while in China, it did not have the same historic or cultural uses and had first been used as a recreational substance. The use of opium had become so well integrated into Indian society that it was not seen as a social problem and rarely caused a debilitating dependency, a situation that continues today despite the enormous population of that nation. Similar to China, North American society experiences problems with most psychoactive drugs because there is no clear cultural consensus on use. Contemporary North American culture allows and even encourages the ingestion of drugs for personal use and for the attainment of quick physical and emotional pain relief. The use of drugs is poorly integrated, with attitudes toward use being ambivalent and inconsistent. People tend to drink one way with members of the family, another way when with business associates, and yet a different way at a party.

Cultural theory also considers the role of media in the development of drug use, misuse, and addiction. Marketing cues may influence the paths that individuals take both toward becoming addicted and moving away from maladaptive consumption and addiction. Beginning in the 1930s, the tobacco industry paid prominent movie stars—such as Gary Cooper, Joan Crawford, Clark Gable, Carole Lombard, Barbara Stanwyck, and Spencer Tracy—$10,000 per year to promote its product (Lum, Polansky, Jackler, & Glantz, 2008). A 2005 study of 6,500 children reported that of the 10 percent who were smokers, nearly 40 percent stated they tried smoking as a result of the way it was portrayed in the movies (Sargent et al., 2005). As well, both tobacco and alcohol consumption rates have been linked to advertising tactics and specific product exposure, which, despite policy changes, continue to target adolescents (Hafez & Ling, 2005; Ota, Akimaru, Suzuki, & Ono, 2008; Snyder, Milici, Slater, Sun, & Strizhakova, 2006; Wilkinson et al., 2009).

All verbal and visual alcohol references were recorded in an examination of 46 hours of televised British professional football (soccer) matches. An average of 111 visual references per hour or about 2 per minute were detected, typically through sponsorship signs in the stadium, on uniforms, and through actual verbal references to alcohol during the broadcast (Graham & Adams, 2013). The average annual number of alcohol ads seen by youth watching television in the United States increased from 217 in 2001 to 366 in 2009, approximately one alcohol ad per day. During the same time period, youth were 22 times more likely to see an alcohol product ad than an alcohol company-sponsored "responsibility" promotion warning against underage drinking and/or alcohol-impaired driving. Exposure to alcohol advertising influences underage drinking and the development of alcohol-related problems (Center on Alcohol Marketing and Youth, 2012). Likewise, a correlation between exposure to cannabis in popular music and early cannabis use among urban American adolescents has been found (Primack, Douglas, & Kraemer, 2009).

Subcultural Theories

Subcultural theories take a slightly different approach than cultural models, though they also view the environment as playing a large role in determining whether a person will drink alcohol or take drugs. However, this model places greater emphasis on the significance of a variety of specific psychosociological variables in determining the extent of the drug use within a specific population. For example, to become a problem drinker, a culture must permit drinking, and heavy drinking at least occasionally. Consumers of alcohol often become conditioned at an early age to expect that alcohol or other psychoactive drugs can do great things for them. Fisher and Harrison (1997) indicated that Irish-Americans were a classic example of this pattern.

Lawson, Peterson, and Lawson (1983) reported that 30 percent of children with parents who were alcohol-dependent themselves developed alcoholism, compared with 5 percent of children with parents who used alcohol moderately and 10 percent of children whose parents abstained. While this is also a potential argument for a genetic model, the fact that those children whose parents did drink but in a non-abusive manner had lower rates of alcoholism than abstainers better supports a subcultural orientation. Lawson (1992) reported that disengaged, rigid families who are conflict-orientated and repressed, along with moralistic families, were the most likely to produce children who later developed an addiction to alcohol.

A distinct subculture that has silently emerged in the 20th century with an above-average consumption of drugs involves post-secondary students. Throughout North America, as well as in Western Europe, high volumes of alcohol consumption and risky single-occasion drinking occur among college and university students. This consumption is associated with considerable harm to both those who consume the alcohol and their fellow students. Male students in particular tend to consume alcohol more often and in higher quantities. Consumption typically occurs during social gatherings for social enhancement, social camaraderie, and tension reduction. Students without family obligations and those living alone, with roommates, or in areas with a high density of students are more likely to consume alcohol in higher quantities and to engage in higher risk behaviour, as are those of greater socio-economic status. Students who consume excessive amounts of alcohol also tend to overestimate the extent of their fellow students' alcohol consumption (LaBrie, Hummer, & Pedersen, 2007; Wechsler, Lee, Kuo, & Lee, 2000; Wicki, Kuntsche, & Gmel, 2010).

A second subcultural theory proposes that there are people who feel alienated from their own particular society, and have no sense of belonging. This alienation prohibits them from feeling bound by society's rules governing drug use, and they therefore have a higher risk of developing a dependence on drugs (Rankin, 1978). Supporting this are recent studies with animals that indicate that leaders of groups are less likely to take drugs than their subordinates (Kuhar, 2002). Both cultural and subcultural theories view the remedy for drug abuse as a unification of cultural norms and societal expectations. Research in this field continually points to an increase in drug use when cultural norms and expectations begin to break down.

There have been a few recent studies conducted that add additional empirical support to this theory. One examined enlisted members of the American Navy and found that they had a far greater use of alcohol than did either civilian members or the general population. Several issues specific to the Navy were found to contribute to problem drinking, according to the study, including the young age of recruits, alternating periods of exertion and boredom within the role, and a culture that emphasizes drinking as a mechanism for bonding, recreation, and stress relief (Ames, Duke, Moore, & Cunradi, 2009). Similarly, the California Department of Health Services (2005) found that smoking overall had decreased over the years in the state except among some very specific subcultures, including Korean men, members of the lesbian, gay, bisexual, and transgender community, and members of the armed forces. Immigrants from India and China were found to be less likely to smoke, though their children born in the United States had a rate of use closer to the mean.

A third variant of subcultural theory arises from the ongoing criminalization of drug use in response to the "War on Drugs," and the complex manner in which social, political, and environmental factors interact to create culture. By criminalizing large segments of specific subgroups because of their use of drugs, criminal activity within these subcultures becomes not only normalized but also creates a sense of social cohesion. Thus, naturalizing illegal activity within these groups and the violation of society's rule of law in this one area erodes adherence to society's rules in general. Further, in groups where production or distribution of illegal drugs has become a primary means of economic survival, social cohesion is created along with ties of loyalty and reciprocity to the group and its behaviours—including violence—rather than to the larger society's rules of conduct. This is further solidified if the subculture is socially vulnerable due to structural and oppressive factors that support drug use within the community. These factors include less education, less access to employment, and greater risk of violence in the community, which is, of course, linked to the greater use and distribution of illegal drugs. Thus, drug issues need to be addressed by policies that attend to social exclusion, such as not being part of broader public discussions, lack of access to existing services, lack of income to satisfy basic needs, and lack of employment options other than in the underground economy (Briones, Cumsille, Henao, & Pardo, 2013).

Deviant Behaviour Theory

Another theoretical explanation that some sociologists have proposed to explain drug use is through deviant behaviour or delinquency. Becker (1963) argues that deviant behaviour is defined as the failure to obey group rules. This orientation emphasizes the fact that many users are individuals who are rejected and separated from the mainstream of society. A person may originally attract attention through some unusual or rebellious act, such as minor crime, public mischief, or illicit drug use, which can also include underage drinking or the use of tobacco. If this behaviour meets with a significant negative reaction from the surrounding society, the individual can be forced into an isolated lifestyle, and drug dependency may result or be maintained and escalate (Topalli, 2005). What is critical to understand is why some behaviour is socially constructed as deviant and who benefits from this definition, as nothing in society has an inherent meaning; rather, it is given meaning. This theory underscores the fact that a diagnosis of alcoholism or drug addiction is a label and a negative subjective judgment made in relation to societal standards of normality. This judgment is contingent on factors that diverge from culture to culture, and the classification of the addicted person can depend on a range of factors, including, but not limited to, age, ethnicity, geographic location, leisure pursuits, sex, sexual orientation, social status, and even the drug of choice. Thus, the notion of deviance is a social construct created by society. It is not a quality of the act a person commits but a consequence of how the dominant group interprets the act and sanctions the persons engaged in the action (Becker, 1963).

The social construction of labels in society occurs mainly through the mass media, which shapes our individual and collective consciousness by organizing and circulating the discrete knowledge individuals have, and the contexts, of their everyday lives (Adoni & Mane, 1984; Goode & Ben-Yehuda, 1994). The media can create a panic by leading citizens to believe that the behaviour of deviants, in this case, drug users, poses a substantial threat to society, such as through a crack cocaine, methamphetamine, or OxyContin epidemic, depending on the era and the context. The larger society then persecutes such drug users, treating them with neglect or hostility—often both. This increases the negative labelling and misrepresentation of the deviant group in the media, as evidenced by the use of the slang term "hillbilly heroin" to refer to OxyContin. Rather than seeing the person who uses drugs as a colleague, friend, or parent, society comes to see the person as an object, an addict. This is how such persons then begin to view themselves, which allows them to engage in additional behaviours labelled as deviant.

The use of marijuana in Jamaican culture, in contrast to its use in continental North America, is an example of differential drug use by culture. Khat is a licit drug in Africa and Arabia and yet was prohibited in Canada with no parliamentary debate. Similarly, coca leaves have been used for thousands of years in South America and can be purchased in markets, much like caffeine in North American. Yet with its refinement and introduction to developed nations, a major drug misuse and abuse problem emerged, often appearing to overwhelm other psychoactive drug issues that in absolute numbers are still a much greater social and health problem.

Marxist Theory

As with Freudian-based psychodynamic theory, Marxist models have been applied to almost every social problem. Marxism has as its central focus the relationship between human labour and capital, the means of production and class struggle that Marx examined from slavery to the age of feudalism, to the establishment of guilds, the predecessors of the union movement of the late 19th and 20th centuries. For Marx, oppression applied to gender, race, and religion, but most importantly, to class. It entailed not just exploitation, but also marginalization. In Marxist philosophy individuals' problems cannot be separated from their environment, or their class status. A Marxist discussing substance abuse would claim that human problems are the direct result of the economic and sociological structure of a culture. Specifically, any society that denies equal opportunities to all citizens or allows one powerful group to exploit less powerful or powerless groups will witness the development of many social problems. These will be most evident in, but not the exclusive domain of, those most greatly disenfranchised. These social problems are the direct result of the stresses and anxieties of an unjust society that does not permit all citizens the right, ability, or opportunity to flourish (Marx, 2004).

Social problems can take many forms: aggression, crime, mental illness, or drug abuse and dependency. The specific problems that a given individual has depend on the environmental circumstances that are prevailing at the time or that exerted a major influence in the past. Thus, personal predisposition can be a factor in determining whether a person develops schizophrenia, an addiction, or becomes physically abusive. The intent of this theory is to take the blame and responsibility that has historically exclusively focused only on the failings of an individual and focus it on those external environmental factors that created the context for the development of drug use or other social issues. This has particular relevance in North America, where an underlying factor in the permitting or prohibiting of drugs was the association of the drug with a threatening foreign culture and/or unruly members of the working class, particularly those who opposed capitalist interests through labour unrest and unionization (Stevens, 2010).

For many critics, the one common concern is how Marxism can address the substance use and abuse of the affluent. For Marx, the one true human need was to work—to labour. He claimed that what differentiates humans from animals is our human spirit, our ability to imagine and create our work and to use our intelligence to devise and understand our purpose. Those who did not have any reason or need to contribute to the means of production turned to drugs in their boredom, in a search for some type of meaning in their lives (Marx, 2004). A variety of studies in the United States have indicated that more affluent adolescents were actually more likely to use alcohol and other drugs than their peers from lower socio-economic communities. Disposable income, disconnected families, and pressure to succeed all contributed to drug use among affluent young people, as did the simple ability to buy fake IDs and the drugs themselves (Wested, 2007). It is also critical to recognize that wealth alone does not insulate people from unjust societal conditions. Marxism is a philosophy, not merely a political idea. Marxists believe that a systems change is required to address problems such as drug abuse. Despite a tendency to be classified and dismissed as a theory of rhetoric, Marxist views do have some validity and a role in providing a global perspective on substance dependency, as well as in critiquing other theoretical perspectives.

The other value of Marxist thought in terms of addiction theory is that it forces us to consider not only demand-side issues but also supply-side issues. Addiction became a moral issue in North America with the intersection of Protestantism and early capitalism. From this arose the notion of renouncing drinking in favour of piety, workplace productivity, and economic gain (Reinarman, 2005). Alcohol consumption was labelled problematic as it was associated with organized labour and its challenge to the status quo of early capitalist enterprises. Dry zones were created around work sites, and company towns outlawed taverns and alcohol (May, 1997; Petersen, 1987).

This is not a historic issue, however, but one that continues in present day. Following is a list of nations the Bush administration deemed as the world's major drug producers or transit hubs and why (Box 2.1). The list contains half of South America's 14 nations, six countries from Central America and the Caribbean, and five from Asia, while there are none from Europe, only Mexico from North America, and Nigeria from Africa. After each nation's name, in parentheses, is their world ranking at the time in terms of their gross domestic product (GDP). GDP is the measure of a nation's income and output in one year. It is the total value of all final goods and services produced in a particular economy within a country's borders in a given year, which, of course, does not include revenues generated from the illicit drug trade. The International Monetary Fund (2008) recognizes the GDP of 179 nations. The average ranking by GDP of the countries on the Bush administration's major drug producers' list is 75, despite the fact that three nations, Brazil, India, and Mexico, place in the top 10 percent. Excluding those three, the mean ranking of the remaining 17 nations drops to 86th, or roughly that of Yemen, whose GDP was $21,818,000 or roughly 66 times less than Canada's, which at $1,436,086,000 ranked 9th in the world in 2007 (United States Department of State, 2008).

Poverty is a complex and pervasive issue worldwide. More than half of the developing world lives in poverty, with over 1 billion people worldwide living on approximately Can$1 a day with another billion earning between $1 and $2. Thus, when there is a chance to become more economically independent or provide for oneself and one's family, it is hardly surprising that many in Third World nations take that opportunity. It is not surprising then to see that the majority of nations in the following list have among the lowest GDPs on the planet. For those who rank higher, such as Brazil, which is 10th, and India, which is 12th, we see nations with great economic disparities and often with a small and newly emerging middle class, which tends to anchor developed nations.

Marxist theory directs us to examine the role that poverty, social exclusion, and the lack of meaning for one's labour play in increasing the risk of addiction through both the demand and supply sides of the drug equation.

BOX 2.1: THE BUSH ADMINISTRATION'S DESIGNATION OF THE WORLD'S MAJOR DRUG PRODUCING NATIONS (GDP)

Afghanistan (117): It grew 93 percent of opium poppy in the world in 2007, which was the second record-setting year in a row. The export value of this harvest was $4 billion, which is more than a third of the country's combined gross domestic product.

The Bahamas (130): It is a transit hub for moving cocaine from South America and marijuana from Jamaica. The country's police force seized $7.8 million in drug-related cash, five vessels, and a plane in 2007. Other officials seized 1,389 pounds of cocaine and approximately 56 tons of marijuana.

Bolivia (102): It is the third-largest producer of cocaine in the world, accounting for an estimated 127 tons. It is also a transit point for cocaine from Peru and a grower of marijuana that is mostly consumed within the country. It is legal to grow up to 29,652 acres of coca leaf for traditional uses, an allotment that the nation's government is discussing increasing in the future.

Brazil (10): Brazil is a major transport hub for cocaine base and cocaine hydrochloride, and, to a lesser extent, a hub for heroin. In 2007 the nation's federal police seized 14 tons of cocaine hydrochloride, 2,019 pounds of cocaine base, 1,076 pounds of crack, 169 tons of marijuana, and 35 pounds of heroin.

Colombia (37): Colombia, the world's number one cocaine supplier, is also a major supplier of heroin and precursor chemicals. In 2007 the government seized 144 tons of cocaine and 350,000 gallons of precursor chemicals. It also destroyed 240 cocaine hydrochloride labs and 2,875 coca base labs.

Dominican Republic (69): It is a major transit country for cocaine and heroin from South America. In 2007 the country's authorities seized approximately 4 tons of cocaine, 226 pounds of heroin, 17,902 units of MDMA, and 1,128 pounds of marijuana.

Ecuador (67): It is a major transit point for cocaine, heroin, and precursor chemicals. In 2007 the government seized 25 tons of cocaine, 397 pounds of heroin,, and 1,631 pounds of cannabis. It also identified cocaine laboratories and plots of coca plants.

Guatemala (76): It is a major transit hub for cocaine and heroin from South America. Although it is not a major producer, poppy cultivation has begun to rise.

Haiti (131): It is a major hub for transportation of cocaine from South America and marijuana from the Caribbean. In 2007 smuggling using small aircraft from Venezuela increased 38 percent, and 29 illicit landing strips were identified. Fast boats also arrive on the southern coast transporting cocaine from South America.

India (12): It is a hub for heroin transport. Drugs are smuggled from Myanmar, and hashish and marijuana are smuggled from Nepal. Most heroin produced within India is used domestically, but an increasing amount is being shipped overseas. India is the only country the international community has authorized to produce opium gum for pharmaceutical uses.

Jamaica (111): It is the largest producer of marijuana and marijuana-derived products in the Caribbean. It is also a major hub for drug transit. Marijuana seizures decreased by 8 percent in 2007 to 46 tons. Cocaine seizures also decreased in 2007.

Laos (139): The country is one of the three that comprise the Golden Triangle. Laos recorded record low levels of opium cultivation in 2007. However, Southeast Asian heroin, amphetamine-type stimulants, and narcotic precursor chemicals still travelled through Laos to other countries in the region.

Mexico (13): Approximately 90 percent of all cocaine consumed in the United States travels through Mexico. The country is also a source of heroin, methamphetamines, and marijuana. In 2007 Mexican officials intercepted more than 52 tons of cocaine, 2,396 tons of marijuana, 643 pounds of opium gum, 656 pounds of heroin, and 1,981 pounds of methamphetamines. Presently the nation has a small civil war underway being fuelled by drug cartels.

Myanmar (101): This totalitarian regime is the world's second-largest producer of opium poppy. Cultivation increased in 2007 after dropping steadily between 1998 and 2006. The increase is slight, however, in comparison with production before 1998. It was one of two countries the United States administration designated as having "failed demonstrably" to meet its counternarcotics agreements over the year.

Nigeria (41): It is home to major drug trafficking networks that move cocaine and heroin to developed countries. Between January and September 2007, Nigerian officials seized 101,272 pounds of cannabis, 571 pounds of cocaine, 189 pounds of heroin, and 450 pounds of psychotropic substances.

Pakistan (47): It is a major hub for transportation of opiates and hashish from Afghanistan. It also saw an increase in poppy cultivation to about 5,720 acres, up from 4,715 acres the previous year. More than 1,482 acres were eradicated. It is part of the Golden Crescent along with Afghanistan and Iran.

Panama (93): Panama is a key transport hub for drugs coming from Colombia. In 2007 the government seized 66 tons of cocaine, including the largest recorded maritime seizure of 17 tons.

Paraguay (107): It is the largest marijuana producer in South America. It is also a transit route for cocaine produced in the Andes. In 2007 the government seized 1,808 pounds of cocaine, 100 metric tons of marijuana, and 18 vehicles.

Peru (54): It is a major producer of cocaine and a large importer of precursor chemicals. In 2007 the government eradicated 27,322 acres of coca. An additional 2,511 were eradicated voluntarily.

Venezuela (35): It is one of the key routes for drugs coming out of Colombia. In 2007 drug seizures in Venezuela dropped, but third-country seizures of drugs coming out of Venezuela rose. It was one of two countries the administration designated as having "failed demonstrably" to meet its counternarcotics agreements (United States Department of State, 2008).

Availability-Control Theory

As with many of the previous models discussed, the availability-control or consumption model was initially built around alcohol use. However, like the others, it can also be equally applied to other psychoactive substances of abuse. In most contemporary societies where alcohol is consumed, some type of control is exercised over its use. Most governments have moved beyond the informal rules that underlie the cultural and subcultural theories and introduced formal substance-control laws.

The most basic law of economics links price to demand. Thus, logically, as the price of alcohol or any other drug increases, consumption should decrease, particularly among those with the least disposable income, which includes teens and young adults. A series of international studies conducted during the 1970s found similar results in the consumption pattern of alcohol across numerous different cultures (Bruun et al., 1975). The availability-control theory of alcohol-related problems asserts that the greater the availability of alcohol in a society, the greater the prevalence and severity of alcohol-related problems in that society. This research confirmed the earlier pioneering work of Ledermann (1956), who postulated that a change in the average consumption of alcohol in a population is likely to be accompanied by a change in the same direction in the proportion of heavy consumers. Since heavy use of alcohol generally increases the probability of physical and social damage, the average consumption should be closely related to the prevalence of such damage in any population. Any measures that may be expected to affect overall consumption, such as those regulating the availability of alcohol, are also likely to affect the prevalence of alcohol problems, and hence should be a central consideration in any prevention programming (Schmidt & Popham, 1978; Skog, 1980).

In the Ledermann distribution equation, while the absolute number of drinkers changes and the proportion of those who actually drink varies, the pattern remains consistent across the different populations studied. Changes in the proportion of the drinking population who are at risk or who may be defined as problem drinkers is directly related to changes in the average alcohol consumption. The higher the average consumption, the greater will be the proportion of drinkers who develop an alcohol dependency. If the attitudes toward alcohol use and intoxication are liberal, then the average consumption is largely dependent on availability. If there are no limits on supply and distribution, the theory states that the main social factor affecting changes in average alcohol consumption will be changes in the relative cost of alcoholic beverages. For example, in Finland, the impact of alcohol tax cuts in March 2004 was significant, resulting in an estimated eight additional alcohol-positive deaths per week, a 17 percent increase compared with the weekly average of 2003 (Koski, Sirén, Vuori, & Poikolainen, 2007). In Norway, a one-hour extension of bar closing hours led to an increase of an average 20 violent incidents on weekend nights per 100,000 people per year (Rossow & Norström, 2012). Likewise, when British Columbia allowed the privatization of liquor stores in 2003, there was a rapid increase in the total number of liquor stores per 1,000 residents. The increase in the number of outlets was followed by an increase of alcohol-related deaths of 3.25 percent for each 20 percent increase in private store density (Stockwell et al., 2011). This supported existing research that had found that the greater alcohol outlet density, the greater alcohol consumption and related harms, including health, injury, crime, and violence (Campbell et al., 2009; Connor, Kypri, Bell, & Cousins, 2010). In contrast, alcohol-related disease mortality declined by 7.0 percent after a 1990 tax increase for spirits and beer in New York State (Delcher, Maldaono-Mollina, & Wagenaar, 2012). It has been estimated that doubling the tax on alcohol in the United States would reduce alcohol-related mortality by an average of 35 percent, traffic crash deaths by 11 percent, sexually transmitted disease by 6 percent, violence by 2 percent, and crime by 1.4 percent per year (Wagenaar, Tobler, & Komro, 2010).

To reduce alcohol-related problems, the average consumption of a group must be changed. Availability-control theory recommends raising the price of alcoholic beverages relative to disposable personal income to reduce the rate of alcohol-related health problems so that those who drink within recommended limits are hardly affected, while heavy drinkers, who cause the most alcohol-related harm, pay the most. Minimum unit pricing and discount bans could save hundreds of millions of dollars every year in health care, crime, and employment costs. Policies that lead to increases in the prices of cheaper drinks available in bars, clubs, and supermarkets promise the greatest impact in terms of crime and accident prevention, primarily by reducing the consumption of 18–24-year-old binge drinkers (Delcher et al., 2012; Meier, 2008). Other methods of reducing consumption include:

- raising the drinking age
- controlling the number of outlets distributing alcohol
- reducing hours of sales
- limiting advertising
- sobriety checkpoints
- lowered legal blood alcohol content (BAC) levels for driving
- administrative licence suspension for those close to the legal BAC limit
- graduated licensing for novice drivers
- screening and brief interventions for risky drinkers (Babor et al., 2003; Chaloupka, Grossman, & Saffer, 2002; Kypri et al., 2006; Patra, Giesbrecht, Rehm, & Bekmuradov, 2012; Wagenaar, Salois, & Komro, 2009)

Canadian addiction policy draws heavily from this theory. Canada has relatively high prices and taxes; it maintains at least partial government retail monopolies in most provinces and territories; the majority of provinces and territories have a minimum purchase age of 19; graduated licensing of drivers is in place in several provinces; and all jurisdictions have comprehensive impaired driving countermeasures. There was a significant decline in drinking and driving incidents between 1980 and 2000, while government revenues from alcohol sales increased from $2.91 billion in 1989 to $5.01 billion in 2007 (Thomas, 2008).

The decrease in Canadian smoking rates has also been directly correlated with the country's high cigarette taxes and restrictions on access in terms of strictly enforcing age of purchase. This includes a program urging retailers to ask for identification of anyone looking less than 25 years of age even though it remains legal to purchase tobacco products at age 19. Similarly, when Utah increased its tobacco tax in 2010 from $0.695 per pack to $1.70, cigarette sales dropped by nearly 10 million packages, or 15 percent of total consumption. It was predicted that approximately 13,000 people would quit smoking after the tax was raised, but actual figures indicate that closer to 19,000 one-pack-a-day smokers had quit. Calls to the state-run tobacco quit line increased by more than 150 percent in the first year the tax increase was instituted (Gehrke, 2011).

Sanctioning the sale of drugs to reduce addiction problems is not a new idea. Even before the great alcohol prohibition experiment, Great Britain attempted to keep its North American colonists in line by restricting activities such as gambling, which was associated with public drinking, and requiring taverns to also provide food and lodging. When extending the model to illicit drug use, society tends to see increases in drug use and drug problems with increases in the availability and distribution network of drugs. The rise in prominence of cocaine can be partially explained by this theory. After Colorado legalized the recreational use of cannabis, it moved from seventh (10.4 percent) to second (12.7 percent) in per capita use in the United States, a 22 percent increase in those acknowledging use of the drug in the month prior to the survey (United States Department of Health and Human Services, 2014). The availability-control theory not only provides a good model of how and why alcohol and other drug-related problems arise, but also provides a series of solutions for dealing with this social issue. However, not only supply but also demand must be decreased if one is to fully respond to both local and global issues of addiction.

Environmental Stress

Even neurobiologists have begun to concede that the environmental context combines with and even shapes genetic factors to influence the development of drinking behaviours and drug use disorders (Enoch, 2011, 2012: Young-Wolff, Enoch, & Prescott, 2011). The studies discussed in the first chapter involving soldiers returning from Vietnam speak directly to the role of the environment in inducing drug use and addiction (Robins et al., 2010; Roffman, 1976).

In the 1960s a device was created at the University of Michigan that allowed rats and other test animals to self-inject heroin. A needle, which was connected to a pump via a tube running through the ceiling of a modified Skinner box (see Figure 2.4), was implanted in the veins of rats, allowing them to inject themselves with the drug simply by pressing a lever. By the end of the 1970s, hundreds of experiments using similar apparatuses had indicated that rats, mice, monkeys, and other captive mammals would willingly self-inject large amounts of various psychoactive drugs, including amphetamines, cocaine, and heroin (Woods, 1978).

FIGURE 2.4: SKINNER BOX

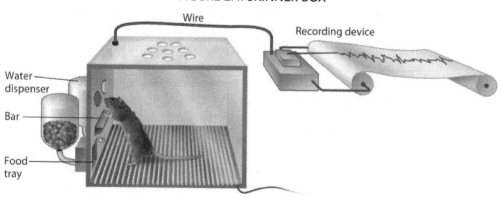

Sources: Lilienfield, Scott O., Lynn, Steven J., Namy, Laura L.; Woolf, Nancy J., *Psychology: From Inquiry to Understanding*, 2nd ed., © 2011. Printed and electronically reproduced by permission of Pearson Education, Inc., New York, New York.

However, when one examines a Skinner box, it is easy to observe that it is a cramped, minimalist environment with few behavioural options available for caged animals, especially ones with implanted needles tethered to self-injection apparatuses. As well, most animals are social creatures, especially rats, and in these experiments they are isolated and removed from direct contact with other members of their species. The question was posed as to whether the animals would self-inject drugs at the same rate in a more natural environment (Goldstein, 1979).

In responding to this question, Canadian psychologist Bruce Alexander truly brought to light the role of stressful social environments in creating addiction. Alexander and his colleagues examined the role of social isolation and stress on drug use in an extensive study undertaken at Simon Fraser University during the 1970s and 1980s. These became known as the "Rat Park" experiments and even served as the subject of a comic book (www.stuart-mcmillen.com/comics_en/rat-park/). Each Rat Park was approximately 200 times larger than a typical Skinner box and featured a peaceful forest scene painted on its plywood walls. Empty tins, wood scraps, wheels, balls, bedding of cedar shavings, and even private spaces that allowed for mating and other social interactions were spread throughout the environment (Alexander, Beyerstein, Hadaway, & Coambs, 1981). The space housed between 16 and 20 rats of both sexes at one time, thus providing companionship without the severe distress caused by overcrowding.

In Rat Park, the rodents had the option of drinking from two water dispensers placed at the end of a tunnel. One contained a morphine solution and the other had no psychoactive substance added. A series of different experiments were designed, including force-feeding heroin to the rats before letting them choose from which dispenser to drink. Regardless of the circumstances, the rats in the open space of Rat Park always consumed less heroin than those in the Skinner box, sometimes up to 20 times less. Some even went through voluntary withdrawal by drinking only the unlaced water. Not all Rat Park inhabitants remained abstinent, but those in the less stressful environment always, without exception, used less heroin. No experimental outcome produced as strong an addiction response in rats living in the natural environment compared to a cage (Alexander, 1985, 1988; Alexander et al., 1981). Alexander concluded that when the stressful social environment was altered, drug use diminished, findings that were subsequently replicated by several other scientists (Bozarth, Murray, & Wise, 1989; Schenk, Hunt, Klukowski, & Amit, 1987; Schenk, Lacelle, Gorman, & Amit, 1987; Shaham, Alvares, Nespor, & Grunberg, 1992). Extrapolating his findings to humans, Alexander stated that people can ignore drugs and avoid addiction even when drugs are plentiful if their environment has limited additional stressors. Much of the research with animals on the creation of addiction and its attribution to biological and psychological processes has involved the forced consumption of substances by animals in isolation. This weakens the foundation of many evidence-informed theories because they fail to acknowledge the importance of the social dimension of addiction.

People do not only use psychoactive drugs because they are available, or allowed by society, but also because they affect both the mind and the body. Psychoactive drugs alter realities, change perception, and impact one's behaviour, both positively and negatively. However, they ultimately produce very rigid modes of behaviour. Thus, addiction is a process, not just an event which means that the temporal and spatial elements of addiction must always be considered. Addiction arises at a particular time and in a particular space and is constantly transforming and developing. Even when we know how a drug operates in the brain, we still need to examine the effect on the social environment of that specific brain function (Oksanen, 2013).

DISCUSSION QUESTIONS

1. Rank the following in order from the most useful to the least useful in terms of explaining drug use:
   (a) the six biological theories
   (b) the six psychological theories
   (c) the six sociological theories
2. What factors did you consider in creating your three lists?
3. Consider your scores from Table 2.1. How do your values and beliefs influence the way you rank the various theories?
4. Using all the theories presented in Chapter 2, draw a theoretical model illustrating why people use drugs. Be creative and briefly explain your model.
5. What overarching ideas guided your creation of this model?

Chapter 3
PSYCHOACTIVE SUBSTANCES OF USE AND ABUSE

Psychoactive drugs can be classified in a variety of ways, one of which is along five pharmacologically related groups or families.

1. Depressants

Depressants slow the body's metabolism and the functioning of both the central and peripheral nervous systems. Mood enhancement occurs because of the disinhibition properties of this drug group. While central nervous system depressants slow brain activity, they do not necessarily depress a person's mood. The following drugs are included in this group:

- barbiturates
- non-barbiturate sedative-hypnotics
- benzodiazepines
- inhalants, including solvents, aerosols, and anaesthetics
- antihistamines
- alcohol

2. Opioids

Like the depressant family, opioids slow brain and central nervous system activity. In addition to their sedative action, opioids also mask pain and can act as cough suppressants. They can be placed into four categories:

- natural
- semi-synthetic
- synthetic
- antagonists, which reverse the respiratory depressant effects of opioids, but which themselves are not psychoactive

3. Stimulants

These substances produce a general increase in central nervous system activity, including mood elevation, increased vigilance, and postponement of fatigue. The following drugs are considered stimulants:

- cocaine
- amphetamines
- Ritalin and related drugs to treat attention-deficit/hyperactivity disorder (ADHD)
- anorexiants
- decongestants
- khat
- bath salts (methylendioxypyrovalerone and mephedrone)
- betel
- nicotine
- caffeine

4. Hallucinogens

Hallucinogens produce generalized disruption in many parts of the brain, with especially profound effects on perception, cognition, mood, and behaviour. Hallucinogens can be placed into four categories:

- LSD-like
- phenylethylamines: mescaline-like psychoative agents
- dissociative anaesthetics (PCP and Ketamine)
- cannabis

5. Psychotherapeutic Agents

These drugs are used to treat persons with specific mental health issues. Rather than increasing, decreasing, or disrupting central nervous system activity as other psychoactive agents do, the primary function of psychotherapeutic agents is to return a user to a homeostatic level. There are three categories of psychotherapeutic agents:

- antidepressants
- antipsychotics
- mood stabilizers

The effect of a drug will depend on the amount taken at one time; the past drug experience of the user; the circumstances in which the drug is taken; the place, the feelings, and activities of the user; the presence of other people; the simultaneous use of other drugs; and the manner in which the drug is taken. Short-term effects are those that appear rapidly after a single dose and disappear within a few hours or days. Long-term effects are those that appear following repeated use over a longer period of time.

Figure 3.1 provides an illustration of the increasing effect of CNS depressants and CNS stimulants as larger amounts are consumed. A person who has not previously used a psychoactive drug begins at a level of homeostasis, or balance. Once a CNS stimulant or depressant is administered, the first step is euphoria, a major reason any drug is administered. A distinct pattern then follows for each. For CNS depressants, including opioids, after euphoria a user will experience relaxation, followed by sedation, drowsiness, stupor, unconsciousness, and potentially a coma state and death if sufficient amounts of the drug are taken. With a CNS stimulant, after euphoria, a user would expect to feel excitation, followed by a state of agitation, irritability, and even violence, physical spasms, convulsions, and—if sufficient amounts of the drug are taken or if the substance is administered for a long enough period of time—coma, and potentially death. Hallucinogens are not illustrated in Figure 3.1 as their primary effect is not the production of euphoria but rather a disconnect between the physical world and the user's perception of it. However, many hallucinogens do have secondary depressant and stimulant effects, and these would follow the same pattern as illustrated in Figure 3.1. Finally, the purpose of psychotherapeutic agents is to bring a user back to a homeostatic or neutral state when they are feeling overly agitated, clinically depressed, or are exhibiting psychotic behaviours.

FIGURE 3.1: EFFECTS OF CENTRAL NERVOUS SYSTEM
DEPRESSANTS AND STIMULANTS

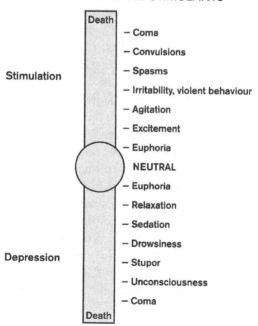

Table 3.13, found at the conclusion of this chapter, presents a summary of the lethal dose levels of several of the drugs from the five different groups that will be discussed in the following sections, while Table 3.14 provides a comparison of what the street cost of a range of psychoactive drugs was in Toronto, Ontario, in 2009.

3.1 DEPRESSANTS
Barbiturates
Non-Barbiturate Sedative-Hypnotics
Benzodiazepines
Inhalants/Solvents
Antihistamines
Alcohol

Barbiturates
Slang: abbots, barbs, barbies, downers, goofballs, idiot pills, sleepers, stumblers
amobarbital (Amytal): blues, blue angels, blue clouds, blue devils
amobarbital (Tuinal): Christmas trees, double trouble, rainbows
pentobarbital (Nembutal): nebbies, yellows, yellow dolls, yellow jackets
secobarbital (Seconal): reds, red birds, red bullets, red devils, seccy

Barbiturates are potent central nervous system depressants that are classified as sedative-hypnotics. Sedatives are used to relieve anxiety and to produce a sense of calm, while hypnotics induce sleep and are used to treat insomnia or produce surgical anaesthesia. Initially developed in the late 19th century, diethyl-barbituric acid was first marketed by Bayer in Germany, giving rise to profound changes in the pharmacological approach to treating psychiatric and neurological disorders at the turn of the 20th century. Within the first decade of that century, barbiturates became widely used to therapeutically treat individuals with serious neuroses and psychoses (now treated with psychotherapeutic agents). Patients would receive intravenous injections, and through the heavy sedation produced, they would be more likely to respond to the suggestions offered through the directive psychotherapy of that era. Those with more severe conditions, such as schizophrenia, were given larger doses to induce calmness and sleep. One barbiturate used for this purpose was sodium pentothal, which would become better known as "truth serum." It was used to sedate prisoners during World War II and have them reveal military facts during the stage of stupor the drug produced. Barbiturates were also used in treating sleep disorders among the general population and for surgical anaesthesia, and were the first effective pharmacological tool for the management of epileptic seizures. Over 2,500 barbiturates have since been synthesized, with 50 being effective and safe enough to be used clinically. These include amobarbital (Amytal), pentobarbital (Nembutal), secobarbital (Seconal), and Tuinal, which is a combination of amobarbital and secobarbital (Table 3.1).

In small doses, barbiturates relieve anxiety, tension, convulsions, and high blood pressure by producing calmness and muscular relaxation through their effects on the neurotransmitter gamma-aminobutyric acid (GABA). Barbiturates can also be used to place persons who have suffered severe physical trauma into a coma-like state to aid in their recovery (López-Muñoz, Ucha-Udabe, & Alamo, 2005).

However, soon after barbiturates were being widely prescribed, many users discovered that these drugs also provided them with a pleasurable intoxicating effect. Larger doses led to impaired judgment, loss of coordination, delayed reaction time, slurred speech, decreased respiration, and impaired short-term memory. These effects made it dangerous to drive a car or perform other complex tasks while consuming these drugs. As well, use of barbiturates during pregnancy has been linked to birth defects and behavioural abnormalities in babies. Despite their widespread use during the first half of the 20th century—70 tons of these drugs were sold in 1936 alone—no barbiturate succeeded in eliminating the main drawbacks: the development of dependence, and death by overdose and through unmanaged withdrawal. The lethality of barbiturates led to them becoming a common method of suicide attempts and part of the lethal mixture employed in some American states that retained capital punishment for the execution of prisoners. Currently, the most common licit use of these psychoactive agents is to prevent and mitigate epileptic seizures, but they continues to be used to lesser degrees for treating essential tremors, severe headaches, migraines, and other types of related pain, as well as some gastrointestinal and asthmatic functional disorders. Phenobarbital is also used in cases of withdrawal syndromes from other sedative-hypnotics with shorter half-lives (López-Muñoz et al., 2005).

It is also important to know that this class of sedative-hypnotics does not produce completely normal sleep as it disrupts the dream cycle. Users may feel tired and irritable even though a sleeping state occurs. Accumulation of barbiturates in body tissue can often occur because of their long half-life and long-term, frequent administration. The resulting chronic intoxication is characterized by impaired central nervous system function, reflected by deficits in attention, memory, judgment, cognitive ability, and fine and gross psychomotor skills, and emotional disorders such as mood swings, depression, and hostility. Physical signs of barbiturate use include glazed eyes, dry skin, rapid breathing, rapid pulse, high blood pressure, cramps, nausea, tremors, and possibly mild to severe convulsions. Mood depression is common with prolonged use, as is aversion to light and noise, insomnia, and some hallucinations. With regular use, tolerance to the effects of barbiturates develops. Tolerance develops more slowly to the harmful effects than to the sleep-inducing or intoxicating effects. Typical overdose for a healthy 77 kg male would be as little as eleven 100 mg pills (see also Table 3.13). As well, with continued heavy use, the difference between an effective dose and a fatal dose narrows, and the risk of fatal overdose increases.

TABLE 3.1: MAJOR BARBITURATES SOLD IN CANADA

Generic Name	Brand Name	Duration of Action	Abuse Potential
amobarbital	Amytal	intermediate	high
amobarbital	Tuinal	short	high
butabarbital	Butisol	intermediate	moderate
butalbital	Florinal, Pronal	intermediate	moderate
pentobarbital	Nembutal	short	high
phenobarbital	Luminal	long	low
secobarbital	Seconal	short	high
talbutal	Lotusate	short	moderate
thiopental	Pentothal	ultra-short-acting	high

Source: Fehr (1987)

Physical and psychological dependence is common with this family of psychoactive agents. Physical dependence on barbiturates can be one of the most life-threatening of all drug dependencies because of the symptoms that appear shortly after abrupt cessation. Withdrawal starts 4–6 hours after the last dose and can last for up to two weeks. Abrupt withdrawal leads to progressive restlessness, anxiety, and possible delirium, delusions, grand mal seizures, and potentially death. Temporary sleep disturbances may lead a user to incorrectly decide that more of the drug is required. There is a high cross-tolerance with other depressants, particularly alcohol. Some alcohol-dependent persons use barbiturates as a substitute for, or in addition to, alcohol. Barbiturates can be legally purchased with a prescription and come in four durations of action: long-acting, intermediate-acting, short-acting, and ultra-short-acting. Usually only the short- and intermediate-acting drugs such as Seconal and Amytal typically appeal to street users (Levinthal, 2012).

Non-Barbiturate Sedative-Hypnotics
Slang: knockout drops
chloral hydrate mixed with alcohol: Mickey Finn
Doriden: doors
Quaaludes: Joe Fridays, lemons, lewds, lovers, Q, Quads, Vitamin Q, soapers, wallbangers

The non-barbiturate sedative-hypnotics are a group of drugs with actions that are very similar to those of the barbiturates. They were first introduced in 1954 as a "safe, non-addicting" alternative to barbiturates, and various types were available as over-the-counter medications for nearly 20 years. However, physical dependence was soon discovered to be a serious problem, and their use became more restricted. Drugs in this group that are controlled substances in Canada are chloral hydrate (Noctec) and paraldehyde, Schedule F (controlled medicine, available by prescription); methaqualone (Dormutil, Mandrax, Parest, Quaalude, Somnafac), Schedule III (restricted but still available on a limited basis by prescription); and meprobmate (Equanil, Miltown, Solacen), Schedule I (narcotic). Other members of this family that may not be legally sold in Canada are ethchlorvynol (Placidyl), glutethimide (Doriden), methyprylon (Noludar), and the most well-known member of this group, methaqualone (Quaalude, Mandrax).

Methaqualone was originally produced as a therapeutic agent as it is an effective anti-malarial agent, but it was soon discovered that it also possessed a very powerful euphoria and sleep-producing effect. By 1972, it was the sixth most frequently prescribed drug in the United States (Falco, 1976). However, like barbiturates, one disturbing side effect was, its disruption of rapid eye movement (REM) sleep. Typically adults have four REM cycles per night. While Quaalude and other non-barbiturate sedative-hypnotics allow a person to obtain the physical rest required while asleep, they can suppress REM sleep. If REM sleep is suppressed for as little as two to three weeks, a person's ability to function begins to deteriorate and he or she can begin to exhibit psychotic-like behaviour (Mirmiran et al., 1983). As well, tolerance is quick to develop, and 2000 mg may be required to induce sleep, which is initially produced by 300 mg of the drug. For a typical 54 kg woman, the lethal range begins at 5400–5500 mg (Carroll & Gallo, 1985).

While North American production was discontinued in 1983, Quaalude remains an available street drug. Case studies have suggested that methaqualone may possess an abuse potential exceeding that of any of the barbiturates. Quaalude is not manufactured or distributed in Canada but continues to be smuggled in and can be used alone or to offset a cocaine, amphetamine, or crystal meth high. At low doses, glutethimide and methaqualone are likely to produce calmness, sedation, drowsiness, relaxation, and lethargy, but they are just as likely to cause anorexia, nausea, and gastrointestinal discomforts. Large doses of these drugs produce a barbiturate-like intoxication. Non-barbiturate sedative-hypnotics are associated with rapid deterioration of vital signs during overdose. However, at high doses, respiratory depression is less marked than with the barbiturates, so the risk of accidental overdose is somewhat lessened. Respiratory depression can be intensified by the simultaneous administration of codeine or any other related CNS depressant. Cardiovascular complications and seizures with these psychoactive agents can be quite severe, with cardiovascular collapse and coma resulting from misuse of these substances. Other common effects include dizziness, lethargy, exacerbation of existing pain, and the above-mentioned reduction of REM sleep, resulting in less dreaming. Effects of long-term use are primarily a continuation of short-term effects because of a buildup of the drug in the body. Even after discontinuation of drug use, a lack of motor coordination, unsteadiness, muscle weakness, visual difficulties, thinking and memory impairment, and slurring of speech, as well as tremors, irritability, and apathy, may remain (Seymour & Smith, 2011).

Development of tolerance to the sleep-inducing effects and to the euphoric and sedative effects is rapid, as it is with barbiturates. If the user wishes to maintain the original intensity of any of these desired effects, the size of the daily dose must be increased. A high degree of cross-tolerance occurs between these drugs and both alcohol and barbiturates. As well, both physical and psychological dependence can occur quickly. Withdrawal, while not as severe as with barbiturates, may also be life-threatening and must be medically monitored. Early withdrawal symptoms tend to occur within 24 hours after the last dose and may include sweating and fever alternating with chills; nausea and vomiting; abdominal cramps; abnormally rapid heart rate; headache; tremors; muscle twitches and spasms; agitation and hyperactivity; insomnia or brief periods of agitated sleep accompanied by nightmares; uncontrollable facial grimaces; psychosis-like syndromes characterized by disorientation, delirium, hallucinations, and paranoid delusions; and grand mal seizures. Some of these symptoms, including grand mal seizures, have abruptly occurred in regular users without their abstaining from the drug. The caution necessary in using barbiturates applies also to the use of all non-barbiturate sedative-hypnotics (Seymour & Smith, 2011).

Benzodiazepines

Slang: benzos, downers, sleep away, tranqs, Zs
Librium: libbys
Rohypnol: forget-me, Mexican valium, roachies, roofies
Valium: foofoo, howards, mother's little helpers, V's, vals, vallies, yellows
Xanax: dogbones, footballs, four bars, X-box, xanny, zanis, zanibars

Benzodiazepines are also referred to as minor tranquillizers, anti-anxiety agents, and anxiolytics-sedatives. All benzodiazepines act by enhancing the actions of a natural brain chemical, gamma-aminobutyric acid (GABA). However, they do not increase the organic synthesis of GABA in any way. The natural action of GABA is augmented by benzodiazepines, which thus exert an extra, often excessive, inhibitory influence on neurons. However, extended use of benzodiazepines can actually decrease the synthesis of GABA in certain areas of the brain.

Benzodiazepines were introduced to replace barbiturates and non-barbiturate sedative-hypnotics in the treatment of anxiety and insomnia, as well as to serve as anti-convulsive agents. These drugs are much safer than previously synthesized sedative-hypnotics as they rarely cause a fatal overdose. The typical lethal range for a 77 kg male is anywhere from approximately 1,000–7,000 5 mg tablets, though it can take fewer for other members of this drug family, such as Serax, to produce an overdose (see Table 3.13). While benzodiazepines are much less likely to produce an overdose compared to either barbiturates or non-barbiturate sedative-hypnotics, overdose is still possible, particularly when benzodiazepines are mixed with another CNS depressant such as alcohol. These drugs are also a major contributor to the accidental poisoning of children and prescription drug–related emergency room visits for adults (Substance Abuse and Mental Health Services Administration, 2013).

The first benzodiazepine-like drug, meprobamate, known as Miltown, was synthesized in 1954. However, the first true benzodiazepine, chlordiazepoxide, was introduced as Librium in 1960. Diazepam, most commonly marketed under the trade name Valium, followed three years later. Since the early 1960s, literally thousands of chemically related compounds have been synthesized and screened for potential as anti-anxiety agents. There are approximately 50 different types of minor tranquillizers in use worldwide, and they have become the most commonly prescribed psychoactive drug in North America, with $336 million spent in Canada alone in 2012–2013. The most common benzodiazepines prescribed in Canada are lorazepam (Ativan, 35.8 percent), zopiclone (Zimovane, 26.0 percent), oxazepam (Serax, 12.5 percent), temazepam (Restoril, 7.7 percent), and alprazolam (Xanax, 5.4 percent) (Morgan et al., 2013). Table 3.2 summarizes the benzodiazepines currently available in Canada, their equivalent strengths, and their primary therapeutic purpose.

Short-term effects from benzodiazepines are variable, depending on the dose, personality of the user, and the user's physical health and anxiety level. They include the following:

- calming hyperactivity tension and agitation
- relaxing muscles and relieving anxiety
- combatting withdrawal effects of other depressant drugs, primarily alcohol
- impairing muscle coordination
- producing dizziness, low blood pressure, and/or fainting
- inhibiting short-term memory

While a normal therapeutic dose produces relaxation and a feeling of well-being, higher doses may produce a state similar to intoxication by alcohol or barbiturates. Excessive use results in drowsiness, lethargy, disorientation, confusion, memory impairment, trance-like episodes, double vision, personality alterations, and other symptoms resembling drunkenness. Benzodiazepines can also sometimes produce unexpected paradoxical effects, such as agitation, insomnia, aggression, rage, and hostility—the very symptoms for which they have been prescribed (Ashton, 2013).

Chronic use of benzodiazepines leads to both physical and psychological dependence. Withdrawal from minor tranquillizers is similar to that from other sedative-hypnotics. Commonly observed effects include tremors; sweating; hypersensitivity to sensory stimuli; blurred vision; tingling sensations; tinnitus (ringing of the ears); insomnia; headache; difficulties in concentration; anorexia; increased lethargy; indifference to one's surroundings; memory, cognitive, and psychomotor impairment; irritability and emotional flatness; disorientation and confusion; sleep disturbances; and gastrointestinal upsets, along with sexual dysfunction and menstrual irregularities.

The withdrawal syndrome ranges in intensity from progressive anxiety, restlessness, insomnia, and irritability in mild cases to delirium and convulsions in severe cases. As with other psychoactive drugs, the intensity of the reaction depends on the dose level, duration of use, and individual user differences. Benzodiazepines can be obtained legally with a prescription. Despite the issue that misuse creates, these drugs do have legitimate therapeutic value and are relatively safe if used for a specific purpose and on a short-term basis, generally not exceeding four weeks. After four weeks of use, physical dependency to the drug is likely to occur, though there have been some reports of physical dependency beginning in as little as two weeks of regular use (Ashton, 2005).

Questions related to Halcion, introduced in 1983 for insomnia, are typical of the debate surrounding the risks and benefits of this family of drugs. Halcion has a very brief onset time and thus is quite effective in producing sleep for those suffering from insomnia. Its effectiveness led to its legalization in over 90 nations worldwide within a decade. However, in 1989, a user who claimed that she became involuntarily intoxicated while taking the drug and unknowingly killed her mother brought a multi-million-dollar lawsuit against the drug's manufacturer, Upjohn Pharmaceutical. The suit never went to trial, though the plaintiff did receive an undisclosed settlement from Upjohn. A minority of other users also reported adverse reactions from the drug, such as increased anxiety, memory loss, hostility, hallucinations, and paranoia, so that warning labels were added to every prescription (Dyer, 1994). Interestingly, during the 1991 Gulf War, both US President George Bush and Secretary of State James Baker were prescribed and consumed Halcion.

With the greater acknowledgement of the sexual violence perpetrated against women in Canada, there has been a parallel concern with the use of Rohypnol or "roofies." Referred to in the media as the date-rape drug, Rohypnol, while not a legal drug for sale in Canada, is legally manufactured and distributed in Mexico and Latin America for severe sleeping disorders and as a pre-anaesthetic medication. Rohypnol has no taste, colour, or odour, and when it is dropped into a beverage, its consumption can cause dizziness, confusion, memory loss, impaired judgment, and prolonged periods of blackout. The formal name for this state is anterograde amnesia. Rohypnol use has been linked to the sexual assault of women who have had the drug dissolved in their beverages without their knowledge. It is manufactured by Hoffman-La Roche and is typically found as a 1 mg olive-green oblong tablet in its licit form, though it is also produced by illegal drug laboratories, primarily in Mexico (United States Department of Justice, 2003a).

TABLE 3.2: BENZODIAZEPINE EQUIVALENCE TO 10 MG DIAZEPAM (VALIUM)

Drug	Half-Life Hours	Equivalent Strength (mg)	Therapeutic Purpose
Alprazolam (Xanax, Xanor, Tafil)	6–12	0.5	a
Bromazepam (Lexotan, Lexomil)	10–20	5–6	a
Chlordiazepoxide (Librium)	5–30	25	a
Clobazam (Frisium)	12–60	20	a, e
Clonazepam (Klonopin, Rivotril)	18–50	0.5	a, e
Clorazepate (Tranxene)	36–200	15	a
Diazepam (Valium)	20–100	10	a
Estazolam (ProSom, Nuctalon)	10–24	1–2	h
Flunitrazepam (Rohypnol)	18–26	1	h
Flurazepam (Dalmane)	40–250	15–30	h
Halazepam (Paxipam)	30–100	20	a
Ketazolam (Anxon)	30–100	15–30	a
Loprazolam (Dormonoct)	6–12	1–2	h
Lorazepam (Ativan, Temesta, Tavor)	10–20	1	a
Lormetazepam (Noctamid)	10–12	1–2	h
Medazepam (Nobrium)	36–200	10	a
Nitrazepam (Mogadon)	15–38	10	h
Nordazepam (Nordaz, Calmday)	36–200	10	a
Oxazepam (Serax, Serenid, Serepax, Seresta)	4–15	20	a
Prazepam (Centrax, Lysanxia)	[36–200]	10–20	a
Quazepam (Doral)	25–100	20	h
Temazepam (Restoril, Normison, Euhypnos)	8–22	20	h
Triazolam (Halcion)	2	0.5	h
Second-Generation Benzodiazepines			
Zaleplon (Sonata)	2	20	h
Zolpidem (Ambien, Stilnoct, Stilnox)	2	20	h
Zopiclone (Zimovane, Imovane)	5–6	15	h
Eszopiclone (Lunesta)	6 (9 in elderly)	3	h

a = treat anxiety; e = anti-convulsant; h = induce sleep
Source: Ashton (2002)

Studies have found that more than one-third of older Canadians have a prescription for at least one benzodiazepine. As licit substances, these drugs are covered by provincial drug insurance plans. The use of benzodiazepines in the older adult population has been associated with an increased risk of falls, fractures, and accidents, as well as contributing to the erroneous diagnosis of Alzheimer's or other forms of dementia. This is in part due to decreasing liver functioning in seniors, which lengthens the time it takes for the body to metabolize the drug. Thus, greater amounts are present in the bodies of older adults for longer periods of time. Older people following a prescription can easily and unintentionally intoxicate themselves and do so on an ongoing basis. Criteria for benzodiazepine use among seniors is that all long-acting versions (with a half-life greater than 24 hours)—diazepam, flurazepam, chlordiazepoxide, and clonazepam—should be avoided. Prescriptions for short- and intermediate-acting benzodiazepines (with a half-life of less than 24 hours) should not exceed the following dosages: alprazolam (Xanax), 2 mg; lorazepam (Ativan), 3 mg; oxazepam (Serax), 60 mg; temazepam (Restoril), 15 mg; and triazolam (Halcion), 0.25 mg (Dionne, Vasiliadis, Latimer, Berbiche, & Preville, 2013).

In this century, benzodiazepine use has increased in many nations worldwide. Easy access via the Internet has also increased the use of these drugs without medical supervision. Unfortunately, many physicians are not well versed in benzodiazepine management, with little expertise in withdrawal in long-term users. Detoxification centres also tend to withdraw patients too rapidly, apply rigid rules and "contract" methods, and provide inadequate support or follow-up without addressing the underlying psychological component that accompanies addiction to these drugs (Ashton, 2013).

Inhalants/Solvents

Slang: air blast, huff, oz, spray
amyl nitrate: aimes, Amsterdam special, boppers, poppers, rush
gammahydroxybutyrate (GHB) and/or gamma butyrolactone (GBL): cherry meth, easy lay, G, Gamma-O, grievous bodily harm, goop, growth hormone booster, jib, liquid ecstasy, liquid E, oxy-sleep, salty water
isobutyl nitrate: quicksilver, rush snappers, whiteout
nitrous oxide: buzz bomb, laughing gas, nox, whippets, whip-its
rubber cement ball that is burned and inhaled: snotball

Inhalants include volatile gases, substances that exist in a gaseous form at body temperature, refrigerants, solvents, general anaesthetics, and propellants (see Table 3.3). Except for nitrous oxide, more commonly referred to as "laughing gas," and related aliphatic nitrates, all inhalants are hydrocarbons. These substances not only have depressant effects, but can also produce minor hallucinogenic effects on the central nervous system. Abuse of volatile hydrocarbons and anaesthetics is not new. Getting high by inhaling ether or nitrous oxide was common in Europe, Great Britain, and North America during the 1800s. Sir Humphry Davy introduced the idea of using "laughing gas" as an anaesthetic before surgery, as well as recreationally. Today this drug can be purchased for recreational use in the form of poppers (amyl or butyl nitrate) or whip-its (nitrous oxide). These highly flammable yellowish liquids are usually sold in small glass screw-top bottles that are popular among some subcultures. The contents are released by crushing or popping the container and inhaling. During this process, oxygen to the brain is partially cut off. In combination with the drug, this produces a relaxed, warm state within 10 seconds that lasts for several minutes.

Widespread acknowledged sniffing of solvents contained in plastic model glues and nail polish removers began during the 1960s and has since been labelled as volatile substance abuse (VSA). The short-term effects of inhalants are dose-related and similar to those of the other central nervous system depressants. At present, there is no objective evidence to support users' claims of subjective effects differing among solvents. The initial effect of inhalation is a feeling of mood enhancement or euphoria, characterized by light-headedness, pleasant exhilaration, vivid fantasies, and excitation. Nausea, increased salivation, sneezing and coughing, loss of co-ordination, depressed reflexes, and sensitivity to light may also occur. In some users, feelings of invincibility may lead to reckless, dangerous, violent, or bizarre behaviour. Physical effects include pallor, thirst, weight loss, nosebleeds, bloodshot eyes, and sores on the nose and mouth (McKim & Hancock, 2013).

Some solvents, such as benzene, can cause reduction in the formation of blood cells in the bone marrow. Others may impair the functioning of the liver while still others may impair the functioning of the liver and kidneys. Contrarily, amyl nitrate and butyl nitrate dilate blood vessels. Deep inhalation or sniffing repeatedly over a short period of time may result in disorientation and loss of self-control, unconsciousness, seizures, or hallucinations, both auditory and visual. There have been some links between the use of these two nitrogen-based inhalants and Kaposi's sarcoma, a rare form of cancer affecting the immune system (Canadian Centre on Substance Abuse, 2006). Long-term exposure to solvents in industrial settings has also been linked to the development of cancer (de Vocht et al., 2009).

Gammahydroxybutyrate (GHB) and gamma butyrolactone (GBL) are two solvents that have recently gained increased attention as they have been identified as potential date-rape drugs. GHB was originally marketed as a surgical anaesthetic and used in Europe for the treatment of insomnia and narcolepsy and as a pharmacological aid for alcoholism. In the United States, it was sold without prescription as a health food and body-building supplement. GBL is a chemical used in a range of industrial cleaners. GBL, when consumed, is actually converted by the body during metabolism into GHB. Adverse effects when consumed in large quantities include hypothermia, dizziness, nausea, vomiting, weakness, loss of peripheral vision, confusion, agitation, and hallucinations. However, when these liquids are introduced into an alcoholic beverage, as little as a teaspoon can produce memory loss and unconsciousness. Within 5–20 minutes, the person who has consumed GHB and alcohol can suffer amnesia, confusion, and seizure-like activity. Ingesting too much GHB can lead to respiratory difficulties and a coma-like state or even death (Brennan & Van Hout, 2014; United States Department of Justice, 2003b).

TABLE 3.3: INHALANT CLASSIFICATION

Class	Examples	Found In
aliphatic/aromatic hydrocarbons (fuels)	benzene	cleaning fluids
	gasoline	gasoline
	hexane	lacquer thinners
	naphtha	lighter fluids
	toluene	model cement
	xylene	
aliphatic nitrates	amyl nitrate	industrial solvents
	butyl nitrate	poppers
esters	amyl acetate	lacquer thinners
	ethyl acetate	plastic cements
ethers	diethylether	anaesthetic
		GHB
gases	nitrous oxide	anaesthetic
		propellant in canned whipping cream
halogenated hydro-carbons	chloroform	aerosol propellants
	halothane	anaesthetics
	perchlorethylene	cleaning fluids
	trichlorethylene	computer duster sprays
ketones	acetone	household cements
	methylethyl ketones	model cement
	methyisobutyl ketone	nail polish remover

Sources: Fehr (1987); International Blue Cross (2002); PRIDE Canada (2001)

Acute physical health effects of solvent use can include abdominal pains, amnesia, mood depression, diarrhea, fatigue/sleepiness, headache/hangover, inattentiveness, irritability, incoordination, loss of appetite, nausea/vomiting, and rapid or irregular heartbeat. Long-term effects include the development of both physical and psychological dependence. Peripheral nerve, liver, and kidney damage, and infertility among male sniffers, have all been documented, as has anxiety, excitability, irritability, restlessness, bone marrow damage, chronic nosebleeds, short-term memory loss, and issues with sleep. Neurological damage also occurs, affecting balance, gait, reasoning, and sensory perceptions such as taste and smell, with the solvent toluene actually destroying the brain tissue of chronic abusers, leading to permanent irreversible brain damage. Solvent abuse has also been reported to cause death through suffocation and by sudden sniffing death (SSD). As a result of inhaling solvents, the cardiac muscle of a user becomes sensitive to the adrenal hormone epinephrine. If a user is suddenly startled and flees, suffers a panic attack, or engages in some other form of vigorous activity, epinephrine is secreted and a dramatic and catastrophic cardiac arrhythmia can occur. The user can die of a heart attack, regardless of age or physical condition. Case studies of sudden sniffing death have also been reported with butane and propane. As solvents are frequently sniffed from a plastic bag, it is also possible for a user to be rendered unconscious by the drug and accidentally suffocate if the bag is not removed from the face (Chenier, 2001; Cruz, 2011).

Regular use of inhalants induces tolerance, making increased doses necessary to produce the same effects. After one year, a glue sniffer may be using several tubes of plastic cement to maintain the effect for the same length of time as was originally achieved with a single tube. Since the body develops a tolerance to the drug, users must increase their dosage if they wish to obtain the same effects, thereby increasing the risk of hazardous health effects. Regular users often become emotionally depressed, lose interest in their surroundings, and experience diminished motivation, and may develop serious and often irreversible neurological damage. Withdrawal symptoms such as chills, hallucinations, headaches, abdominal pains, muscular cramps, and delirium tremens (DTs) have been reported, though the latter is not commonly observed. The constant sniffing of solvents can also lead to vapours remaining within the body or saturating the skin or clothing of the user. If a match is lit to smoke a cigarette or joint, a user can set himself or herself on fire (McKim & Hancock, 2013).

Volatile substance misuse is most often associated with young males, but women of childbearing age are also known to abuse solvents. When used during pregnancy, inhalants pass from the mother across the placenta into the bloodstream of the developing fetus. Chronic solvent use can prematurely terminate a pregnancy in the initial 20 weeks of development. It can also produce fetal solvent syndrome, which is similar to fetal alcohol spectrum disorder (FASD). Solvents can significantly reduce the amount of oxygen available for transfer to a developing fetus, producing brain damage that affects learning, memory, higher-level judgment, and decision-making abilities throughout the life cycle. Fetal solvent syndrome is evident in low birth weight, low levels of muscle tone, congenital facial abnormalities, a head size too small for a newborn's body size, and blunted fingers. Chromosome damage is also possible. The inhalants most commonly associated with fetal solvent syndrome are nitrous oxide, toluene, and trichloroethylene, though benzene, petroleum ether, xylene, and methanol have also been linked to the disorder (Bowen, 2011).

A major reason solvents are so problematic is because of their accessibility and availability. Solvents can be legally purchased by anyone, and a variety of different inhalants can be found in every household. As well, there is no restriction on possession, and only retail merchants can truly control access by limiting the purchase of a solvent. The second major concern is age of use. The majority of users range in age from 8 to 16, with an average age of 12 to 13, although there are adult sniffers. Inhalants provide a cheap, widely available means of achieving intoxication. In addition to enhancing mood, these substances tend to decrease the intensity of negative feelings such as anxiety, depression, inferiority, or boredom. Solvents tend to be an early experimental drug, though young, poor, adolescent males and young members of isolated Indigenous communities in Canada tend to use solvents to a greater extent than members of other populations. However, solvents are an even greater problem outside North America, particularly in developing nations, though recently increasing numbers of adults in the United States have been seeking treatment for solvent abuse (National Institute on Drug Abuse, 2010).

Antihistamines

Slang: tripelennamine mixed with pentazocine (Talwin): T's and blues

Antihistamines, first used in the 1940s, have many therapeutic uses. Over 40 different types are available that are

- effective in combatting the symptoms associated with certain types of allergic reactions, such as hay fever (phenyltoloxamine [Sinutab]; tripelennamine [Ro-Hist]; pheniramine [Triaminic]), though they have no value in fighting the common cold virus;
- used as anti-nauseants in the treatment of ailments such as motion sickness (Gravol);
- used in sleeping aids (diphenhydramine [Benadryl, Nytol, Sominex]);
- valuable as anti-spasmodics (diphenhydramine [Valdrene]); and
- useful in treating persons with excessive stomach acid (cimetidine [Tagamet]).

The extent of the usefulness of these psychoactive drugs is typically not realized, but in the adult Canadian population, the prevalence of rhinosinusitis alone is

5.7 percent of women and 3.4 percent of men (Chen, Dales, & Lin, 2003). In the United States, simple allergic diseases are responsible for 3.5 million lost workdays and 2 million missed school days. Students suffering from a combination of allergies, asthma, and sinusitis, creating even greater health issues, are estimated to miss more than 10 million school days. In adults, these conditions result in more than 73 million days of restricted work activity (Kay, 2000).

At therapeutic doses, common effects of the antihistamines include drowsiness; dizziness; and mild impairment of CNS function, perception, concentration, and psychomotor abilities that is further enhanced by the use of alcohol or other sedative-hypnotics. Other effects include lethargy, mood enhancement, gastrointestinal discomfort, and appetite suppression. Higher doses can further enhance mood or cause minor hallucinatory effects, especially when mixed with alcohol or other CNS-depressant drugs. When antihistamines are used regularly at therapeutic dose levels, adverse effects are generally mild and tend to be similar to short-term low-dose effects. With chronic regular use, however, the effectiveness of the drugs appears to diminish, though physical dependency can still occur. Regular topical application of certain antihistamines can cause allergic skin rashes, impaired coordination, confusion, disorientation, muscle twitching, and tremors (McKim & Hancock, 2013). Among older individuals, extended ongoing use can lead to the diminishment of natural histamine in the CNS. This can lead to dementia-like symptoms, though these lessen once the antihistamine is no longer being administered (Tannenbaum, Paquette, Hilmer, Holroyd-Leduc, & Carnahan, 2012).

Tolerance to the sedative effects of the antihistamines develops with regular use as the liver increases its ability to metabolize the drug. If an antihistamine is regularly used for its psychoactive effects, users may become physically and psychologically dependent. Antihistamines produce little euphoria, and what is produced rapidly decreases with regular use. As with other psychoactive drugs, children can be more easily accidentally poisoned, with as few as 87 tablets of Nytol being lethal for a 54 kg person. However, the use of antihistamines by women to combat morning sickness has not produced any issues during pregnancy or developmentally. Likewise, all antihistamines are considered safe to use while breastfeeding, as minimal amounts are excreted in the breast milk and do not cause any adverse effects to the infant (Seto, Einarson, & Koren, 1997; So, Bozzo, & Inoue, 2010).

Second-generation antihistamines, now widely available for over-the-counter purchase, are more effective in relieving allergy symptoms while producing far fewer depressant and sedative effects. Antihistamines with anti-inflammatory properties are currently being studied for use not only with allergies, but also with skin conditions and a range of inflammatory ailments. Nevertheless, older types of antihistamines remain widely available and do produce drowsiness. They can be used as mood-altering agents or to enhance the effects of other CNS depressants, and thus their abuse potential remains moderate (Simons & Simons, 2011).

Alcohol

Slang: 2-4, 26 ouncer, booze, brewski, browns, brown pop, fire water, forty pounder, hooch, grog, kegger, mickey, shots, snort, suds, vino

The most commonly abused psychoactive drug worldwide is ethyl alcohol: ethanol. It is the waste product formed when yeast utilizes sugar as an energy source during fermentation, and it has been associated with a contributing factor in more than 230 diseases. It is estimated to be the third most common cause of disability-adjusted life years lost, at 4.6 percent globally, and responsible for 3.8 percent of all global deaths (Rehm et al., 2009). As alcohol production has been possible for thousands of years, well before even the simplest of human technologies, alcohol must occasionally have been available to pre-human primates and prehistoric man. It is unlikely that enough occurred naturally to be incorporated into religious and social custom, and probably no widespread use developed until fruits and grains came under cultivation, leading anthropologists to believe this was one factor that led to the development of agrarian society. This would have occurred approximately 10,000 years ago, and there are many indications that the early growth of agriculture owes much to the effects of alcohol.

Alcohol indirectly stimulates dopamine release in the ventral striatum of the brain, which is a key component of the central nervous system's reward system. The neurobiology of alcohol involves several neurotransmitters, though the importance of GABA and glutamate, another neurotransmitter, has been increasingly emphasized. It is believed that alcohol may inhibit both GABA and glutamate terminals in the ventral tegmental area (VTA) of the brain, which in turn amplifies the release of dopamine (Paul, 2006; Ticku, 1990).

Alcohol content varies from product to product, as illustrated in Table 3.4. Nevertheless, a drink is a drink is a drink—1.5 oz. of liquor, a 12 oz. bottle of beer (5 percent alcohol), a 5 oz. glass of table wine (12 percent alcohol), and a 4 oz. glass of fortified wine all contain the same amount of ethanol (Figure 3.2). They affect human physiology in a consistent manner as measured by blood alcohol content (BAC), though there are distinct differences between men and women (Table 3.5). Differences in effects from person to person produced by beverage alcohol do not generally result from the type of drink consumed, but rather from the person's size, previous drinking experiences, and rate of consumption. A person's feelings and activities or the presence of other people also play a role in the way the alcohol affects behaviour.

Alcohol is a depressant drug that produces disinhibition in the user and anaesthetic effects on the brain. Short-term effects include relaxation, impaired coordination, slowing down of reflexes and mental processes, changes in attitude, and increased risk taking to the point of bad judgment, including dangerous driving or working with machinery. A significant minority of pedestrians killed by motor vehicles are legally intoxicated at the time of the collision (Dultz & Frangos, 2013). Drinking heavily over a short period may produce a poisoning effect commonly referred to as a hangover, which includes headache, nausea, shakiness, and possibly vomiting beginning 8–12 hours after drinking has ceased. A hangover is the body's reaction to too much alcohol. In part it is related to poisoning by alcohol and other components of the drink, and in part it is the body's response to withdrawal from alcohol and dehydration. Hangovers are typically associated with binge drinking, which is accompanied by unique issues, including alcohol poisoning, short-term memory loss, unplanned sexual activity, suicidal ideation, and injury and death from engaging in high-risk behaviour (King, de Wit, McNamara, & Cao, 2011).

TABLE 3.4: ALCOHOL CONTENT OF VARIOUS FORMS OF BEVERAGE ETHANOL

Beverage	Concentration of Alcohol (Percent by Volume)
"light" beer	2.5–4.5
regular beer	5
malt liquors	6.5
table wine	8–14
fortified wines (sherry/port/vermouth)	16–20
ciders	5–12
sake	14–16
spirits (gin, vodka, whiskies, rum, cognac)	40
regular liqueurs	16–56
cream and egg-based liqueurs	16–18

FIGURE 3.2: STANDARD DRINK CHART

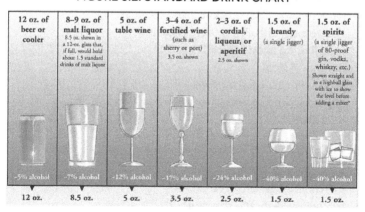

Source: National Institute on Alcohol Abuse and Alcoholism (2005, p. 24)

TABLE 3.5: BLOOD ALCOHOL CONTENT

Lean Body Weight		Female Number of Drinks									
Pounds	Kilos	1	2	3	4	5	6	7	8	9	10
100	45.4	50	101	152	203	253	304	355	406	456	507
125	56.7	40	80	120	162	202	244	282	324	364	404
150	68.1	34	68	101	135	169	203	237	271	304	338
175	79.4	29	58	87	117	146	175	204	233	262	292
200	90.8	26	50	76	101	126	152	177	203	227	253
225	102.1	22	45	68	91	113	136	159	182	204	227
250	113.4	20	41	61	82	101	122	142	162	182	202
Lean Body Weight		Male Number of Drinks									
Pounds	Kilos	1	2	3	4	5	6	7	8	9	10
100	45.4	43	87	130	174	217	261	304	348	391	435
125	56.7	34	69	103	139	173	209	242	278	312	346
150	68.1	29	58	87	116	145	174	203	232	261	290
175	79.4	25	50	75	100	125	150	175	200	225	250
200	90.8	22	43	65	87	108	130	152	174	195	217
225	102.1	19	39	58	78	97	117	136	156	175	195
250	113.4	17	35	52	70	87	105	122	139	156	173

Note: Milligrams of alcohol in mL of blood; rate of elimination 15 mg per hour.

Source: Sinclair (1998)

Regular, long-term use of alcohol has been associated with damage to every human organ system:

- Blood
    anaemia
    easy bleeding or bruising
- Bones
    interference with formation of bones
    reduced bone mass (thickness and volume)
    interference with absorption of calcium
    contribution to osteoporosis
- Endocrine System
    decrease in male testosterone level
    impotence and decreased sperm production
    infertility
- Heart
    hypertension
    increased risk of stroke
    increased cholesterol level
    irregular heartbeat (arrhythmias)

- Liver
  - alcoholic fatty liver disease
  - alcoholic hepatitis
  - cirrhosis (scarring of the liver due to death of liver cells)
  - cancer
- Lungs
  - interference with immunity system leads to higher incidence of pneumonia or tuberculosis
- Muscles
  - disruption of the body's mineral balance can produce inflammation of the muscles
  - swelling, tenderness, weakness linked to degenerating muscle fibres
- Neurological
  - seizures or convulsions
  - dementia
  - loss of balance
  - damage to peripheral nerves
  - loss of supportive tissue in the brain resulting in deterioration of attention span, concentration, problem solving, planning, learning, verbal fluency, and short-term memory
  - Wernicke-Korsakoff syndrome and other forms of dementia
- Pancreas
  - pancreatitis
  - pancreatic cancer
- Stomach
  - gastritis
  - ulcer irritation (corrosion of the stomach wall)
  - esophagitis (chronic heartburn)

(Azodi, Orsini, Andrén-Sandberg, & Wolk, 2011; Babor, Higgins-Biddle, Saunders, & Monterra, 2001; Beier, Artel, & McClain, 2011; Malik et al., 2008; Maurel, Boisseau, Benhamou, & Jaffe, 2011; White, Altmann, & Nanchahal, 2002).

Along with these issues, alcohol is a leading preventable cause of cancer deaths, including breast, esophagus, colon, gastric, liver, mouth, pancreatic, rectal, throat, and testicular cancer, leading to an average early mortality of nearly two decades (Ferrari et al., 2007; Heinen, Verhage, Ambergen, Goldbohm, & van den Brandt, 2009; Lachenmeier, Kanteres, & Rehm, 2009; Zhang et al., 2007). Binge drinking and alcohol misuse also regularly result in physical and emotional injury, assaults, and various forms of trauma. While there has been a documented benefit against coronary heart disease from moderate alcohol consumption, it does not apply equally to the entire population but only to those with a specific cholesteryl protein (Mukamal, 2012), nor does it mitigate the other body systems that are negatively affected.

As well, there is the irreversible damage that occurs as a result of a woman's drinking during the course of her pregnancy, that of fetal alcohol spectrum disorder. FASD is a collective term rather than a diagnostic category, which includes Fetal Alcohol Syndrome (FAS), Alcohol-Related Neurodevelopmental Disorder (ARND), and partial FAS (pFAS). FASD is the leading cause of developmental disability, affecting 9 out of every 1,000 Canadian infants. Estimates of the annual cost of fetal alcohol spectrum disorder in Canada is in the $1.3–$2.3 billion range. FASD, along with prenatal alcohol exposure (PAE), impacts each child differently, though there are commonalities within different diagnostic categories. As alcohol freely crosses the placenta from mother to child, the risks for the unborn child increase the more a pregnant woman drinks, though at this time, no safe level of drinking has been established. Primary disabilities from FASD include impairments in attention, verbal learning, and executive functioning as the direct result of damage as well as an increased risk of childhood leukemia. Secondary disabilities are deficits not evident at birth but that arise from primary disabilities and interaction with the environment, such as mental health and addiction issues, conflict with the law, and difficulties with education, employment, and family relationships. Drinking alcohol during pregnancy may lead to cognitive impairment; heart, face, joint, and limb abnormalities; lower birth weight; hyperactivity with shorter attention spans; poor self-concept; depression; and aggression. The disabilities created by FASD are not minimized with time and continue to create difficulties for and marginalize individuals throughout their adult lives (Burnside & Fuchs, 2013; Denys, Rasmussen, & Henneveld, 2011; Jones, 1986; Kully-Martens, Treit, Pei, & Rasmussen, 2013; Latino-Martel et al., 2010; Rutman & Van Bibber, 2010).

Chronic alcohol consumption blunts the biological clock's ability to synchronize daily activities to light and disrupts natural activity patterns. It continues to affect the body's clock, or circadian rhythm, even days after the drinking ends. Other than regulating sleeping and waking, the circadian rhythm also affects physiological functions, such as hormonal secretions, appetite, digestion, activity levels, and body temperature. Ongoing disruption of the body's natural clock increases the risk of developing cancer, heart disease, and depression.

Regular use of alcohol induces tolerance, making increased doses necessary to produce the same effects (Hasler, Smith, Cousins, & Bootzins, 2012). When tolerance develops, alcohol-dependent people may drink steadily throughout the day without appearing to be intoxicated. As these persons may continue to work reasonably well, their condition may go unrecognized by others until severe physical damage develops or until they are hospitalized for other reasons and experience alcohol withdrawal symptoms. Tolerance is lost if the drinker abstains, but is quickly regained once alcohol consumption resumes. A person tolerant to the effects of alcohol is also tolerant to the effects of many other CNS-depressant drugs. Physical and psychological dependence are common among alcohol abusers.

When an alcohol-dependent person stops drinking, he or she will experience withdrawal symptoms ranging from mild to severe. Withdrawal may consist of shakes or tremulousness (nearly always evident 0–48 hours after cessation of drinking), anxiety and agitation, flushing of the skin, sweating, sleeplessness, and restlessness. Seizures may occur during the first 48 hours, with a peak frequency between 13 and 18 hours, and may continue up to five days after alcohol consumption ends. This can be followed by hallucinations, intense psychomotor agitation, and acute anxiety. Delirium tremens (DTs) can start suddenly and usually peak three days after the last drink. Paranoia and disorientation to time, place, and person are also common, as is intense restlessness, fever, and profuse sweating (Dziegielewski, 2005).

Combining alcohol with antihistamines, marijuana, benzodiazepines, barbiturates, or other depressants can intensify the combined effects to a potentially lethal level. Although extremely large doses of alcohol can kill by suppressing the brain's autonomic nervous system's control over breathing, this rarely happens as a drinker typically passes out before a lethal dose can be taken or vomits before all of the ingested alcohol can be absorbed. The lethal blood alcohol level (BAL) for humans is approximately 0.5 percent, although heavy drinkers with an enhanced tolerance to the drug have been known to survive considerably higher levels. The phases of an alcohol overdose consist of confused thinking, poor judgment, mood swings, poor concentration, marked muscle coordination problems, slurred speech, nausea and vomiting, anaesthesia (sleepiness), memory lapses, and finally respiratory failure, coma, and, as with excessive amounts of any CNS depressant, possibly death.

Ironically, under the Canadian Food and Drugs Act, alcohol remains classified as a food. This is partially because when the liver metabolizes alcohol, it produces energy. This is a result of the high caloric content of the various forms of ethyl alcohol. A regular beer typically has 120 calories, a half glass of wine, 80–120 calories, while 1 oz. of spirits falls at approximately 80 calories per serving. Legally sanctioned, socially accepted, and easily accessible, alcohol is one of society's most destructive psychoactive substances.

3.2 OPIOIDS
Natural Opioids
Semi-Synthetic Opioids
Synthetic Opioids
Antagonists

These drugs are also referred to as narcotics, opiates (opium derivatives), narcotic analgesics, and opioid analgesics, though "opioids" is the most inclusive term. Opioids are found in nature and occur in both a synthetic and semi-synthetic form. They mimic endogenous endorphins neurotransmitters, which occur naturally in the body. The use of opium is described in the writings of the Sumerians as early as 4000 BCE. The ancient Greeks knew about the uses of poppy juice, or opion, and described the occurrence of tolerance and depend-ence. During the Middle Ages, the plant was used by Arab physicians for sed-ation, analgesia, and relief of dysentery, and Arab traders are thought to have introduced this psychoactive drug to the Far East at that time. The majority of opium currently harvested for licit use by Canadians comes from Afghanistan, Tasmania, and Turkey. These poppy fields are owned by international pharma-ceutical corporations and are under strict government control.

Opium from the Asian poppy *Papaver somniferum* is eaten or smoked. While many opioids are injected intravenously—the popular perception of the way to administer this substance—they may also be smoked, or taken orally or across mucous membrane. Opioid analgesics can be classified with CNS depressants, as both slow CNS functioning. However, along with their disinhibiting charac-teristics, opioids also remove the emotional reaction to pain. They do not elimi-nate pain; rather, they mask it and assist people in dealing with its psychological component (Zhao et al., 2007). Opioids also slow down the gastrointestinal tract and act as a cough suppressant, as one of their primary effects is depression of the medulla oblongata, which is responsible for controlling cardiac, respiratory, and vasomotor centres. Opioids, like all psychoactive agents, are metabolized mainly in the liver. Excretion occurs largely via the kidneys, although some metabolites are excreted in the feces. Elimination is usually complete in a few hours, although a few members of this family of drugs, notably methadone and buprenorphine, are metabolized and excreted much more slowly.

Opioids are used medically to relieve acute pain as a result of disease, surgery, or injury; in the treatment of some forms of acute heart failure; and in the control of diarrhea. They are of also of great value in the control of chronic pain in the later stages of terminal illnesses, such as cancer, where dependence and dose levels are no longer an issue. However, they are not in-tended for long-term use for chronic pain relief due to injury or non-terminal illness. Opium customarily produces an exaggerated feeling of well-being and a temporary release from anxiety. Despite their media portrayal, opioids are relatively benign in comparison with other psychoactive agents. The most harmful long-term implication of opioid use is often the lifestyle users main-tain, which is primarily a result of the global prohibition against heroin. Per-haps because of this, the non-medical use of prescribed opioids has increased dramatically in Canada over the past decade. Doctors grapple with balancing the pain-masking benefits of opioids with the risk of creating dependency if they are overused or misused (Nosyk et al., 2012). With illicit use, particularly injection drug use, abscesses, cellulitis, liver disease, HIV, hepatitis C, and possible brain damage may result from infections associated with unsterile injection techniques. Pulmonary complications, including various types of pneumonia, may also result from an unhealthy lifestyle, as well as the depres-sant effect of opioids on respiration. Emboli—small, undissolved particles or air bubbles—may block small blood vessels in the lungs, brain, heart, or other organs. With chronic use, weight loss, reduction in testosterone, and suppression of the immune system are common. A Canadian study also found that the greater the daily dose level of those using opioids, the greater the risk for road trauma (Goodman, 2013; Levinthal, 2012).

Tolerance to the many effects of opioids, including respiratory depression, analgesia, sedation, nausea, and enhancement of mood, develops within days of continuous use, though overdose remains a concern. If administration is intermittent, however, little change in drug sensitivity is observed. However, regular users become both psychologically and physically dependent on opioids. With their powerful mood-enhancing and anxiety-relieving effects, opioids have a high psychological dependence liability (Dziegielewski, 2005). Opioids cross the placenta, as do all other psychoactive drugs, and thus withdrawal has the same physical effects on the fetus as it does on the drug-using mother. During pregnancy, withdrawal from opioids has been associated with placental abruption, which could be life-threatening for the woman. When an infant is born to a mother who is dependent on opioids, there is a recognizable withdrawal syndrome, known as called Neonatal Abstinence Syndrome (NAS). If untreated, NAS can be fatal. However, no long-term cognitive effects have been observed, unlike with alcohol or solvent use during pregnancy (Jansson & Velez, 2012).

Opioids affect endorphins in the brain, the body's natural pain maskers, along with GABA and dopamine. The binding of opioid drugs to endorphin receptors reduces the excitability of neurons, which is likely the source of the euphoric effect and reduction of pain sensation. The euphoric effect appears to involve the GABA-inhibitory inter-neurons, which reduce the amount of GABA released. This in turn reduces the amount of dopamine released. By inhibiting this inhibitor, opioids increase the amount of dopamine produced and the amount of pleasure felt. However, a complicated relationship exists between the opioid receptor system and the dopamine system, with blockage of one or the other interfering with but not completely removing the reinforcing effects of opioids on the brain. This is partially responsible for some of the odd physiological effects observed, such as when tolerance to euphoria develops, but there is no equivalent tolerance to respiratory depression. Altering endorphin levels in the brain creates respiratory depression, along with euphoria, sedation, decreased gastrointestinal motility, spinal analgesia, sedation, dyspnea (shortness of breath), tolerance, withdrawal, dysphoria during withdrawal, and ultimately dependency. Changes in brain biochemistry resulting from the use of opioids are not temporary. Both chronic and, in some cases, limited use of drugs can produce long-lasting changes in brain neurochemistry, as well as in cell development and structure (Trescot, Datta, Lee, & Hansen, 2008).

Patterns of purposeful drug-seeking behaviour associated with opioids are difficult to break, and the relapse rate is significant. Withdrawal from opioids, which may begin as early as a few hours after the last administration, produces uneasiness, chills, nausea and vomiting, stomach cramps and diarrhea, insomnia, fever, irritability, restlessness, excessive sweating, and crawling skin sensations known as parasthesia (Gevirtz, Frost, & Kaye, 2011). These symptoms are accompanied by a substantive craving for the drug. Withdrawal symptoms typically start from 8 to 16 hours after the last administration of the opioid, and the shorter the half-life of the drug, the quicker the onset of symptoms. The worst symptoms peak in intensity between 36 and 72 hours after cessation of drug use. The primary withdrawal syndrome typically lasts from five to eight days, though a much longer period with milder symptoms is not unusual. Some bodily functions do not return to normal levels for as long as six months, depending on how long the drug was administered. Sudden withdrawal by heavily dependent users who are in poor health has occasionally been fatal. However, opioid withdrawal is much less dangerous to life than are alcohol, barbiturate, and non-barbiturate sedative-hypnotic induced withdrawal syndromes. Overall, the symptoms are similar to an extremely severe, exceedingly painful, long-lasting case of the flu. With opioids, overdose is of much greater concern than withdrawal. An overdose of opioids is indicated by the combination of pinpoint pupils, depressed respiration, and ultimately coma. Death almost always results from respiratory depression within a few hours of administration, although late complications such as pneumonia, pulmonary edema, or shock can also be fatal.

Canada currently ranks second only to the United States in per capita consumption of prescription opioids. The rate of dispensing high-dose opioid formulations increased, from 781 units per 1,000 population in 2006 to 961 units per 1,000 population in 2011 (23 percent), with the number of cases of overdose increasing in tandem with the increase in dispensing (Gomes, Mamdani, Paterson, Dhalla, & Juurlink, 2014).

Opioids can be categorized into the following groups:

- Natural opioids or opioid alkaloids: derived directly from opium or dried poppy juice, including codeine (methylmorphine), morphine, and opium
- Semi-synthetic opioids: chemically modified versions of opioid alkaloids like codeine or morphine, which are typically more potent than the natural form of the drug, including heroin, hydromorphone (Dilaudid), and oxycodone (Percocet and Percodan)
- Synthetic opioids: produced to mimic the effects of natural opioids with only minimal structural similarities to opium, including fentanyl, hydrocodone (Novahistex DH), meperidine (Demerol), methadone, and propoxyphene (Darvon)

As well, there is a subgroup of non-psychoactive drugs known as *opioid antagonists*, which, when administered, counteract the effects of opioids, primarily respiratory depression, though they have also been used for other therapeutic purposes. These include naloxone (Narcan), naltrexone (Revia), and pentazocine (Talwin).

Natural Opioids

Codeine (methylmorphine)
Slang: AC/DC, Captain Cody, cody, coties, dreamer, fours, nods, school boy, syrup, sizzurp (codeine, antihistamine, Sprite, and dissolved Jolly Rancher candy)

Codeine is derived from the opium poppy. It is a drug of comparatively low potency used in cough syrups and in preparations containing non-opioid pain suppressants such as Aspirin. In Canada, low doses can be bought without a prescription. Discovered in 1832, codeine is often used by opioid-dependent persons when more potent drugs are unavailable as it is metabolized into morphine by the liver. It is also partially subject to non-medical use because of its ready availability. Dependence, tolerance, and withdrawal are similar to that experienced by a morphine abuser, though much less intense. Due to potential negative effects, codeine is no longer recommended for use in Canada by children under the age of 12 or by breastfeeding mothers, who metabolize the drug quickly. As with other, more potent opioids, a toxic reaction to codeine includes dizziness, confusion, extreme drowsiness, and shortness of breath or difficulty breathing, and if the dose is high enough, seizures (Health Canada, 2013a).

Morphine
Slang: dreamer, first line, God's drug, M, Miss Emma, Mr. Blue, monkey, morph, mud, Murphy, white stuff

Like codeine, morphine is a natural substance derived from the opium poppy. It is used clinically for pain management, especially continuous dull pain, and is considered the prototypical narcotic analgesic. It has recently also been used during trauma care and to reduce the risk of the development of post-traumatic stress disorder (PTSD) in those who have experienced serious injury, such as in combat (Holbrook, Galarneau, Dye, Quinn, & Dougherty, 2010).

Discovered in 1803, it has the second-greatest dependency liability after heroin (see Table 3.7). Morphine inhibits GABA neurons via the opioid receptors, resulting in an increase in dopamine input and enhancing a sense of euphoria. Most commonly injected, it can also be smoked, inhaled, or swallowed. As morphine is not as lipid soluble as heroin, codeine, or methadone, onset of action is not as prompt. Drowsiness and mental clouding occur at doses higher than those required for pain relief. Lethargy and impaired concentration and cognition are also common with the use of this psychoactive agent (Julien, Advokat, & Comaty, 2008).

Opium
Slang: A-bomb (when mixed with cannabis), aunti, Aunti Emma, big O, black pill, Chinese molasses, Chinese tobacco, dream stick, dreams, God's medicine, joy plant, midnight oil, O

Opium is a crude resinous preparation obtained from the unripened seed pods of the opium poppy. It has an unpleasant odour and bitter taste that frequently produce nausea when it is consumed. Morphine comprises approximately 6–12 percent of the bulk of crude opium, with codeine comprising 0.5–1.5 percent. Opium is smoked because of its euphoric properties, while clinically it can be used to treat diarrhea and dysentery. However, it has been largely replaced as an analgesic by other naturally occurring, semi-synthetic, and wholly synthetic substitutes, such as morphine, hydromorphone, and meperidine. Nonetheless, a highly purified form of opium marketed as Pantopan is still occasionally used when a person cannot tolerate morphine. Dependence and tolerance are much lower and less marked with opium than with morphine.

"Doda" is the term used for ground dried poppy pods or poppy heads. These grounds are either eaten or, more often, added to water or tea for their therapeutic effects, primarily among members of the Southeast Asian community. In the past, doda could be purchased as a spice in East Indian markets across Canada. Known as "the poor man's heroin," these leftovers of opium production induce relaxation and calm rather than the euphoric effect of most other members of this family of psychoactive substances. The drug does not enter Canada in its powder form, but as legally imported dried flowers for flower arrangements. The tea version is often so mild that it is not classified as a narcotic. However, despite its low levels of opium, it is still possible to become physically and psychologically dependent on doda.

Semi-Synthetic Opioids

Buprenorphine
Slang: bupe, orange guys, subs, subbies

Buprenorphine is derived from thebaine and acts as a partial opioid agonist. It produces less sedation than methadone and morphine, which are full opioid agonists, while decreasing cravings for other opioids and preventing opioid withdrawal. The effects of buprenorphine peak 1–4 hours after the initial dose. Adverse effects are similar to those of other opioids, and include nausea, vomiting, and constipation. In intravenous polydrug use, usually with benzodiazepines, administered to produce a euphoric effect closer to that of heroin when heroin is not accessible, severe respiratory depression and death have been reported. Buprenorphine is well tolerated and safe to use during pregnancy. However, Neonatal Abstinence Syndrome can occur, as with all opioids (Srivastava & Kahan, 2006).

The primary use for buprenorphine is as an alternative to methadone in the maintenance and treatment of opioid dependence. It is typically used in combination with naloxone (page 136) to create Suboxone, which, if taken sublingually, will safely stave off the withdrawal effects of opioids, as it is neutralized by the liver. If taken intravenously, however, it will trigger an immediate withdrawal reaction, as it bypasses the liver and proceeds directly through the blood-brain barrier to the CNS. Buprenorphine has a much lower risk of overdose than methadone and is also more effective in tapering as it has less severe withdrawal effects. While buprenorphine is safer for use than methadone for individuals at risk for respiratory depression, such as elderly patients and those taking benzodiazepines, it is far more expensive. The therapeutic dose range is 8–16 mg daily (Kahan, Srivastava, Ordean, & Cirone, 2011).

Heroin (diacetylmorphine or diamorphine)

Slang: Aunt Hazel, Bart Simpson, big H, big Harry, black tar, blue velvet, bobby brown, brown crystal, dust, H, hardball (mixed with cocaine), horse, junk, Mexican Mud, nickel deck, scag, smack, speedball (mixed with cocaine), red chicken, spider

Heroin, derived from the German *heroisch*, meaning "powerful," was synthesized in 1874 in England from morphine but was not marketed until 1898 by Bayer in Germany. Heroin is a powerful semi-synthetic opioid analgesic, which is much more potent than morphine in its psychoactive effects. Like so many other drugs, it was initially marketed as presenting no addiction risk. This, of course, was later demonstrated to be grossly incorrect, but not until it was in wide use as a cough syrup and to decrease chest pain from pneumonia and tuberculosis (Levinthal, 2012).

Through its ability to widen blood vessels, heroin provides a feeling of warmth. The euphoria it produces has been regularly described as an orgasmic-like high, along with a feeling of detachment from life. Although it has only ever been used by a very small percentage of persons and regularly ranks among the drugs least used by Canadians, it remains widely publicized due to the lucrative drug trade and the continuing controversy over its medical use. Heroin is a highly effective pain masker. It has been approved on a limited basis for managing the severe pain associated with terminal illness and for limited use when methadone is not effective. Physical effects may include restlessness, vomiting, nausea, fatigue, dry mouth, and a warm, heavy feeling throughout the body. Other physical effects are constipation, increased urination, contraction of the pupils, itchy skin, and slowed breathing. With larger doses, pupils contract to pinpoints, the skin becomes cold, moist, and bluish, and breathing slows or even stops, thereby causing death. Long-term effects can include pulmonary complications, constipation, menstrual irregularities in women, and reduction in reproductive hormone levels for both men and women (Trescot et al., 2008).

Tolerance to heroin develops rapidly with regular use, and both physical and psychological dependence occurs. Overdose is generally due to users injecting pure or minimally cut heroin rather than the typical dose, which tends to be diluted with substances such as sugar, baking soda, or baby powder. Withdrawal symptoms usually appear 4–5 hours after the last dose and can be quite severe. They often last seven to ten days and include severe anxiety, insomnia, increased perspiration, chills, shivering, and tremors. The pain of withdrawal has been said to be more like that of bone cancer than of severe flu. However, as previously stated, while highly unpleasant, withdrawal from heroin is much less life-threatening than withdrawl from heavy use of alcohol, barbiturates, or non-barbiturate sedative-hypnotics. Heroin is used primarily by intravenous injection, though it can also be smoked, inhaled, swallowed, and administered by skin-popping. Due to its extremely high dependence liability, it is one of the few drugs that is globally prohibited (Sproule, 2004).

Hydromorphone (Dilaudid)
Slang: D's, delats, dillies, hospital heroin, hydro, juice, M2s

Synthesized in 1936, hydromorphone is also a morphine derivative. It is a potent analgesic used to mask severe pain and to suppress the cough reflex. It can be administered both orally and intravenously, though the latter tends to produce pain and tissue irritation when the drug is used chronically. Dilaudid produces less nausea, vomiting, and drowsiness than morphine but more intense respiratory depression. This drug has a pain-masking potential that is seven to eight times that of morphine. Tolerance and physical dependence develop, with withdrawal symptoms similar to a severe, long-lasting flu. Psychological features of withdrawal are depression, anxiety, insomnia, and loss of appetite, combined with periods of agitation. As well, a smaller amount of hydromorphone is required to produce an overdose when compared with other opioids. Its pharmacodynamic profile, including onset of action and time to peak levels, is similar to heroin, and in double-blind experiments—situations when neither user nor experimenter are aware of what substance is being administered—the effects of hydromorphone could not be distinguished from heroin (Fulton, Barrett, Stewart, & MacIsaac, 2012).

An extended-release form of hydromorphone hydrocholoride, manufactured by Purdue Pharma (2004), is also available. Marketed as Palladone, it too is a controlled substance and is available in 12 mg, 16 mg, 24 mg, and 32 mg capsules. It is intended only for adults with long-term constant, chronic pain. However, as with any extended- or gradual-release drug, if it is chewed or crushed, the drug is released much faster than intended. A significant euphoric reaction can then be obtained and a risk of overdose occurs.

Oxycodone (Percodan)/OxyContin (oxycodone HCl controlled-release)

Slang: blue, cotton, hillybilly heroin, kicker, killers, O's, OC, Ox, Oxy, Oxycoffin, Oxycotton, Percs

Oxycodone, first produced in 1938, is created by modifying codeine. It is a white, odourless crystalline powder used to treat moderate to severe pain. It has powerful mood-enhancing, analgesic, and sedative effects. It is available alone or in combination with non-opioid analgesics, such as acetylsalicylic acid (Percodan) or acetaminophen (Percocet). Administration is exclusively oral. Oxycodone has the potential to produce powerful physical dependence in users because of its potent effects.

OxyContin was developed in 1995 by Purdue Pharma. It was made available in Canada in 1996 as a time-release version of oxycodone for use in the management of moderate to severe pain when a continuous, around-the-clock analgesic is needed for an extended period of time. OxyContin was originally intended for use with individuals who had already developed a level of opioid dependency for chronic pain, and thus it has the potential to lead to death through respiratory depression among non-tolerant individuals, even if used properly. However, it soon became a drug of choice for prescribing general practitioners not only for its analgesic effects, but also because it was initially marketed as being non-addictive. OxyContin, however, has a potency 16 times greater than a single Percocet. Issues also arose with this opioid when, rather than being administered as intended, it was instead crushed and injected or simply chewed and then swallowed, leading to a rapid release of the opioid properties that were intended to be gradually released and producing a potent psychoactive effect. This altered method of administration has led to issues with diversion and increased reports of overdose and death. Over a five-year period, of the people coming to the medical withdrawal service of the Centre for Addiction and Mental Health in Toronto, Ontario, for the treatment of opioid dependence, those having a problem with OxyContin increased steadily from fewer than 4 percent to 55 percent (Sproule, Brands, Li & Catz-Biro, 2009). Saskatchewan, Ontario, and the Atlantic provinces stopped providing provincial funding for the drug except in cases of cancer or palliative care, as did Health Canada. To mitigate public concern, OxyContin was replaced by its manufacturer with OxyNeo, which provides similar pain management but is more difficult, though not impossible, to alter and administer in an unintended manner. However, the patent on OxyContin has now expired, which allows other drug manufacturers to produce their own generic version of this opioid.

A major component of the OxyContin controversy was its marketing. Heavily promoted by Purdue Pharma as being a safe opioid, it became one of the top-selling prescription drugs in North America. Sales in Canada increased from $3 million in 1998 to $243 million in 2010, the height of the controversy regarding its safety and misuse. At the University of Toronto, the textbook *Pain Management*, paid for and copyrighted by Purdue, was distributed free to students. Early versions of the book claimed that continuous-release opioids like OxyContin had low abuse potential, and a later edition stated that physicians had an ethical duty to consider opioids for non-cancer patients. Purdue's financial ties to the Canadian medical community are extensive. Of 49 experts on a panel that produced new practice guidelines on using opioids to treat non-cancer patients, 12 were receiving speaking or consulting fees of more than $5,000 a year from Purdue or other pharmaceutical companies. Western University's Dr. Morley-Forster reported that her pain clinic in London received $200,000 from Purdue in one year (Blackwell, 2011).

Synthetic Opioids

Fentanyl

Slang: Apache, China girl, Chinatown, dance fever, friend, goodfella, great bear, jackpot, king ivory, murder 8, Tango and Cash, TNT

First developed in 1959 for use as a general anaesthetic, fentanyl is a synthetic drug primarily prescribed to provide physical and emotional relief from acute pain, principally for palliative care patients or those with long-term chronic pain who experience breakthrough pain when using other opioids. It has rapid onset and short duration of action. It is thus primarily administered transdermally to make its use more convenient for those who are severely ill, with each patch designed to slowly release the potent substance over 72 hours. However, sublingual spray and lollipop versions that transfer the pain-masking properties via mucous membrane are also available for cancer patients. Fentanyl is quickly metabolized through the liver and has no active metabolites. Within 72 hours, approximately 75 percent of fentanyl is excreted, primarily through urine. Fentanyl is a highly selective opioid agonist that works mainly at the μ-opioid receptor in the central nervous system, with some activity at the delta and kappa receptor sites. It is approximately 80–100 times more potent than morphine (Grape, Schug, & Schug, 2010). A noticeable increase in illicit use of fentanyl coincided with the prohibition of OxyContin in jurisdictions across North America.

Hydrocodone (Novahistex DH)
Slang: vikings

Hydrocodone, synthesized in 1955, which is more potent than codeine, is the psychoactive component of Vicodin. It was initially intended for use as a cough suppressant, an antitussive. However, high doses can produce euphoria and sedation, and it quickly became used as a pain-masking agent with substantive abuse potential. Dependence to hydrocodone is greater than to codeine, with tolerance also occurring much more rapidly. The severity of the withdrawal reaction ranges between the reactions produced by codeine and by morphine (Walsh, Nuzzo, Lofwall, & Holtman, Jr., 2008).

Meperidine (Demerol)
Slang: peth

One of the earliest synthesized opioids, meperidine was first made available in Germany in 1939, just prior to World War II. It is effective as a short-acting oral analgesic. It can also produce central nervous system excitement at high doses, manifested by muscle twitches, tremor, and agitation. It remains widely used in clinical settings, though with chronic administration metabolites can accumulate and give rise to toxic reactions. Meperidine produces both physical and psychological dependence similar to that of morphine, though tolerance is slower in developing. Withdrawal begins in 3 hours, peaks in 8–12 hours, and ends in four to five days. There is little nausea, vomiting, and diarrhea, but muscle twitching, restlessness, and anxiety are much worse than with morphine.

Methadone
Slang: dollies, done, fizzies, juice, meth, my drink, the drink

Methadone is a white crystalline powder or colourless crystals. While available in tablet form, it is administered in a liquid form in its current primary global use in harm reduction. Methadone is a long-acting analgesic with properties similar to those of morphine. Its synthesis began prior to World War II in the laboratories of the German pharmaceutical company IG Farben as an alternative to opium-based analgesics. It is unlike morphine in that it is highly effective when administered orally. As it is excreted slowly, it is effective for up to 24 hours. Methadone is currently used primarily as substitution therapy for opioid-dependent individuals as it produces morphine-like actions and cross-tolerance but does not produce euphoria for opioid users when given orally. However, tolerance and withdrawal do occur in methadone users, though its development is much slower than with other opioids. Without other forms of intervention, chronic users eventually become both psychologically and physically dependent on methadone. Ternes and O'Brien (1990) claimed that a street heroin user can be placed on methadone and then weaned off within 10 days, yet there are Canadians who have been receiving methadone for more than 20 years with no indication of cessation. Methadone is no longer used exclusively with those moving away from heroin use.

Its use has been expanded to replace opioids in general, including less potent opioids. While methadone is very effective, it requires careful adherence to dosing guidelines and close monitoring because its long half-life increases the risk of overdose. Methadone provides a helpful tool for reducing some components of craving and risk of relapse to opioids. However, a minority remain at risk of cue-induced cravings (Fareed et al., 2010).

Methadone's side effects include weight gain (due to lowered metabolism), dental issues (due to decreased salivation), constipation, numbness in extremities, sedation, and, for some, hallucinations. Long-term use will also create sexual dysfunction due to decreased testosterone levels in males, as occurs with chronic use of any opioid. Those in methadone maintenance programs may thus require testosterone supplements as treatment adjuncts (Samaan, 2014). An interesting unintended side effect is methadone's ability to kill leukemia cells that anti-cancer drugs commonly used in conventional therapies failed to kill (Friesen, Roscher, Alt, & Miltner, 2008).

Propoxyphene (Darvon)
Slang: none known

Propoxyphene is a mild analgesic used to relieve mild to moderate pain as an alternative to codeine. Synthesized in 1955, dependency on, tolerance to, and withdrawal from Darvon are similar to the effects produced by codeine. Darvon has one-half to two-thirds the potency of codeine when administered orally. It is sold alone or in combination with acetylsalicylic acid (ASA) and was regularly among the top 10 most-prescribed substances in North America in the latter half of the 20th century. Abuse is minimal as high doses produce dizziness, skin rashes, skin irritation, and, if injected, the risk of toxic psychosis.

Antagonists

Naloxone (Narcan)
Slang: no street use

Naloxone is a pure antagonist, with no pain relief or psychoactive properties. Naloxone's primary therapeutic use is to reverse the opioid-induced respiratory depression that is commonly observed in cases of overdose. However, this drug will not reverse the respiratory depression caused by high doses of other psychoactive drugs. Naloxone begins working within 30 seconds of injection. It can also be used in the control of seizures induced by meperidine or propoxyphene. Some communities are now distributing naloxone kits at the request of substance users to allow them to self-administer should they experience a drug overdose. When Naloxone is administered to an opioid-free individual, there is little or no discernible effect other than occasional mild dysphoria. When orally administered, naloxone can also improve symptoms of opioid-associated constipation, which is common in those using opioids to address issues of chronic pain (Meissner, Schmidt, Hartmann, Kah, & Reinhart, 2000). Suboxone, a safer though more expensive alternative to methadone, is a combination of four parts buprenorphine to one part naloxone.

Naltrexone (Revia)
Slang: no street use

Naltrexone is an antagonist with properties similar to those of naloxone, but with a much longer duration of action. As with naloxone, even after prolonged use its discontinuation does not produce any withdrawal effects, respiratory depression, gross behavioural effects, or euphoria. Naltrexone is very efficient at suppressing the effects of heroin. This allows it to be used as a protective drug with heroin users, as Antabuse and Temposil once were used with alcohol-dependent persons. While some clinical trials have demonstrated the positive value of naltrexone as a protective drug, others have shown that it is not totally effective in this function as cravings continue during naltrexone maintenance (Krystal, Cramer, Krol, Kirk, & Rosenheck, 2001). For those for whom external incentives to stay away from drugs are important, such as health care professionals or business executives, naltrexone therapy has been very effective. Naltrexone also received attention as an anti-alcohol-craving drug and has also been touted for use with persons who have impulse control disorders, such as problem gambling and kleptomania (Kirchmayer, Davoli, & Verster, 2003; Litten & Allen, 1998).

Pentazocine (Talwin)
Slang: tall, T's and Blues (mixed with antihistamines), kibbles and bits, one and ones, poor man's heroin, ritz & T's, T's & R's (mixed with Ritalin)

Pentazocine, synthesized in 1962, is a weak opioid antagonist with moderate analgesic properties, though it is more accurately classified as an agonist-antagonist rather than a pure antagonist. Pentazocine was created to relieve pain without producing a dependence or leading to abuse, as does use of other narcotic analgesics. Tolerance can develop, though it is slower than with most opioids. Talwin has no cross-tolerance with any other opioid. Withdrawal effects include abdominal cramps, chills, hypothermia, vomiting, and both a physical and psychological craving for the drug. Unfortunately, when combined with the antihistamine tripelennamine hydrochloride, such as Benzoxal, and injected, a heroin-like effect is produced. This combination is referred to as "T's and Blues." Combining Talwin with Ritalin produces a similar effect. Attempts have been made to prevent this mixing by adding naloxone (see above) to create Talwin Nx, but this has not completely stopped the practice.

TABLE 3.6: CLINICAL FEATURES OF OPIOIDS

Drug	Clinical Dosage (milligrams)		Duration of Onset (minutes)		Dependency Liability
	Injection	Oral	Injection	Oral	
Morphine	10	60	30–60	90–120	high
Codeine	—	32–65	—	90–120	moderate
Heroin	5	60	30–60	90–120	high
Dilaudid	1.5	7.5	30–60	90–120	high
Percodan	—	30	—	30–60	high
Meperidine	75	300	30–60	60–120	high
Methadone	—	20	—	60–120	high
Talwin	60	180	30–60	90–120	low

Source: Fehr (1987); Ternes & O'Brien (1990)

TABLE 3.7: DURATION OF VARIOUS OPIOIDS COMPARED WITH MORPHINE

Drug		Duration
Hydromorphone	(Dilaudid)	slightly shorter
Meperidine	(Demerol)	shorter
Methadone	(Dolophine)	same
Oxymorphone	(Numorphan)	slightly shorter
Pentazocine	(Talwin)	shorter

Source: Krogh (1995)

3.3 STIMULANTS
Cocaine
Amphetamines
Drugs to Treat Attention-Deficit/Hyperactivity Disorder
Anorexiants
Decongestants
Khat
Bath Salts (methylendioxypyrovalerone and mephedrone)
Betel
Nicotine
Caffeine

Central nervous system stimulants are drugs that increase the activity of both the central and autonomic nervous systems. Mood enhancement occurs because of these changes. Upon initial ingestion there is euphoria, followed by excitement and then agitation. Higher doses produce irritability, violent behaviour, spasms, convulsions, and, in infrequent extreme cases, death. More common and frequent short-term effects include enhanced concentration, increased vigilance, increased blood pressure, increased strength, reduced fatigue, reduced appetite, and feelings of power. While all stimulants increase alertness, they exhibit considerable differences in the nature of their individual effects and relative potencies.

Cocaine

Slang: Angie, base (crack), baseball (crack), bazooka (mixed with cannabis), beam me up Scotty (mixed with PCP), Bernie's Flakes, big C, blow, C, bone-crusher (crack), coke, crack, flake, hardball (mixed with heroin), hunter, jelly, king's habit, line, nose candy, nose powder, Peruvian lady, snow, snowflake, speedball (mixed with heroin), stardust, white horse, Yale

Cocaine, though chemically not related to amphetamines, has CNS actions so similar that it has been classified as a stimulant. In Canada, though, it has remained improperly criminally classified as a narcotic. At the close of the 19th century, cocaine hydrochloride was the world's newest wonder drug, touted as a cure for everything from morphine addiction to tuberculosis. It was a component of wine approved by the Vatican and a variety of patent medicines, including cough drops for children, and, of course, a soft drink to counter the evils of consuming alcohol. Cocaine is a mixture of a local anaesthetic and a central and sympathetic nervous system stimulant. It produces its psychoactive effect by directly inhibiting the reuptake of dopamine in the CNS. This increases the availability of dopamine in the synapse and increases dopamine's action on postsynaptic neurons, producing enhanced mood along with euphoria. Cocaine's effect is usually quite short, prompting the user to repeatedly administer cocaine to re-experience its intense subjective effects.

Cocaine concentrates its effects on the reward areas of the brain, which are rich in dopamine synapses. When cocaine is present in the synapse, it binds to the uptake pumps and prevents them from removing dopamine from the synapse. This leads to greater levels of dopamine in the synapse, and, as a result, there are increased impulses that activate the brain's reward system. With continued use of cocaine, the body relies upon this drug to maintain rewarding feelings. The person is no longer able to feel the positive reinforcement or pleasurable feelings of other basic rewards such as food, water, or sex. It has also been discovered that the brain's dopamine system is related to mental health issues and that any negative changes that occur during adolescence due to drug use may not be reversible later in life, including alterations that lead to lifelong cravings for psychoactive drugs (European Monitoring Centre for Drugs and Drug Addiction, 2009a).

There are 250 different coca plants, though cocaine hydrochloride, the powder form of the drug, is extracted primarily from the leaves of the *Erythroxylon coca* bush. This particular coca plant grows on the eastern slopes of the Andes, mainly in Peru and Bolivia, though two other varieties are also used for cocaine production: one from the Amazonian basin and the other from Colombia. Global acreage of coca bush cultivation in 2008 was estimated to be between 156,900 and 220,000 hectares, down from the peaks of the beginning of this century (Figure 3.3).

Traditionally, inhabitants of the Andes mixed coca with ash or lime and placed it in the mouth like chewing tobacco. The juice was allowed to trickle into the stomach and served as a mild stimulant to facilitate heavy labour at high altitudes. Its cultivation for medicinal purposes—such as stomach upset, colic, nausea, diarrhea, headache, dizziness, toothache, ulcers, asthma, and fatigue—dates to the beginnings of recorded history in South America. Coca leaves are also a source of vitamin B and vitamin C. Cocaine was also used extensively as an anaesthetic for eye operations, dentistry, and facial surgery, and remained a preferred local anaesthetic in a few circumstances in Canada until the beginning of the 21st century. Currently some coca is still legally grown in Peru and Bolivia for processing into de-cocalized flavouring agents that are sold to international manufacturers of soft drinks. It remains widely available throughout markets in the Andes, with no restrictions on the sale of coca tea, leaves, or mints (American Council for Drug Education, 1997; European Monitoring Centre for Drugs and Drug Addiction, 2008; Weil, 1978).

The extraction process to produce illicit cocaine powder is a very toxic one. It entails mixing coca leaves with a host of toxic chemicals, including kerosene, gasoline, acetone, potassium permanganate or potassium hydroxide, and/or toluene, and then placing the mixture into a press and crushing it to obtain a thick paste. The mixture is then treated with hydrochloride or sulphuric acid to remove further impurities, resulting in crystalline cocaine powder: cocaine hydrochloride. The few legal importers of cocaine, particularly those using it for medical purposes, do not use such a harsh refinement process. Cocaine may be smoked, sniffed (snorted), or injected directly into the veins or rubbed along the gums. To obtain crack from cocaine powder (cocaine hydrochloride), all one needs to do is to add a weak base, such as a combination of baking soda and water. Crack and cocaine are the same substance, but in different forms. Crack is cocaine that can be smoked, while cocaine hydrochloride is not heat-soluble except with significant modification. The absorption of crack is so rapid that a user can experience the drug effect within 8 seconds. This rapid delivery to the brain and equally efficient excretion is a major cause of crack cocaine abuse.

FIGURE 3.3: TREND OF COCA CULTIVATION IN
THE ANDEAN REGION, 1990–2011

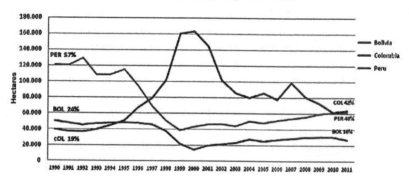

Source: Briones, Cumsille, Henao, & Pardo (2013)

Short-term effects of cocaine are similar to those produced by the body's own adrenaline. A naive or infrequent user of cocaine will feel and exhibit a variety of effects, such as enhanced mood, self-confidence and self-esteem, increased energy, increased sex drive, decreased appetite, increased concentration, garrulousness (talkativeness), increased alertness, increased motor activity, anxiety, and rapid respiration. Cocaine also increases body temperature and heart rate, and is a vasoconstrictor, leading to a rise in blood pressure and consequently increasing the risk of stroke. High doses can cause cardiac arrhythmia, hypothermia, seizures, and, unlike any other stimulant, respiratory depression. Vomiting also brings its own risk of death by aspiration. With larger doses the user will experience stronger and more frequent "highs," exhibit bizarre, erratic, and sometimes violent behaviour, and even paranoid psychosis during periods of sustained administration. Symptoms subside when administration is discontinued, but periods of severe depression may persist. The risk of convulsions increases with larger doses and sometimes a sensation of something crawling under the skin is perceived. With long-term use, cocaine, when snorted, can cause tissue damage in the nasal passages due to its irritating properties. When smoked over the long-term, cocaine can also cause damage to the lungs and to the pleasure-perceiving portions of the brain. Chronic cocaine use has also been linked to such diverse problems as memory loss and renal failure. Death from overdose can occur either from cocaine alone or in combination with other substances that affect the respiratory control centre in the brain. As cocaine has anaesthetic properties, it is very dangerous when combined with CNS depressants such as alcohol, barbiturates, or heroin, as it has the increased potential to produce death through respiratory arrest. Anorexia and weight loss, gastrointestinal disturbances, and impotence have also been observed in chronic users, as well as stiffer arteries, higher blood pressure, thicker heart muscles, increased risk of aneurysms, strokes, seizures, and hemorrhaging in tissues surrounding the brain. Cocaine-dependent individuals appear aged compared to their peers, and their mortality rates are up to eight times higher than in the healthy population of equivalent age. Psychological and physiological changes typically associated with old age, such as cognitive decline, brain atrophy, glaucoma, and immunodeficiency, occur in middle-aged cocaine-dependent individuals, with the annual rate of gray matter volume loss in cocaine-dependent individuals almost twice that of healthy non-users (Ersche, Jones, Williams, Robbins, & Bullmore, 2013; Kozor et al., 2014; Sproule, 2004).

Over the course of a single binge, cocaine users become less sensitive to the mood-enhancing effects of the drug and consequently tend to increase the dose in an attempt to compensate for the decreased effect. This acute tolerance has been demonstrated in laboratory situations as well. Their sensitivity to the drug can, however, be restored with a period of abstinence. The powerfully reinforcing effects of cocaine, both as a euphoriant and as a treatment of post-drug craving, are overwhelming for many users. Experiments with laboratory animals suggest that cocaine has among the strongest behaviourally reinforcing qualities of all psychoactive drugs. Rats, given the choice, have selected cocaine over food, water, and access to a sexual partner. Cocaine dependence can have devastating effects on the lives of individuals, not only because of the pharmacological effects of the drug, but also due to its cost. Upon abrupt discontinuation of drug administration, abstinence symptoms similar to those associated with amphetamine withdrawal are observed. Symptoms—including fatigue, severe mood depression, lethargy, and irritability—are commonly referred to as the "crash," which can also include abdominal and muscle cramps, dehydration, and a general apathy. As well, information about the risks associated with cocaine use and pregnancy have been widely publicized. Cocaine, like most psychoactive drugs, is transferred across the placenta, and its use may cause placental abruption, the premature detachment of the placenta from the uterus. This can cause bleeding, pre-term birth, and, in severe cases, fetal and maternal death. Women who use cocaine have a significantly greater chance of giving birth prematurely, with the fetus suffering withdrawal symptoms. However, unlike with alcohol and solvents, there is no fetal cocaine syndrome other than the issues arising from the withdrawal process (Ahmed & Koob, 1997; Dziegielewski, 2005; Manzardo, Stein, & Belluzzi, 2002).

Between 450 and 600 kg of coca leaf are required to produce 1 kg of cocaine hydrochloride paste. A typical Colombian farmer receives on average from $1 to $2 per kilo of coca leaf, while the actual cost of a kilo of cocaine paste is between $600 and $1,000. By the time the drug has been transported to port to be smuggled out of the country, the price can range from $5,000 to $10,000, with a markup of 50 percent by the time the drug reaches Central America, and another 50 percent on its reaching the Mexico-US border. A typical kilo that has been successfully smuggled into the United States retailed for approximately $30,000 in 2010, with a gram of refined cocaine having an average market price of $165, though there is great variance across the country. However, as the kilo of paste has also undergone chemical alteration that decreases its purity while increasing its weight, a kilo that initially cost as little as $600 at source can now have a street value of over $300,000, or a five hundred-fold increase in value along the network. The majority of profit is made at the end of the process. Thus, approximately 1 percent of profit is seen at the source, 10 percent in transit, and 66 percent at the point of final distribution (Briones et al., 2013).

More than 90 percent of all cocaine smuggled into the United States is of Colombian origin and transits through Mexico. Cocaine trafficking remains the most lucrative source of income for organized criminal groups in Central America, and intensified competition has increased the level of violence in the region. While much has been written about the escalation of murders in Mexico, there is concern throughout Central America. The national murder rate in Honduras continues to be one of the highest on record (International Narcotics Control Board, 2014).

There is a belief that the crack form of cocaine is less expensive. In reality, powder cocaine can be less expensive by total weight, though crack can be purchased in smaller units (see Table 3.14). As with all illicit drugs, there is a huge range of purity of street samples of cocaine. Purity is typically between 5 and 35 percent cocaine, though some seized samples have been found to be more than 80 percent pure. This accounts not only for the variance in price but also for the different reactions users obtain, from mild euphoria to cardiac arrest.

Amphetamines

Slang: amp, beans, bennies, black and white, black beauty, black cadillacs, black mollies, brain pills, bumblebees, crank, dexies, lid poppers, pep pills, splash, truckers, uppers, wake-ups
methamphetamine: blade, crystal, crystal meth, dust, glass, ice, ice cream, quartz, Scooby Snax, speed, Tina, weak, yaba, yellow barn

Amphetamines are a group of drugs whose action on the body resembles that of adrenaline. They are chemically related to the naturally occurring catecholamine neurotransmitter substances norepinephrine and dopamine. Amphetamines not only block the dopamine reuptake transporter but also lead to reverse transport of dopamine via the dopamine reuptake transporter. Amphetamines are used to raise energy levels, and reduce appetite and the need for sleep, while providing feelings of clear-headedness and power. Amphetamines initially attracted favourable clinical attention because of their reported ability to elevate the mood of clinically depressed persons and to reduce the appetite of the obese. One form of amphetamines, benzedrine inhalers, became popular for the relief of nasal congestion. Amphetamine effects on non-mental state and mood are in many respects similar to those of cocaine: first, relief from fatigue, increased ability to concentrate, and improved physical performance, then euphoria, followed later by depression and fatigue during the withdrawal phase. Amphetamines have been given to combat pilots regularly since World War II, and it is estimated that 200 million amphetamine tablets were distributed to military personnel during that conflict to fight battle fatigue. It had previously been believed that the dependence liability of amphetamines was low, and therefore they have historically been sold widely without prescription as decongestants and, in the United States, as appetite suppressants and legal stimulants (McKim & Hancock, 2013).

Although the first synthesis of amphetamines occurred in 1887, the physiological effects of these compounds were not fully appreciated until the late 1920s. At that time it was reported that these compounds could constrict blood vessels, increase blood pressure, and dilate the bronchial tubes. Between 1935 and 1945, the mood-altering and stimulant properties of amphetamines were recognized, and they were subsequently used to treat overeating, depression, narcolepsy, Parkinson's disease, hyperactivity in children, and the sedation caused by some anti-epileptic drugs (Sproule, 2004).

Methamphetamine, an illicit amphetamine, originally referred to as "speed," has become a public health concern. Methamphetamine enjoyed popularity in Canada in the 1970s, but because of the harsh toll it took on the body it was a relatively short-lived phenomenon. However, it re-emerged during the rave era and became known as "the poor man's cocaine." The fact that it could be relatively easily created from chemicals also gave it a greater breadth of manufacturing potential than cocaine, which has to be imported. Methamphetamine, like all amphetamines, is a white, odourless, bitter-tasting crystalline powder whose use can lead to memory loss, aggressive behaviour, violence, and paranoid and psychotic behaviour if abused. Part of this behaviour is because its use allows an individual to remain awake for extended periods of time, thus not needing to sleep and, in turn, not dreaming. The prolonged lack of REM sleep and subsequent lack of dreaming are associated with paranoid and psychotic behaviour. Long-term use of methamphetamine is also associated with cardiovascular and neurological damage and, when injected, the associated risks of using unsterile needles (United States Department of Justice, 2003c).

Crystal meth is a synthesized from of methamphetamine that can be smoked, thus creating a fast, intense stimulant response similar to that of crack cocaine, with a much longer duration of 6 to 12 hours. Among the reasons for its popularity is that initially users experience an increased and intensified sex drive, along with feelings of enhanced sexual pleasure. This is because the use of this drug can release up to 12 times as much dopamine in the CNS as eating one's favourite food or engaging in non-drug-enhanced sex. This effect dissipates, though, with as little as six months of regular use. There is no known behaviour that humans engage in that releases even close to the amount of dopamine that is released through the use of this psychoactive substance (United States Department of Justice, 2003c).

The long-term use of crystal methamphetamine has also been associated with aggressive and violent behaviour. Short-term effects are like any CNS stimulant: disturbed sleep, hyperactivity, decreased hunger, irritability, confusion, anxiety, and paranoia. Long-term physical effects can include damage to the heart and cardiovascular system; liver, kidney, and lung damage; memory impairment; mood swings; malnutrition; decrease in the body's ability to produce sufficient levels of dopamine for normal functioning, leading to psychotic symptoms and increased risk of schizophrenia; and possible premature death through prolonged use. As well, the toxic ingredients used to synthesize the drug lead to severe tooth decay, labelled "meth mouth." Teeth become blackened and rot to the point where they fall out or need to be pulled because of damage to the gums and roots (Canadian Centre on Substance Abuse, 2005; Li et al., 2014; Werb, Kerr, Zhang, Montaner, & Wood, 2010; Westover & Nakonezny, 2010).

Regular use of amphetamines induces tolerance to some effects, making increased doses necessary to produce them. Tolerance does not develop to all effects at the same rate; however, it does rapidly develop to the mood-enhancing effects, necessitating an increase in dosage. While a therapeutic dose averages 30 mg, doses of up to 1 g of methamphetamine have been given to tolerant users without them demonstrating any exaggerated effects. Cross-tolerance between amphetamines and other amphetamine-like CNS stimulants has been clinically observed, though there does not appear to be cross-tolerance with cocaine due to their disparate chemistries. Both physical and psychological dependence occur with chronic amphetamine use. Animals made dependent on amphetamines and then withdrawn from them will work very hard to get more of the drug, and will keep trying approximately twice as long as similar animals made dependent on heroin and then withdrawn from it. The most common symptoms of withdrawal among heavy users are fatigue, long but disturbed sleep due to disrupted REM cycles, irritability, strong hunger, abdominal and muscle cramps, apathy, and moderate to severe depression, which may lead to suicidal behaviour. Fits of violence have also been frequently observed. These disturbances can be temporarily reversed if the drug is taken again, with the syndrome itself usually subsiding after several days of abstinence (Levinthal, 2012).

Drugs to Treat Attention-Deficit/Hyperactivity Disorder
Slang: Diet Coke, kiddie cocaine, kiddie speed, r-ball, silver bullet, smarties, vitamin R, west coast, kibble and bits, one and ones, poor man's heroin, ritz & T's, T's & R's (mixed with Talwin)

The Ciba Geigy company synthesized methylphenidate (Ritalin) during the 1940s to break a patent held by a rival pharmaceutical manufacturer of stimulants. Ritalin was initially marketed to treat chronic fatigue, depression, and narcolepsy, and to offset the sedating effects of other medications, including barbiturate overdose (Alexander & Stockton, 2000). Presently, Ritalin, Concerta, methylphenidate extended release (Biphentin), atomoxetine (Strattera), and dextroamphetamine (Adderall) are commonly used to treat attention-deficit/hyperactivity disorder (ADHD) in children and some adults. ADHD is a congenital condition that can be misdiagnosed in children with a behavioural or conduct disorder. There is still no objective diagnostic criteria for ADHD in terms of physical symptoms, neurological signs, brain scan findings, or biochemical imbalances detected in a blood test. Rather, ADHD is described as a pattern of inattention and/or hyperactivity, impulsivity, and behavioural symptoms that lasts for at least six months to a degree that interferes with a child's development. It entails disruptions in more than one environment, so not only school but also home or peer interactions must be impacted. These stimulants have the capacity to increase the attention span of both children and adults with and without ADHD. This has led some to label medicine for this condition as "sit down and shut up" drugs. However, increases in academic performance have been repeatedly documented once this drug is taken as prescribed (Grizenko, Cai, Jolicoeur, Ter-Stepanian, 2013).

It is proposed that those with ADHD have a net deficit of dopamine in their CNS, though the exact cause or causes have yet to be determined. In contrast to amphetamines, ADHD drugs are not taken up into the dopamine terminal. Rather, they block the transport mechanism and prevent the reuptake of dopamine from the sending neuron, thus allowing more dopamine to flow across the synaptic cleft to activate surrounding neurons. This increased flow of dopamine allows the brain to carry on its executive functions as would a normally functioning brain, counteracting the effects of ADHD. The question of what effect ADHD drugs have on a misdiagnosed child or adult whose executive brain functions are working properly has not been addressed. The label of ADHD can easily be applied to children who do not fit other medical criteria, including highly intelligent children who are restless and bored in a school system developed to teach the average child. However, critics contend that there is as great a chance of underdiagnosing as overdiagnosing ADHD, and thereby failing to assist a child who could benefit from the drug. Those with untreated ADHD have a greater chance of underachieving academically, increased drug use in adulthood, and engaging in unlawful behaviours (European Monitoring Centre for Drugs and Drug Addiction, 2009a; Fusar-Poli, Rubia, Rossi, Sartori, & Balottin, 2012; Lee, Humphreys, Flory, Liu, & Glass, 2011).

There is no question that Ritalin and related medications are effective, as they aid not only those with ADHD but also those who suffer from seizures (Santos, Palmini, Radziuk, Rotert, & Bastos, 2013). The controversy is not with the drug, but by and how widely whom it should be used. The Ontario Ministry of Health and Long Term Care (2010) states that 5–12 percent of school-aged children—8–10 percent of boys and 3–4 percent of girls under 18—have ADHD. Over two-thirds continue to meet the diagnostic criteria into adolescence and 60 percent into adulthood. However, some have questioned whether some children diagnosed with ADHD are actually afflicted with fetal alcohol spectrum disorder. There is also a trend now to treat adults who are unable to focus or concentrate. University students are also attempting to obtain a competitive academic edge by using these drugs to decrease fatigue and enhance their focus during exams.

ADHD is the most commonly diagnosed children's mental health disorder globally. From 1990 to 1997 in Canada, there was more than a 500 percent increase in the number of Ritalin prescriptions written, with a greater likelihood of a prescription being obtained when some type of family disruption occurred, such as a divorce (Strohschein, 2007). In the United States, use in children jumped 46 percent from 2002 to 2010 (Chai et al., 2012), likewise rising in Canada from 1994 to 2007 (Brault & Lacourse, 2012). During the same period, advertising by drug companies for this drug also rose. In the United States, the Food and Drug Administration has cited every manufacturer of a major ADHD drug, including Adderall, Concerta, Focalin, Vyvanse, Intuniv, and Strattera, for false and misleading advertising since 2000 (Schwarz, 2013).

As with any psychoactive agent, the use of ADHD drugs has a range of negative side effects, such as loss of appetite, nervousness, tics, Tourette's syndrome, cardiac arrhythmia, increased blood pressure, rash, dry mouth, and abdominal pain (Sumnall, Woolfall, Cole, Mackridge & McVeigh, 2008). The use of Ritalin and related stimulants has been also been shown to delay physical growth (height and/or weight) and development in children (Faraone, Biederman, Morley, & Spencer, 2008). More troubling, however, is the work of Breeding and Baughman (2003), who have linked 160 cardiovascular deaths between 1990 and 1997 to the use of Ritalin, and the fact that in 2004, Eli Lilly attached a suicide ideation warning when it released Strattera. These drugs should never be given to preschool-aged children, especially as clinical trials of many ADHD drugs have not been designed to assess for either rare adverse events or long-term safety and efficacy (Bourgeois, Kim, & Mandl, 2014).

Anorexiants
Slang: preludes, slims

Diethylpropion and fenfluramine are examples of lesser amphetamines that have been regularly prescribed over short periods of time to assist with weight reduction and treat clinical obesity, replacing the more potent amphetamines that were used as anorexiants prior to the early 1970s. Fenfluramine in particular does not produce nearly as much CNS stimulation as the rest of the amphetamines, and, in fact, causes drowsiness in some users. However, its excessive use has become associated with cardiovascular problems, especially when used in combination with phentermine. However, in general, anorexiants are not drugs of choice among illicit users, but large doses may be consumed as a last resort if more potent stimulants are unavailable. Examples of anorexiants include phentermine (Ionamin), diethylpropion (Tenuate), fenfluramine (Ponderal), and phenmetrazine (Preludin).

Decongestants

Slang: pseudococaine, robo-tripping

Drugs used as decongestants have chemical structures similar to those of the other amphetamines, though these have a much lower dependency liability. Like other CNS stimulants, they constrict blood vessels and thereby relieve nasal and sinus congestion. For this reason, they are found in many cold and allergy medications, often in combination with an antihistamine. The family of decongestants consists of phenylpropanolamine (PPA), ephedrine, and propylhexedrine (PE). In 2001, all prescription and over-the-counter medications containing phenylpropanolamine were withdrawn across North America, due to its potential to produce severe cardiovascular consequences if overused. PPA was found in such common substances as Alka Seltzer Plus, Dexatrim, Triaminic products, Robitussin, and Contact cold medicines. Not surprisingly, PPA, when used beyond recommended limits for extended periods of time, produced health risks associated with all stimulants, such as cardiovascular disease, including high blood pressure, heart attacks, strokes, and seizures (Sproule, 2004).

When given at therapeutic doses for the management of nasal or sinus congestion, hypertension is unlikely to be a problem except in the most sensitive of patients. However, when these drugs are self-administered as stimulants, a high dose is often taken because of their relatively weak CNS effects. This greatly increases the risk of hypertension, even in young, healthy users. The most severe reactions, those of stroke, seizures, and kidney failure, tend to occur in users of combination products. Deaths, although rare, have been reported. However, the major concern was with pseudoephedrine and related decongestants, used as precursor chemicals in the illicit synthesis of methamphetamine. Some jurisdictions require the presentation of identification before products containing these drugs can be bought and limits on how much can be purchased in a given time period.

Khat

Slang: Abyssinian tea, African salad, Arabian tea, Bushman's tea, cat, Catha, chat, Flower of Paradise, oat, Somalia tea

Khat/qat leaves were chewed by warriors in Western Africa and the Arabian Peninsula to fight fatigue, and even Alexander the Great instructed his soldiers to use khat prior to engaging in battle. While a relatively new drug of misuse and abuse in North America, its use dates back to ancient Egypt where it was used alongside alcohol. Khat is a fundamental part of social and cultural traditions in some parts of Yemen and East Africa, with use by 85 percent of adult males in some communities. Worldwide, this small shrub, whose formal name is *Catha edulis*, is the most popular stimulant from the monoamine group. It is native to East Africa, and widely cultivated in Yemen, Somalia, Kenya, and Ethiopia. Khat leaves contain cathine and cathinone, which are chemically similar to amphetamine. Among many Islamic nations, its use is considered much more acceptable than other drugs, including alcohol, with as many as 5 million daily users throughout the Horn of Africa (Khatib, Jarrar, Bizrah, & Checinski, 2013; Spinella, 2001).

Khat has crimson-brown leaves that turn yellow-green and leathery with age. Its use in Canada increased with the influx of Somali refugees and immigrants. In Eastern Africa and Southern Arabia, where it is most commonly used, it is a social drug, consumed by chewing the leaves or brewing them in tea, though it can also be smoked. Like all stimulants, khat use temporarily dispells perceptions of hunger, fatigue, and depression while enhancing concentration and motor activity. Users report that khat provides energy and a euphoric feeling, with short-term stimulant effects similar to those of several cups of coffee. There have been some health concerns, though, about khat's ability to suppress appetite, prevent sleep, increase respiration, and lead to hyperactive behaviour, followed by withdrawal effects featuring a general malaise (Nasrulla, 2000). As well, along with short-term effects such as constipation, dizziness, insomnia, loss of appetite, migraine headaches, and stomach upset, long-term effects such as liver, kidney, lung, and cardiovascular damage have been reported among chronic users. Ongoing use of this natural CNS stimulant can also produce negative cardiovascular and gastrointestinal effects, anxiety, insomnia, disorientation, tremors, aggression, paranoia, hallucinations (visual as well as auditory), and delusions. Withdrawal is typically accompanied by depression. Some chronic khat users have been reported to suffer permanent brain alteration, including symptoms similar to those associated with Parkinson's disease and, in severe cases, paranoid psychosis. While recreational use is not associated with significant impairment, physical and psychological dependency to the substance is possible (Carvalho, 2003; Nencini, Ahmed, & Elmi, 1986; Khatib et al., 2013; Spinella, 2001).

Khat is a legal substance in much of Europe and in the regions where it is grown, and it accounts for more than one-third of Yemen's economic output. It was also a legal commodity in Canada until 1997. However, on May 14, 1997, it became criminalized and was moved from the Food and Drug Act to the Controlled Substances Act, making possession and importation of this substance illegal. In the first two months of criminalization, the RCMP made over two dozen seizures totalling approximately 750 kg of the drug. Ironically, when the traffickers boarded their planes, they were importers who generally had declared their possession of khat as it was a legal substance. However, as they flew across the Atlantic, their property suddenly became illegal. In 1997, when it was still a licit substance, it typically cost $40–$60 a bundle. When it became an illicit drug, the price quickly doubled (Dubey, 1997) (see also Table 3.14). Most khat currently enters Canada via the Netherlands and the United Kingdom. This too will change, as the United Kingdom joined Canada and the United States in prohibiting the drug in 2014. Despite ongoing prohibition, khat continues to flow into Canada. Seizures of the drug have fluctuated over the years, with over 20,000 kg captured in 2005, 14,000 kg in 2006, 23,000 kg in 2008, and 19,000 kg in 2009, with the majority confiscated at Toronto Pearson International Airport (Royal Canadian Mounted Police, 2006, 2010).

Bath Salts (methylendioxypyrovalerone and mephedrone)

Slang/brand names: Arctic blast, blue silk, charge, cloud 10, gold rush, hurricane Charlie, ivory snow, ivory wave, kamikaze, lunar wave, meow meow mystic, ocean burst, plant fertilizer, pure ivory, purple wave, red dove, scarface, snow leopard, stardust, vanilla sky, white knight, white lightning, wicked X, zoom

Bath salts are not intended as a relaxing additive for bathing but rather are one of several designer drugs or legal highs that have emerged in the 21st century, primarily in an attempt to avoid legislation prohibiting other potent stimulants and hallucinogens. They have been placed into a broader classification of new psychoactive substances (NPS), which are not controlled by the 1961 United Nations Single Convention on Narcotic Drugs or the 1971 United Nations Convention on Psychotropic Substances. The substances include both synthetic compounds, such as synthetic cannabinoids, synthetic cathinones, and piperazines, and traditional plant-based psychoactive substances, such as khat (*Catha edulis*), kratom (*Mitragyna speciosa*), and *Salvia divinorum* (Briones et al., 2013).

Bath salts are most closely related to khat. Its psychoactive property is derived from the same source, cathinone, though the synthetic version is much more potent. While cathinone was synthesized by pharmaceutical companies in the late 20th century, its derivatives did not become broadly used within the drug trade until the beginning of this century. It also shares some pharmacological similarity with methylenedioxymethamphetamine (MDMA/ecstasy) but with less hallucinogenic and more stimulant properties closer to the effects of methamphetamine. In a study of the rewarding and reinforcing effects of methylendioxypyrovalerone (MDPV), rats showed self-administration patterns and escalation of drug intake nearly identical to methamphetamine (Cameron, Kolanos, Solis, Glennon, & Felice, 2013; Cameron, Kolanos, Verkariva, Felice, & Glennon, 2013; Kyle, Iverson, Gajaogowni, & Spencer, 2011).

Bath salts are typically sold in 50–500 mg packets. The price ranges from $25 to $50 per 50 mg packet, though as little as 5–10 mg can produce a psychoactive effect. This drug can be administered orally, across mucous membrane, via inhalation, or by injection. The energizing and often agitating effects occur because of increased levels of dopamine, which also increase a user's heart rate and blood pressure. This surge in dopamine creates feelings of euphoria, increased physical activity, heightened sexual interest, a lack of hunger and thirst, muscle spasms, sleeplessness, and, when sleep does occur, disrupted dream cycles. Behavioural effects include erratic behaviour, teeth grinding, lack of recall of how much of the substance has been consumed, panic attacks, anxiety, agitation, severe paranoia, hallucinations, psychosis, self-mutilation, and behaviour that can be aggressive, violent, and, in extreme cases, move beyond suicidal ideation to suicidal action. Overdose is possible due to heart and blood vessel problems. This drug lacks any type of regulation, leading to inconsistency in the amount of the psychoactive ingredient between brands. In 2012 the government of Canada made it illegal to possess, traffic, import, or export methylendioxypyrovalerone unless authorized by regulation (Antnowicz, Metzger, & Ramanujam, 2011; Ross, Reisfield, Watson, Chronister, & Goldberger, 2012; Wieland, Halter, & Levine, 2012).

Betel
Slang: none known

The betel plant is an evergreen and perennial creeper, with glossy heart-shaped leaves and a white flower cluster. It belongs to the *Piperaceae* family, which includes pepper and kava, and acts as a mild stimulant when administered orally. Betel quid is a combination of betel leaf, areca nut, and slaked lime, though in some cultures, spices are also added for additional flavour. Tobacco is also commonly added, and this product, known as *gutka*, can be readily purchased in foil packets/sachets and tins. It is consumed by placing a pinch of the mixture in the mouth between the gum and cheek, and gently sucking and chewing. The excess saliva produced by chewing may be swallowed or spit out as with chewing tobacco. Betel quid, while uncommon in North America, is regularly used by over half a billion people, mostly throughout Southeast Asia and the Indian subcontinent, making it the fourth most commonly used psychoactive drug after caffeine, alcohol, and tobacco. It is used as a mouth freshener and a taste enhancer, for impotence and gynecological problems, for parasitic intestinal infection, and for indigestion and prevention of morning sickness. It remains most commonly employed, however, as a mild stimulant euphoric because of the amount of psychoactive alkaloids it contains. Chewing betel quid increases the capacity to work, causes a hot sensation in the body, and heightens alertness. It is commonly used among lower socio-economic groups to avoid boredom and to suppress hunger. Long-term use has been linked to increases in precancerous lesions on the outside and inner lining of the mouth and esophagus, and oral cancer of the lip, mouth, and tongue, and pharynx (Floraa, Mascie-Taylorb, & Rahmanc, 2012; Gupta & Ray, 2004; Lin, Jiang, Wu, Chen, & Liu, 2011; Nair, Bartsch, & Nair, 2004).

Nicotine
Slang: butts, cigs, coffin sticks, smokes

Nicotine, in combination with its agent of delivery, tobacco, causes more premature death than any other psychoactive agent in Canada and throughout the world. It remains actively marketed globally, with a specific focus on youth, specifically young women (American Cancer Society, 2009). It is such a toxic substance that a few drops of pure nicotine placed on the tongue will quickly kill a healthy adult, while there are sufficient toxic remnants in the filter of a typical cigarette to make a child ill should he or she consume it. A lethal dose of nicotine for adults is approximately 60 mg, but very small amounts—as low as 4 mg—can produce severe illness. Tobacco smoke consists of some 500 compounds, including tar, ammonia, acetaldehyde, acetone, benzene, toluene, benzoapyrene, dimethylnitros-amine, methylethylnitrosamine, naphthalene, carbon monoxide, and carbon dioxide.

Nicotine is the psychoactive agent found in tobacco that makes its use a compulsive behaviour, and it occurs naturally in only three species of tobacco plants: *Nicotiana tabacum*, *Nicotiana rustica*, and *Nicotiana persica*. This psychoactive agent is produced by these plants so that insects do not eat their leaves, thus acting as a natural insecticide. All three species contain between 0.6 and 0.9 percent nicotine, though some tobacco manufacturers have been accused of artificially increasing the amount of nicotine in cigarettes to enhance smokers' physical dependency and thus increase sales (Land et al., 2014). Tobacco originated in the Ecuadorean and Peruvian Andes mountain range, where it had been growing for at least 5,000 years before the Incas began to use it. By about the 1st century, tobacco was widely used in culturally specific ways throughout North and South America. Tobacco was one of the first plants Europeans brought back to Europe, where it quickly became popular among the elite classes. They began to inhale the smoke and demand an increased supply from the Americas. Europeans taught the Ottomans how to cultivate and cure tobacco, though over time, the Turks perfected their own approach to growing, curing, and smoking tobacco through a hookah. The distinct flavour and intensity of Turkish tobacco led to a billion-dollar business, which in turn has led to significant health and social costs (Gately, 2001).

Nicotine stimulates the release of dopamine in the nucleus accumbens, a major part of the brain's reward system. Habitual smokers continually stimulate the nucleus accumbens, thereby causing dependence due to the complex activation of the core and shell of the nucleus (Balfour, 2002). Research indicates that opioid receptors, GABA B, cannabinoid C_1, and dopamine D_2, are all involved in the creation of nicotine dependence (Berrettini & Lerman, 2005). Nicotine is a mild stimulant that in cigarette smoke is delivered, along with the tar, in the form of tiny particles suspended in the gaseous phase. The drug is absorbed rapidly from the lungs and can reach the brain within 8 seconds. As cigarette smoke acidifies the saliva, the drug is not efficiently absorbed orally. Smokers do not absorb much nicotine unless they inhale the smoke, though nicotine can be effectively absorbed across the oral or nasal mucosa if the drug is administered in the form of chewing tobacco or snuff. The elimination half-life of nicotine is approximately 30–60 minutes. Frequent smokers often light their next cigarette before all of the nicotine from the previous one is cleared from the body. When they do, the drug can accumulate in the tissues over the course of a day's regular use (McKim & Hancock, 2013).

Nicotine is a central nervous system stimulant that increases heart rate, pulse rate, and blood pressure; depresses the spinal reflex; reduces muscle tone; decreases skin temperature; increases acid in the stomach; reduces urine formation; precipitates a loss of appetite; increases adrenaline production, and stimulates, then reduces, brain and nervous system activity. In non-smokers, small doses, even less than one cigarette, may produce an unpleasant reaction that includes coughing, nausea, vomiting, dizziness, abdominal discomfort, weakness, and flushing.

For both men and women, regular smoking reduces life expectancy by 5–10 years (Woloshin, Schwartz, & Wlech, 2008). Long-term effects of smoking and nicotine ingestion include narrowing or hardening of blood vessels in the heart and brain, leading to an increased risk of heart attack or stroke in all age groups; shortness of breath; more respiratory infections, such as colds and pneumonia; chronic bronchitis; oxygen deprivation of all body tissues; and a risk of cancer of the lungs, mouth, larynx, esophagus, skin, bladder, kidney, pancreas, stomach, gastric system, breasts, bowel, blood, head, neck, and cervix. Smoking tobacco has also been associated with stomach ulcers, impotence, increased risk of brain hemorrhages and brain damage, cognitive decline and memory loss, increased risk of developing chronic obstructive pulmonary disease (COPD), emphysema, progression of multiple sclerosis symptoms, and risk of thrombosis in users of birth control pills (Boffetta & Straif, 2009; Borchers et al., 2009; Freedman et al., 2007; Healy et al., 2009; Hunt, van der Hel, McMillan, Boffetta, & Brennan, 2005; Richards, Jarvis, Thompson, & Wadsworth, 2003). Table 3.8 provides examples of possible outcomes from the risk of chronic tobacco use.

TABLE 3.8: OUTCOMES OF SMOKING

Roll of Two Dice	Outcome Probability	Disease Outcome
2	1/36	NO DISEASE
3	2/36	Cancer of the lips
4	3/36	Cancer of the mouth
5	4/36	Stroke
6	5/36	Emphysema
7	6/36	Lung cancer
8	5/36	Bronchitis
9	4/36	Heart disease
10	3/36	Ulcers
11	2/36	Wrinkles
12	1/36	Cancer of the tongue

Source: Hall & Vander Bilt (2000)

Nicotine crosses the placenta, and women who smoke during pregnancy tend to have smaller babies and are more likely to give birth prematurely. They also have a greater number of stillbirths, and deaths among their newborn babies—sudden infant death syndrome (SIDS)—are also more common than for non-smokers, as is the risk of having a child who develops ADHD (Thapar et al., 2003). In 1997, Dr. Michael Moffat of the University of Manitoba found that Indigenous infants were three times as likely to die from sudden infant death syndrome, and that exposure to cigarette smoke was a major contributing factor. Infants living in the homes of smokers are more prone to respiratory infections and problems. Swedish researchers Montgomery and Ekbom (2002) found that children of women who smoked during pregnancy were more likely to develop diabetes later in life than children of non-smoking mothers. There is also a greater risk of birth defects among children born to smoking versus non-smoking mothers, including cardiovascular/heart defects, musculoskeletal defects, limb reduction, missing/extra digits, clubfoot, facial defects, eye defects, orofacial clefts, gastrointestinal defects, and undescended testes (Hackshaw, Rodeck, & Boniface, 2011).

Tolerance to nicotine does develop and is most clearly reflected in the many short-term symptoms that are either not present or greatly reduced while the chronic user is smoking. Regular smokers quickly become less sensitive to the effects of nicotine, as well as to those of carbon monoxide and the constituents of tar. Tolerance develops particularly rapidly to the nausea and dizziness experienced by the first-time smoker. Smokers generally report that the first cigarette of the day produces the most intense effects. This phenomenon suggests the rapid development of tolerance during the day, and its equally rapid loss at night.

A significant long-term effect of smoking is physical and psychological dependence upon tobacco. Both are commonly observed when daily use exceeds 10 cigarettes. Particular emotional states and environmental events, even after some months or years of abstinence, can precipitate craving for a cigarette. Nicotine, in the first-time smoker, produces primarily aversive effects. The initiation of a smoking habit, therefore, is highly dependent on psychosocial factors, although biological factors also play a role. Signs of tobacco dependence include a history of several unsuccessful attempts to reduce consumption even though a serious tobacco-related physical disorder is present, and the appearance of withdrawal symptoms while abstaining. The feeling of relaxation that regular smokers often report when smoking is also partially due to the body's dependence on nicotine and the staving off of withdrawal effects. Physical dependence on nicotine leads to a variety of withdrawal symptoms when a smoker attempts to stop. A person in the early stages of withdrawal may experience anxiety, irritability, increased appetite, mild confusion, emotional depression, difficulty concentrating, anger, sleeping problems, and changes in blood pressure and pulse rate (Levinthal, 2012).

Those who use smokeless tobacco may avoid the problems associated with inhalation but are far from risk-free. Not only is there an enhanced risk of oral cancer, but, even in casual users, there is a loss of sensitivity to salty, sweet, and bitter foods. Along with a discolouration of teeth comes the risk of damage to both teeth and gums, leading to gum disease and loss of teeth. As well, the nicotine in either chewing tobacco or snuff leads to an increased chance of heart attacks and stroke (Rodu & Jansson, 2004).

In a study of people using multiple psychoactive drugs, it was discovered that a majority found cigarettes more difficult to quit than their primary drug of choice (Kozlowski et al., 1989) Approximately 1,000 people seeking alcohol or drug treatment at the Ontario Addiction Research Foundation's Clinical Institute during the 1980s were asked to compare quitting smoking with the difficulty of quitting their alcohol or other drug dependency, the strength of their strongest urges, and the pleasure they derived from use. The researchers found that

- 74 percent of respondents indicated that cigarettes would be at least as hard to give up as alcohol or the other drugs that they were in treatment for.
- 57 percent said cigarettes would be harder to give up.
- heavy smokers, who smoked within 10 minutes of waking or more than 20 cigarettes per day, were much more likely to find quitting cigarettes at least as difficult as avoiding alcohol or drugs.

- 28 percent of the cocaine users said that cigarette urges were stronger.
- alcohol users were approximately four times more likely than drug users to report that their strongest urges for cigarettes equalled or exceeded those for alcohol.
- smoking was consistently rated as less pleasurable than alcohol or other drugs.
- almost 60 percent of the alcohol users found cigarettes less pleasurable.
- 96 percent of cocaine users derived more pleasure from cocaine.
- approximately 95 percent of all smokers in the study who had stopped relapsed at least once.

Second-hand smoke (SHS) is primarily composed of sidestream smoke emitted from the smouldering tip of a cigarette and partially from exhaled mainstream smoke. It contains a complex mixture of approximately 4,000 chemical compounds in the form of gases and particulate matter, and has been classified as a human carcinogen and an indoor air pollutant. Hirayama's (1981) ground-breaking research examined the effects of second-hand smoke on non-smokers. He studied 265,000 Japanese persons over 14 years and found a statistically significant relationship between the mortality rates of non-smoking wives of heavily smoking husbands. Non-smoking women married to smoking husbands were twice as likely to die from lung cancer than those married to non-smoking spouses. This relationship has since been observed in 11 different studies (Douville, 1990; Doyle, 1987). A meta-analysis reported that pregnant women exposed to second-hand smoke are 23 percent more likely to experience stillbirth and 13 percent more likely to give birth to a child with a congenital malformation. However, it is still unclear if there are times during a woman's pregnancy when she is more vulnerable. It is thus strongly recommended to prevent second-hand smoke exposure in women both before and during pregnancy (Leonardi-Bee, Britton, & Venn, 2011). Second-hand smoke also increases the risk of coronary heart disease by approximately 30 percent (Barnoya & Glantz, 2005), exacerbates the asthma of non-smokers (Eisner et al., 2005), and increases the risk of dementia and breast cancer (Llewelyn, Lang, Langa, Naughton, & Matthews, 2009). World-wide, 603,000 deaths were attributable to second-hand smoke in 2004, which was about 1.0 percent of worldwide mortality. This included 379,000 deaths from heart disease, 165,000 from lower respiratory infections, 36,900 from asthma, and 21,400 from lung cancer. These findings should not be overly surprising, given that environmental tobacco smoke (ETS) contains more contaminants than mainstream smoke, including up to 3 times more tar, 31 times more 4-aminobiphenyl, 40 times more ammonia, 10 times more benzene, 5 times more carbon monoxide, 3 times more cadmium, 2 times more phenol, and up to 6 times more nicotine (Oberg, Jaakkola, Woodward, Peruga, & Pruss-Ustun, 2011).

There is now also concern about third-hand smoke (THS), which consists of tobacco smoke pollutants found in SHS that have settled on the surfaces of an indoor space and are later re-emitted into the air. THS includes particulate matter that has accumulated on surfaces and in dust, or has become trapped in carpets, upholstery, fabrics, and other porous materials commonly found in indoor environments. THS consists of nicotine, 3-ethenylpyridine (3-EP), phenol, cresols, naphthalene, formaldehyde, and tobacco-specific nitrosamines, and can persist months after smokers have left the environment. Given the persistence of high levels of nicotine on indoor surfaces, including clothing and human skin, THS is an unappreciated health hazard whose implications are not yet fully understood (Matt et al., 2011).

Despite nicotine being the most lethal of all psychoactive drugs, it does have some potential uses other than for killing insects. Research that began at Duke University, in Durham, North Carolina, the heart of the American tobacco belt, as well as subsequent work at the University of Vermont College of Medicine, has found that nicotine may be beneficial in combatting Alzheimer's and other memory-degrading diseases. Nicotine has also been shown to alleviate some symptoms of Tourette's syndrome, Parkinson's disorder, and arthritis; calm hyperactive children; and relieve some anxiety disorders (American Association for the Advancement of Science, 2000; Chen et al., 2010; Finckh, Dehler, Costenbader, & Gabay, 2007; Ritz et al., 2007; Thacker et al., 2007). As well, indigenous peoples throughout the Americas have historically used tobacco for specific cultural and religious purposes. Smoke from ceremonial tobacco is used in traditional healing ceremonies, as smoke represents and accompanies prayers as they ascend toward the creator.

The positive news for those who have smoked for extended periods of time is that on cessation of tobacco use, the body begins to recover almost immediately. Within the first day, carbon monoxide levels drop in the body and the oxygen level in the blood returns to normal. Only one week after quitting, lung capacity begins to increase and bronchial tube inflammation and heart attack risk both decrease, while the senses of both taste and smell begin to recover. By the three-month mark, lung functioning typically improves by one-third, while within six months, coughing, sinus congestion, and feelings of tiredness all improve. One year after quitting, risk of smoking-related heart attack decreases by 50 percent. After a decade, the same holds true for death from lung cancer. And after 15 years, the risk of death from smoking-related heart attack is the same as a non-smoker (Health Canada, 2007). However, those who stop smoking do gain weight. Nicotine suppresses leptin, a hormone in the brain that controls appetite, just as cocaine and amphetamines do. Once nicotine ingestion is ended, leptin is more readily released, increasing one's appetite. Increased eating will result in weight gain unless activity levels increase correspondingly. As nicotine artificially suppresses appetite, it is not surprising that on cessation an average increase of 4.5 kg in body weight after 12 months of abstinence persists, most of which occurs within the first three months after quitting. While more than 10 percent of those who quit will put on as much as 9 kg, 16 percent of quitters actually lost weight (Aubin, Farley, Lycett, Lahmek, & Aveyard, 2012).

Caffeine

Slang: coffee: cup of joe, cup of tar, java, joe, mud

While alcohol is the most commonly abused psychoactive drug in the world, caffeine is the world's most used psychoactive drug, with estimates of 120,000 tons consumed globally each year. Over 80 percent of Canadians consume caffeine on a regular basis, with an estimated 15 billion cups of coffee alone sold annually in Canada. Historically, there is evidence that tea was known to the Chinese about 3000 BCE, and well-documented reports exist of its use in the first few centuries of the common era. Coffee plants evolved in Ethiopia and coffee was well established in the Arab world by the 7th century, though it did not gain popularity in Europe until nearly 1,000 years later (Weinberg & Bealer, 2001).

Caffeine, in its pure form, was first isolated from coffee in 1820. Presently, caffeine-containing beverages and food constitute such a large portion of a normal diet that the psychoactive substance is wrongly thought of more as a nutrient than as a drug by some. The active ingredient in caffeine is methyl-xanthine, and it is derived from any of several plants:

- seeds of *Coffea arabica* and related species (coffee)
- leaves of *Thea sinensis* (tea)
- seeds of *Theobroma cacao* (cocoa, chocolate)
- leaves of the South American mate plant *Ilex paraguariensis* (yerba mate)
- kola nuts from the tree *Cola acuminata* (cola drinks)

In 1964 it became illegal to add caffeine to any non-prescription substance except cola beverages in Canada, though not in the United States. During the mid-1990s, a large range of caffeine-enhanced beverages were introduced to American consumers looking for an added physical lift, including bottled water. Caffeine taken in beverage form begins to reach all tissues of the body within 5 minutes. Peak blood levels are reached in about 30 minutes. Half of a given dose of caffeine is metabolized in about 4 hours, more rapidly in smokers and less rapidly in newborn infants, women in late pregnancy, and sufferers of liver disease. Normally, almost all ingested caffeine is metabolized. Less than 3 percent appears unchanged in urine, and there is no day-to-day accumulation of the drug in the body.

Due to its tendency to constrict cerebral blood vessels, caffeine is used in combination with other drugs to combat migraine and other cerebrovascular headaches associated with high blood pressure. However, contrary to popular belief, caffeine is not effective in ameliorating headaches due to other causes, and in some cases, it may even exacerbate pain. In other medical uses, caffeine is employed to counteract certain symptoms, such as respiratory depression associated with CNS-depressant poisoning, and also as

- a respiratory stimulant in babies who have had apnea episodes (periods when spontaneous breathing ceases);
- an emergency bronchodilator in asthmatic children;
- a substitute for methylphenidate for children with attention-deficit/hyperactivity disorder;
- an anti-fungal agent in the treatment of skin disorders;
- an aid in fertility because of its ability to enhance sperm mobility; and
- a mild stimulant for an assortment of medical problems.

Much of the caffeine that is taken out of coffee, approximately 2 million pounds a year, is bought by the soft drink industry and added to soft drinks and energy drinks. Agents used to remove caffeine include methylene chloride, ethyl acetate, and effervescence plus water. Generally, ginger ales, club sodas, tonic waters, root beers, and most fruit-flavoured drinks contain no natural or added caffeine. If caffeine is added, it must be listed on the label. Pepper beverages, such as colas, commonly contain caffeine (Goulart, 1984). Table 3.9 summarizes the amount of caffeine various products contain.

TABLE 3.9: CAFFEINE CONTENT

Product	Caffeine (milligrams)
Stimulants (standard dose)	
Caffedrine capsules	200
NoDoz tablets	100
Vivarin tablets	200
Pain Relievers (standard dose)	
Anacin	32
Excedrin	65
Midol	65
Plain aspirin, any brand	0

Diuretics (standard dose)	
Aqua-Ban	200
Permathene H Off	200
Pre-Mens Forte	100

Cold Remedies (standard dose)	
Coryban-D	30
Dristan	32
Triaminicin	30

Weight-Control Aids (daily dose)	
Dexatrim	200
Dietac	200
Prolamine	280

Chocolate	
Hershey's Chocolate Bar	9
Hershey's Kisses	1
Hershey's Special Dark	31
Hershey's with Almonds	8
Kit Kat	6
Zingos Mints	15

Beverages	Ounces	Caffeine (mg)	mg/ounce
7-Up	12	0	0
A&W Creme Soda	12	29	2.42
Afri Cola	12	100	8.33
Arizona Green Tea	16	40	2.5
Barq's Root Beer	12	22	1.83
Cherry Coke	12	34	2.83
Cherry RC Cola	12	43.2	3.6
Chocolate Milk	8	5	0.63
Coca-Cola C2	12	34	2.83
Coca-Cola Classic	12	34	2.83
Coca-Cola Zero	12	34.5	2.88
Coffee (brewed)	8	107.5	13.44
Coffee (decaf, brewed)	8	3.5	0.44
Coffee (decaf, instant)	8	2.5	0.31
Coffee (drip)	8	145	18.13

Diet Dr Pepper	12	41	3.42
Diet Mountain Dew	12	55	4.58
Diet Pepsi-Cola	12	36	3
Diet Sunkist Orange Soda	12	42	3.5
Diet Vanilla Coke	12	45	3.75
Dr Pepper	12	41	3.42
Espresso	2	100	50
Hot cocoa	8	14	1.75
Jolt Cola	12	72	6
Lipton Brisk	12	9	0.75
Monster	16	140	8.75
Mountain Dew	12	55	4.58
Mountain Dew Amp	8.4	75	8.93
Nestea Lemon Iced Tea	12	16	1.33
Nestea Sweet Iced Tea	12	26	2.17
Pepsi One	12	55	4.58
Pepsi-Cola	12	38	3.17
Red Bull	8.3	80	9.64
Red Flash	12	40	3.33
Rockstar	24	150	6.25
Royal Crown Cola	12	43.2	3.6
Snapple Decaffeinated Lemon Tea	12	4.5	0.38
Snapple Diet Lemon Tea	12	31.5	2.63
Snapple Ginseng Tea	12	7.5	0.63
Snapple Lemon Tea	12	31.5	2.63
Snapple Lemonade Iced Tea	12	13.5	1.13
Snapple Mint Tea	12	31.5	2.63
Snapple Raspberry Tea	12	31.5	2.63
Snapple Sun Tea	12	7.5	0.63
Sprite	12	0	0
Starbucks Double Shot	6.5	120	18.46
Sunkist Orange Soda	12	41	3.42
Surge	12	51	4.25
TAB	12	45	3.75
Tea (brewed, imported)	8	60	7.5

Tea (brewed)	8	30	3.75
Tea (green)	8	15	1.88
Tea (iced)	8	47	5.88
Tea (instant)	8	30	3.75
Vanilla Coke	12	34	2.83
Wild Cherry Pepsi	12	38	3.17
XS	8.4	85	10.12
XTZ Chai	12	154	12.83

Source: Energy Fiend (2009)

When taken even in moderate amounts, such as one or two cups of brewed or percolated coffee, caffeine can produce stimulant effects on the central nervous system similar to those of small doses of amphetamines. This can include producing mild mood elevation, feelings of enhanced energy, increased alertness, reduced performance deficit due to boredom or fatigue, postponement of feelings of fatigue and the need for sleep, and a decrease in hand steadiness, suggesting impaired fine motor performance. Small doses of caffeine can also increase motor activity, alter sleep patterns (including delaying the onset of sleep), diminish sleep time and reduce the depth of sleep (including altering REM patterns), while also increasing respiration, blood pressure, and metabolism (McKim & Hancock, 2013).

Like steroids, caffeine is stored in intracellular sites in the body. While low to moderate daily doses of caffeine do not appear to produce harmful effects in healthy adults, higher daily consumption of approximately 1000 mg of caffeine for a healthy 80 kg male 20–40 years of age—less for women, older persons, lighter persons, and especially children—can result in caffeinism. This is characterized by irritability, anxiety, restlessness and agitation, headache, light-headedness, rapid breathing, tremor, muscle twitches, increased sensitivity to sensory stimuli, light flashes, tinnitus, gastrointestinal upset, abnormally rapid and irregular heartbeat, and disrupted sleep. Chronic long-term caffeine misuse has been linked with ulcers, persistent anxiety, raised cholesterol levels, and depression. It can also decrease potassium levels in the body, which, if prolonged, can negatively affect nerve and muscle cells. Three or more cups of coffee per day or its caffeine equivalent has also been recently linked to bone loss in older women. Caffeine also crosses the placenta, and high levels of consumption have been linked with fetal arrhythmia as the fetus does not yet possess the enzymes necessary to metabolize caffeine. Caffeine effects appear with decreasing doses as a person becomes older; intake should thus decrease with age. The marketing of energy drinks and energy pills has seen a subsequent rise in the number of emergency room admissions and hospitalizations due to caffeine overdoses, which were rare until this century (Gupta & Gupta, 1999; Jabbar & Hanly, 2013; Kerrigan & Lindsey, 2005; McCarthy, Mycyk, & DesLauriers, 2006). The consumption of caffeinated alcoholic beverages has also become a health and safety concern because of the increasing number of incidents of automobile collisions and physical and sexual violence arising from the use of this hybrid substance (Brache & Stockwell, 2011; Price, Hilchey, Darredeau, Fulton, & Barrett, 2010; Weldy, 2010). Substantially lower doses can prove problematic to children, for, like nicotine, caffeine can also be used as an insecticide, though it is less potent (Thomson, Draguleasa, & Tan, 2015).

Tolerance develops to most of caffeine's effects, with clinical experiments demonstrating that tolerance to the cardiovascular effects of caffeine can develop within four days. Consumption of 350–600 mg of caffeine on a regular basis causes physical dependence. There is also evidence that users may develop a mild psychological dependence on caffeine, as manifested by the well-recognized morning coffee habit. Clearly, factors such as taste and aroma are important as reinforcers, since coffee drinkers cannot always be persuaded to switch to tea (and vice versa).

Interruption of the regular use of caffeine produces a characteristic withdrawal syndrome, particularly an often-severe headache that can be temporarily relieved by ingesting caffeine. Absence of caffeine also makes regular users feel irritable, lethargic, anxious, and fatigued. Withdrawal can begin between 3 and 48 hours after the last administration of caffeine. Relief from these withdrawal effects is often given as a reason for ongoing use of caffeine.

3.4 HALLUCINOGENS
LSD-Like Hallucinogens
Phenylethylamines: Mescaline-Like Hallucinogens
Dissociative Anaesthetics
Cannabis

The term "hallucinogen" is applied to any psychoactive substance that is administered to produce radical changes in a person's mental state, an effect that entails distortions of reality, including, but not limited to, sensory hallucinations. Many hallucinogens are synthetic creations manufactured in laboratories, but there are also approximately 100 species of plants that can produce hallucinogenic effects, along with the secretions of a variety of amphibians. Biological substances that can create hallucinations include seeds, mushrooms, fungi, and flowers, plus certain forms of toad slime and venom. While central nervous system depressants and stimulants initially produce euphoria with ingestion, hallucinogens cause a distortion in the way the brain perceives stimuli and thus how the user relates to the physical environment. The neurotransmitter serotonin is most closely identified with hallucinogens. Cannabis, though, is linked with anandamide, which is one explanation for why marijuana works in a distinct manner on the CNS from other hallucinogens (Gonzalez-Maeso et al., 2007).

Hallucinogens may be administered orally, inhaled, injected, and, in the case of LSD, absorbed transdermally. Drugs categorized under this heading produce sensations of separation from self and reality, as well as unusual changes in thoughts, feelings, and perceptions, including delusions and illusions, but without typically creating delirium. Illusions and delusions may include a loss or confusion of body image, altered perceptions of colour, distance, and shape, and an apparent distortion, blending, or synthesis of senses whereby one sees sounds and smells colours. These agents can also produce severe anxiety and panic. Physical effects for one grouping of hallucinogens, phenylethylamines, are similar to those produced by amphetamines: rapid pulse, dilated pupils, arousal, excitation, impaired motor coordination, and muscle weakness. Contrarily, two categories—dissociative anaesthetics and cannabis—have secondary effects much more closely related to central nervous system depressants. Occasionally hallucinogens can also produce convulsions. In low doses, hallucinogens produce a spectrum of effects according to the properties of the particular drug and the individual user's sensitivity to them. Users may experience dissimilar reactions to the same drug on different occasions, finding the effects sometimes pleasant and at other times disturbing and threatening. Flashbacks, or Hallucinogen Persisting Perception Disorder (HPPD), usually visual in nature, have been reported to occur months or even years after even a single experience with a hallucinogen. They are generally quite disturbing and can be potentially dangerous, depending on what the person is doing when they occur. They may even precipitate or intensify already existing anxieties or psychoses in some users (McKim & Hancock, 2013).

For the majority of hallucinogens, with the exception of cannabis, long-term effects are purely psychological. Hallucinogens interfere with the chemicals in the body involved in processing cognitions and emotions. Dramatic changes can take place, ranging from mild euphoria to extremely disturbing and distressing perceptions. Tolerance to hallucinogens develops within days, so even if users take the drug regularly, after three to four days, no effects are felt. As a result, physical dependence does not develop. As there is no physical dependence, there are no withdrawal reactions, even with long-time users. Thus, these are not fully addicting agents, again with the exception of cannabis. Chronic users may become psychologically dependent, however, with all the associated problems of that state (Levinthal, 2012).

From the late 1950s to the early 1970s, researchers explored the use of several different hallucinogens to treat the existential anxiety, despair, and isolation associated with advanced-stage cancer, and with addiction, primarily alcoholism. Those studies described critically ill individuals undergoing psychospiritual revelations, as had early shamans, often with powerful and sustained improvement in mood and decreased anxiety, as well as a diminished need for pain medication. Despite promising initial results, inconsistent outcomes and the spectre of these being illicit substances precluded ongoing research (Grob et al., 2011; Smart, Storm, Baker, & Solursh, 1967). This century has seen a resurgence of interest in using different hallucinogens, such as ibogaine, Ketamine, LSD, and MDMA, in attempts to treat anxiety, depression, and PTSD, as well as addiction (Jerome, Schuster, & Yazar-Klosinski, 2013; Krebs & Johansen, 2012; Parrott, 2014).

Hallucinogens can be classified into one of four groups (see also Table 3.10):

1. LSD-like, with no secondary psychoactive effects:
   • d-lysergic acid diethylamide (LSD)
   • psilocybin
   • dimethyltryptamine (DMT)
   • morning glory seeds
2. Phenylethylamines, mescaline-like, with secondary stimulant effects:
   • mescaline (peyote)
   • methylenedioxyamphetamine (MDA)
   • 3,4-methylenedioxymethamphetamine (MDMA)
   • paramethoxyamphetamine (PMA)
   • 2,5-dimethoxy-4-methylamphetamine (DOM or STP)
   • trimethoxyamphetamine (TMA)
   • nutmeg
   • ibogaine
   • jimson weed
3. Dissociative anaesthetics, hallucinogens that possess anaesthetic effects along with secondary CNS-depressant effects:
   • phencyclidine (PCP)
   • Ketamine
4. Cannabis, which includes marijuana, hashish, and hash oil. Along with hallucinations and memory loss, cannabis products also produce CNS-depressant effects. Synthetic cannabis recently emerged as a new form of psychoactive substance. It is produced by spraying chemicals on inert plants or those with minor hallucogenic properties to replicate the effects of highly potent delta-9-THC.

LSD-Like Hallucinogens

Known as indolealkylamines, this family bears similarity to serotonin, 5-hy-droxytryptamine, one of the transmitter substances that occurs naturally in the brain.

d-Lysergic Acid Diethylamide (LSD)

Slang: acid, aeon flux, barrels, Beavis & Butthead, big D, black star, black sunshine, black tabs, blotter, blue vials, California sunshine, chocolate chips, fields, golden dragon, heavenly blue, instant zen, lens, Lucy in the Sky , microdots, Might Quinn, pink panther, purple hearts, royal blues, sunshine, Syd, tabs, twenty-five, wedding bells, windowpane, yellow sunshine, zen

LSD is a colourless, tasteless, odourless semi-synthetic drug derived from a fungus that grows on rye and other grains. It was discovered in 1938, though its effects were not truly appreciated until 1943 when research scientist Dr. Albert Hoffman, a future Nobel committee member working for the Sandoz pharmaceutical company, accidentally ingested a small quantity (250 mcg) while attempting to create a new heart stimulant drug. This small amount was five times the amount required to produce hallucinations, and the effects produced were quite surprising.

LSD is the most powerful of all known hallucinogens. A dose as small as 0.05 mg (50 mcg) may produce changes in perception, mood, and thought. The initial effects of this drug are felt in less than an hour, generally last from 8 to 12 hours, and then gradually taper off. Shortly after ingestion, LSD can produce a variety of physical symptoms, which include increased heart rate and blood pressure, elevated body temperature, reduced appetite, nausea, vomiting, abdominal discomfort, rapid reflexes, motor incoordination, relaxed bronchial muscles, and pupillary dilation (Smart, Storm, Baker, & Solursh, 1967). However, it is among the hallucinogens that is being examined for potential therapeutic uses for cluster headaches and anxiety, and as a cure for addiction, though in lower doses than recreational users administer (Krebs & Johansen, 2012; Sewell, Halpern & Pope, 2006).

LSD diminishes the user's capacity to differentiate the boundaries of one object from another and of the self from the environment. For some, this is a pleasant sensation, but for others, the feeling of loss of control may result in a panic reaction. In rare cases, a long-term psychotic reaction has resulted from a single episode of use, although a predisposition for psychotic or schizophrenic behaviours is believed to have existed prior to drug use in these cases. A user may experience several different emotions at the same time or swing rapidly from one mood to another. Hearing and vision may be intensified or merged, and one's sense of time may also be affected. Impairment of short-term memory often occurs (United States Department of Justice, 2003d).

TABLE 3.10: TABLE OF HALLUCINOGENS

Common Name	Chemical Name or Active Ingredients	Street Name(s)	Usual Dose *	Appearance	Source	Distinctive Features
LSD	lysergic acid diethylamide	acid, blotter, window pane	0.05-0.15 mg	white crystals dissolved in water and dropped onto blotting paper, tablets, or sheets of gelatine; or in capsules	semi-synthetic from ergot source or synthetic	potent in very small doses
psilocybin	psilocybin	magic mushroom, shrooms, mushrooms	4-10 mg	white crystals (pure form) or mushrooms	psilocybin and concybe	effects similar to those of LSD
DMT	dimethyltryptamine	business man's lunch	50-60 mg	white crystals (pure form) or powdered plant	*Piptadina peregrina* or synthetic material	short period of intoxication
morning glory seeds	erigine, isoergine	heavenly blue, pearly gates	100 ground seeds	brown seeds	*Rivera corymbosa; Ipomoea violacea*	similar to LSD but much less potent
peyote (mescaline)	mescaline cactus	button, mesc (pure form)	300-500 mg	white crystals or ground peyote buttons	*Lophophora williamsil* (peyote cactus) or synthetic	effects are LSD-like at low doses
MDA	methylenedioxy; amphetamine	love drug	100-150 mg	white crystals (yellow or brown if impure)	synthetic	fewer perceptions and distortions than with LSD
MDMA	methylenedioxy methamphetamine	ecstasy	100-150 mg	similar to MDA	synthetic	similar to MDA
PMA	parameth-oxyamphetamine	death drug	50-70 mg	white crystals; pink or beige powder or chunks if impure	synthetic	pronounced hallucinogenic and stimulant effects; toxic
DOM	2.5-dimethoxy-4-amphetamine	STP	1-5 mg	white crystals	synthetic	mescaline-like effects
TMA	trimethoxy amphetamine		150-200 mg	yellow or beige powder	synthetic	mescaline-like effects, hostility at high doses
nutmeg	myristicin		5-10 g	coarse brown powder	*Myristica fragrans*	toxic side effects, slow recovery
PCP	phencyclidine	angel dust, hog, horse, tranquilizer	5-15 mg	white crystals, or in tablet or capsule form	synthetic	unpredictable depressant, hallucinogenic effects

Source: Fehr (1987)

Another potential after-effect of LSD use is Hallucinogen Persisting Perception Disorder (HPPD), more commonly referred to as a flashback, a spontaneous reoccurrence of the sensations that occurred during a prior drug experience. A flashback can be experienced days, weeks, or even years after the last ingestion of LSD, though the likelihood of reoccurrence diminishes with time. The effects range from pleasant to severely anxiety-producing. Chronic LSD use has also been associated with amotivational syndrome, apathy, disinterest in the environment and with social contacts, and also with a general passive attitude toward life, though it does not appear to produce chromosomal damage. While there are no known deaths directly attributable to the pharmacological effects of LSD in humans, there have been many reports of deaths due to LSD-associated accidents and suicides, including one that was the antecedent event for the creation of the Ontario Substance Abuse Bureau during the 1990s.

One of the most famous and enduring urban drug legends involves LSD. A warning flyer is directed toward parents concerning *blue star tattoos*. The warning appeals to parents to be aware of a small piece of paper containing a blue star about the size of a pencil eraser. This paper is supposedly soaked with LSD, and it can be absorbed through the skin. On the paper there may be other brightly coloured tattoos of cartoon characters, such as Superman, Bart Simpson, Mickey Mouse, Donald Duck, or an assortment of other Disney characters. The message goes on to say that young lives have already been taken and to forward the message on to other concerned parents and professionals. However, there has yet to be one verified case anywhere of blue star tattoos, even though the warning has been circulating for over 40 years (www.lycaeum.org/drugs/other/tattoo/).

Psilocybin
Slang: Alice, boomers, fungus, magic mushrooms, Mexican mushrooms, shrooms, Simple Simon

Psilocybin is the active ingredient in the *Psilocybemexicana* mushroom and some of the other psilocybe and conocybe species. It was historically used in religious ceremonies in southern Mexico by indigenous peoples, including the Hopi, and continues to be used by the Yaqui Indians as part of their seeing ceremony, though no formal therapeutic uses for this drug have been documented. Psilocybin and the related drug psilocin are derivatives of tryptamine, and are chemically related to both LSD and DMT (dimethyltryptamine), though roughly 100 times less potent and with a shorter duration of effects. The threshold level to create a psychoactive response is 250 mg. In pure form, psilocybin is a white crystalline material, but it may also be distributed in crude mushroom preparations, intact dried brown mushrooms, or as a capsule containing a powdered material of any colour. It is usually taken orally but may also be injected. Doses of the pure compound generally vary from 4–10 mg, although amounts up to 60 mg are not unusual (Levinthal, 2012).

The initial effects of this drug are felt approximately 30 minutes after ingestion and usually last several hours, with the peak occurring 2–4 hours after administration. The short-term effects of psilocybin include an increase in blood pressure, heart rate, and body temperature. Initially, the user experiences nausea, vomiting and intestinal cramping. Later, distortions of visual stimuli and pseudo-hallucinations are likely to occur. They are accompanied by further distortions of time, space, and body image; heightened sensory awareness; synesthesiae (the perception of the melding of the senses); and a loss of boundaries between oneself and the environment. While users claim to gain insight into themselves and experience a greater sense of creativity, use of this drug impairs concentration, attention, cognition, and memory. As well, past events may be vividly recalled. Although bad trips (analogous to an acute psychotic reaction) may occur, deaths due directly to a psilocybin overdose have not been reported. As well, there have been no reports of long-term physical harm, though glucose production increases throughout the brain when used. This psychoactive substance has negligible abuse potential, and there is a low risk of physical dependence. Individuals with mental health issues, however, should avoid this drug, as it can exacerbate existing conditions and heighten feelings of fear and confusion. Like LSD, psilocybin is one of several hallucinogens being touted as an option to treat anxiety, cluster headaches, depression, and addiction (Grob et al., 2011; Sewell et al., 2006; United States Department of Justice, 2003e).

Dimetheyltryptamine (DMT)
Slang: businessman's special, businessman's trip, Dimitri, snakes

DMT, similar to psilocybin in its effects, was historically used by the Santo Daime and the Uniao do Vegetal, South American First Nations groups who lived along the Amazon basin prior to the arrival of Europeans. It was ingested in a brewed form known as *ayahuasca*, or *yage*, meaning either "vine of the dead" or "vine of the souls." DMT is also naturally excreted by the human pineal gland and is believed to play a role in dreaming and possibly near-death experiences and other mystical states. When used recreationally, this uncommon drug is typically consumed in combination with marijuana, which is soaked in a solution of DMT and then dried and smoked in a pipe or cigarette. DMT can also be made into a tea and consumed orally. Anxiety reactions and panic states are more frequently associated with DMT than other hallucinogens, probably because of the unexpectedly rapid onset of its effects and their intensity. The effects of DMT also disappear much more rapidly than those of other members of this family, typically within 30–60 minutes after administration. DMT also acts as a monoamine oxidase inhibitor (MAO). MAO inhibitors are antidepressants that can interact with a variety of drugs and foods, such as red wine and old cheese, and these combinations can produce hazardous and potentially fatal results (Cakic, Potkonyak, & Marshall, 2010; Riba et al., 2011).

Morning Glory Seeds
Slang: flying saucers, heavenly blues, pearly gates

The predominant active ingredient in morning glory seeds, lysergic acid amide (LSA), is a natural alkaloid that is chemically related to LSD, but is approximately one-tenth as potent. The seeds, if eaten whole, usually pass through the digestive tract with little effect upon the user. When seeds are chewed, effects begin after approximately 30–90 minutes and again are similar to those of LSD. Depending on the variety of seeds, an estimated 300 would produce effects equivalent to those of a .02–.03 mg dose of LSD. However, LSA can be extracted and injected to produce a faster and more intense experience (Schiff, 2006).

Morning glory seeds are packaged commercially and sold legally throughout North America. Many varieties have been treated with insecticides, fungicides, or other chemicals that are poisonous, with some varieties specially treated to induce nausea if eaten. As with all members of this subgroup of hallucinogens, no known deaths have occurred as a direct result of the psychoactive properties of LSA. LSA can also be a component in what is termed "synthetic highs," or herbal highs, drugs that produce psychoactive effects using a series of ingredients not fully regulated by current drug laws. Examples of such products that can be purchased on the Internet or in head shops include Strawberry Fields, Bliss Extra, Druids Fantasy, Dionysos, Mind Broadening, BC2, Shrooms, and SSrooms.

Phenylethylamines: Mescaline-Like Hallucinogens
Most phenylethylamines, while sharing the psychoactive effects produced by the LSD family of hallucinogens, are actually more closely related to the neurotransmitter norepinephrine than serotonin. Though considerably weaker than LSD, in equal doses they produce similar sensory and psychological effects. However, phenylethylamines cannot be used to prolong the hallucinogenic effects of LSD once the maximum effects are reached and tolerance occurs.

Phenylethylamines also bear a structural relationship to amphetamines. At high doses, these drugs can produce agitation and marked stimulation of the peripheral nervous system, manifested in both an abnormally accelerated heart rate and high blood pressure. Like most members of the LSD family, the majority of drugs in the mescaline family are produced only for the street user in illicit laboratories. Their simple molecular structure has made it easy to produce large numbers of derivatives. However, unlike most members of the LSD-like hallucinogens group of psychoactive agents, use of some members of this family of drugs has led directly to deaths.

Mescaline

Slang: big chick, blue caps, britton, buttons, cactus, cactus head, half moon, mesc, mescal, moon, topi

Mescaline is the only entirely natural alkaloid in this drug family, though it too can be synthesized. Mescaline is prepared from the Mexican peyote cactus and the San Pedro cactus found in Ecuador and Peru. It has historically been used in religious ceremonies of Native cultures in Mexico, such as the Aztecs, and the Southwestern United States. It is currently recognized as the legal sacrament of the Native American Church (NAC) of North America and is used in the church's formal ceremonies. The NAC expanded throughout the United States and into Canada in the early part of the 20th century, bringing peyote with it. Even though peyote was not an illegal substance, RCMP and local police engaged in extensive surveillance of Canadian reserves to determine if peyote was being used. Their concern was not with the use or abuse of peyote, but with its power to unite First Nations in response to the oppression and subjugation they endured under the reserve system (Dyck & Bradford, 2012).

In using the drug psychoactively, the heads or buttons of the cactus are dried and then sliced, chopped, or ground and sometimes placed into capsules. Peyote can also be smoked, and occasionally users inject it. It is considerably less potent than LSD but can be much more powerful than marijuana. At low doses, from three to six peyote buttons or 300–500 mg of mescaline, effects appear slowly and last from 10 to 18 hours. Physical effects include dilation of pupils, an increase in body temperature, some muscular relaxation, nausea, and vomiting. The common psychological effects include euphoria, heightened sensory perception, visual hallucinations (which users generally realize are imaginary), perceived alterations of one's body image, and difficulty in thinking. Accounts of mystical or religious experiences have been regularly reported with use of this psychoactive substance and have been highlighted in both television and movies. High doses can cause headache, hypotension (low blood pressure), cardiac depression, and slowing of the respiratory rate, despite its secondary stimulant properties. Hallucinations typically begin 1–2 hours after administration. There have not yet been any reports of harmful dependence or withdrawal reactions among those who, like the NAC, use peyote on a regular basis in a formal, culturally specific process and where use is neither indiscriminate nor irresponsible (Halpern, Sherwood, Hudson, Yurgelun-Todd, & Pope, 2005).

Methylenedioxyamphetamine (MDA)

Slang: love drug, love trip

MDA is a serotonin-releasing chemical related both to mescaline and to the amphetamines. It produces both LSD-like hallucinogenic effects and stimulant effects. It is customarily swallowed, but may also be sniffed or injected. When MDA is taken orally, the effects are first perceived after approximately half an hour and may last up to 8 hours. It can be found as a white to light-brown powder and sometimes as an amber liquid. For many users, low doses of MDA, from 60–150 mg, are reported to artificially produce a sense of peacefulness and emotional closeness to others. For this reason, it has been labelled the "love drug." Users generally report a sense of well-being along with heightened tactile sensations, intensification of feelings, a heightened level of consciousness, and increased self-insight. Physical effects, which become more pronounced as dosage increases, include dilation of pupils, increased blood pressure, increased body temperature, profuse sweating, and dryness of the nose and throat. Doses of 300–500 mg all produce significant amphetamine-like effects, including hyperactive reflexes, hyper-responsivity to sensory stimuli, hypothermia, and agitation. Hallucinations, seizures, and respiratory insufficiency due to spasms of chest muscles can also potentially occur. These serious physical reactions require immediate medical treatment as MDA-associated deaths and near-deaths have been regularly reported (McKim & Hancock, 2013).

MDA has no therapeutic uses at this time, though little medical research has been conducted with this drug. The long-term effects and dependence-liability of MDA are largely unknown, with no evidence yet reported of physical dependence occurring. Most problems arise with MDA as a result of a substitute and less desirous drug such as PCP, PMA, or PMMA being sold as MDA. Use and distribution of MDA has waned with the emergence and increased popularity of MDMA. In studies with animals, long-term use of MDA created damage through serotonin depletion. It also caused damage to axons and nerve terminals, which can have protracted effects on behaviour. This suggests that even moderate doses of the drug may pose risks (Baumann, Wang & Rothman, 2007; Harkin, Connor, Mulrooney, Kelly, & Leonard, 2001).

3,4-Methylenedioxymethamphetamine (MDMA)

Slang: Adam, b-bombs, Bermuda triangle, bickie, blue kisses, blue lips, blue nile, California sunrise, clarity, E, ecstasy, elephants, euphoria, Eve, love pill, M & M's, molly, rolling, running, Scooby snacks, snowball, speed for lovers, swans, thizz, X, XTC, yuppie psychedelic

MDMA is more commonly referred to as ecstasy and was first manufactured in 1912 by the German pharmaceutical company Merck. There is a belief that

"Molly" (a current slang term for the drug) is a pure form of MDMA. However, given the illicit nature of this substance, purity remains an issue. Overdoses occur not because of its enhanced purity, but rather because "Molly" often consists of a harsher substance, typically paramethoxyamphetamine (PMA) or paramethoxymethamphetamine (PMMA).

MDMA is a derivative of oil of sassafras and oil of nutmeg and was synthesized by chemists looking for amphetamine-like drugs to help suppress appetite. Its effects are similar to those of MDA, but those of MDMA are typically milder and do not last as long. In the mid-20th century there was some experimental use of the drug by some psychiatrists to facilitate psychotherapy. It was even briefly called "the penicillin of the soul" when it was claimed to assist in overcoming neuroses, increasing self-confidence, and inducing feelings of euphoria. Through the release of serotonin, it decreases activity in the amygdala, a region of the brain associated with the fear response, and increases activity in the prefrontal cortex, where higher level brain processing occurs. However, there were inconsistent outcomes with the drug, and its subsequent emergence as a street drug, particularly in association with raves, has led to a restriction of its clinical use. Despite this, a US study is currently attempting to determine if MDMA can assist in the treatment of PTSD. With the increasing recreational use of ecstasy, more information has come to light regarding the drug's pharmacology and toxicology. Its primary use is to induce feelings of warmth, closeness, diminished anxiety, empathy, peacefulness, energy level, and a positive "vibe" for several minutes to several hours, with peak effects occurring 2–4 hours after ingestion (Centre for Addiction and Mental Health, 2001).

Psychotherapy patients in clinical trials involving the drug have reported a variety of physical side effects, including sweating, blurred vision, fluctuations in blood pressure, loss of appetite, and stiffness of the bones. Chronic ecstasy use produces a range of side effects in doses as small as 30 mg, though a typical tablet contains 75–125 mg. These effects range from teeth grinding, dehydration, anxiety, insomnia, fever, and loss of appetite to more substantive issues including hyperthermia, uncontrollable seizures, high blood pressure, anxiety, paranoia, and depression caused by a sudden drop in serotonin levels in the days following use, which has led to the new slang term "Suicide Tuesdays." It has also been shown to interfere with memory formation, with regular users achieving lower academic outcomes than non-users, but also lower scores than users of only alcohol or cannabis. Serotonin levels may not return to pre-use levels for up to two years among those who chronically use this drug. Ongoing use has also been demonstrated to cause long-lasting damage to brain areas critical for thought, as excessive amounts of MDMA can damage nerve cells that use serotonin to communicate in areas of the brain where conscious thought occurs. Reported fatalities have been attributed to the pressure the drug can produce on the heart and respiratory system, though absolute numbers remain very low and are often a result of hyperthermia and dehydration on hot, crowded dance floors, as MDMA does not have an established lethal dosage level. Persons most vulnerable to the negative effects of MDMA are those with pre-existing heart disease, epilepsy, diabetes, or mental health issues (Bolla, McCann, & Ricaurte, 1998; Martins & Alexandre, 2009; Rogers et al., 2009; Zakzanis & Young, 2001).

The global nature and environmental destructiveness of psychoactive drugs is well illustrated in the production of MDMA. Currently, the production of sassafras oil, the source of MDMA, has been linked to the devastation of old growth forests in southwest Cambodia. Sassafras oil from the Cardamom mountain area of Cambodia is more than 90 percent pure, and the desire to access this limited resource has resulted in the mass harvesting of trees, which has severely damaged the local ecosystem. Illicit factories can be found throughout the region, and the influx of workers into the camps has led to a depletion of wildlife in the area as well as the pollution of the rivers from chemical runoff from the distilled oil. These rivers flow into the rest of Cambodia though the Mekong and Sap rivers. Thus, not only is the flora and fauna from the immediate area being killed off, but the entire nation's water system is being polluted (United Nations Office for the Coordination of Humanitarian Affairs, 2008).

Paramethoxyamphetamine (PMA) and Paramethoxymethamphetamine (PMMA)

Slang: chicken powder, chicken yellow, death, double-stacked, Dr. Death, green rolex, killer, mitsubishi, mitsubishi double-stack, red death, red mitsubishi, white mitsubishi

PMA and PMMA are hallucinogenic stimulants with effects similar to those of mescaline and ecstasy (MDMA). Once absorbed into the system, PMMA is metabolized to PMA. PMA both increases the release and decreases the reuptake of serotonin, and can inhibit monoamine oxidase. The physical effects usually include greatly increased pulse rate and heart rate, high blood pressure, increased and laboured respiration, highly elevated body temperature, erratic eye movements, muscle spasms, nausea and vomiting, tachycardia, and hallucinations. At the same dose as MDA, PMA can be fatal because of the way it interferes with blood pressure, body temperature, and pulse rate, leading to renal failure, convulsions, coma, and death far more frequently than other hallucinogens. Only a slight chemical modification is required to alter the safer MDA to the more toxic PMA. This can lead to increased profits for dealers as it is cheaper to produce PMA than MDMA. Fatalities are most often reported from MDA or MDMA use when PMA has mistakenly and inadvertently been taken, as there is no way to discern between the two without a chemical test. This increase in fatalities is in part because, while the amphetamine component of PMMA and PMA is much more potent and longer lasting than that of MDMA, there is a delayed onset of effects. Individuals who believe they have taken MDMA may double dose when the initial onset of effect is slow, further increasing the risk of overdose (Lurie et al., 2012).

2,5-Dimethoxy-4-methylamphetamine (DOM)
Slang: STP-serenity, tranquillity and peace, super terrific psychedelic

DOM, known as "STP" on the streets, is chemically related to mescaline and amphetamines. It was originally synthesized in an effort to find a treatment for schizophrenia in 1964. Typically administered orally, it is considerably more potent than mescaline, but less potent than LSD at equivalent dose levels. Physical effects can include sleeplessness, dry mouth, nausea, blurred vision, sweating, flushed skin, and shaking, while at low doses it also acts as an amphetamine. Exhaustion, confusion, excitement, delirium, and convulsions may also occur with large doses. Severe adverse reactions—the "bad trip"—are frequent, and the effects of the drug may last from 16 to 24 hours. Although there have been no official reports of deaths directly attributable to STP, users who have already experienced psychological disturbances may suffer a prolonged psychotic reaction. Tolerance to DOM develops within three days, and thus there have been no reports of physical dependence on this hallucinogen. It is produced in laboratories specifically for the illicit drug market as there are no current medical uses for this substance (Hans, 2010).

Trimethoxyamphetamine (TMA)
Slang: Christmas trees, true mon amis, tutor marked assessment

TMA is an infrequently encountered hallucinogen that also has stimulant effects. TMA is more potent than mescaline and may be taken orally or injected. After approximately 2 hours, the user experiences intensified auditory and tactile sensations and mescaline-like hallucinations. TMA also produces some unusual effects as the size of the dose is increased. However, the amount required to produce an effect is very close to the toxic level. The mescaline-like effects observed at lower doses of TMA tend to be replaced at higher doses by such behaviour as unprovoked anger and aggression. TMA is prohibited in most nations, making its production subject to clandestine synthesis and producing a drug with varying quality and thus inconsistent effects (Freeman & Alder, 2002).

Nutmeg
Slang: none known

The known active ingredient in nutmeg, myristicin, is chemically related to TMA. To obtain a psychoactive effect, nutmeg kernels may be eaten, ground, or powdered, with the powder form typically snorted. Nutmeg may produce feelings of depersonalization and unreality. Low doses may also produce mild, brief euphoria, light-headedness, and CNS stimulation. At higher doses, there may be rapid heartbeat, excessive thirst, agitation, anxiety, acute panic, vomiting, and hallucinations. The effects begin slowly, last several hours, and are most often followed by excessive drowsiness. Recovery from nutmeg intoxication is slow and involves an extremely physically unpleasant hangover effect. Although nutmeg is readily available, it is generally only used when other hallucinogens are not obtainable and by groups who are unable to obtain other types of psychoactive drugs. Despite its innocuous association with Christmas, nutmeg abuse is possible and there have even been reported cases of fatal poisoning (McKim & Hancock, 2013; Stein, Greyer, & Hentscehl, 2001).

Ibogaine
Slang: Ibo, Indra

Ibogaine is a naturally occurring psychoactive alkaloid found in the root of the shrub *Tabernanthe iboga*, which grows in the rainforest of western Central Africa. As it can produce visual hallucinations during a waking dream-like state, it has been historically used at moderate doses as a shamanic drug. At high doses, it can mimic a near-death experience and has therefore became an integral part of coming-of-age rituals to help young men prepare for the responsibilities of adulthood. At low doses, it is purported to have aphrodisiac properties. Ibogaine is prohibited in some countries as its use has been linked to cardiac arrest and seizure even several days after its last use. However, it is not banned in Canada, where ibogaine hydrochloride (Ibo HCl) has been assessed for its utility in the treatment of addiction. Ibogaine is listed as a natural health product by Health Canada, so it is not presently governed by regulatory guidelines. This has allowed its use in pharmacological treatment programs as a primary or adjunct drug to eliminate dependency on opioids, stimulants, and alcohol (Alper, Lotsof, & Kaplan, 2008; Maas & Strubelt, 2006).

Ibogaine is a white powder and is therapeutically administered in capsule form, with effects beginning within 40–60 minutes. At doses of 3–5 mg per kg of body weight, ibogaine has a mild stimulant effect. At greater doses—those of 10 mg per kg of body weight or more—users are more likely to experience visual hallucinations, enhanced mood, and a sense of calm and euphoria. The peak experience lasts approximately 2 hours, producing a dream-like state. However, ibogaine use can also induce anxiety, apprehension, mental confusion, and neurotoxicity, commonly witnessed in the form of ataxia, which consists of dizziness and muscle incoordination. Nausea and vomiting are also common responses to high doses, as both ibogaine and its primary metabolite noribogaine are toxic. Its use is not recommended for those with an existing mental health condition as ibogaine works not only as a moderate opioid receptor agonist (which is why it may aid in opioid withdrawal), but also as a serotonin reuptake inhibitor (which explains its hallucinatory effects) (Alper, Lotsof, Frenken, Luciano, & Bastiaans, 1999; Kubiliene et al., 2008).

Jimson Weed
Slang: devil's apple, devil's weed, locoweed, stink weed

Jimson weed (*Datura stramonium*) was again in the headlines at the beginning of the 21st century in Central Canada because of misuse. Jimson weed is native to South America. It was introduced to North America sometime during the 1800s and now grows wild throughout the continent. The psychoactive components of jimson weed are atropine and hyoscyamine, members of the alkaloid family, which are also active ingredients in belladonna, another poisonous plant. The large, jagged, bitter-tasting leaves produce vivid hallucinations if dried and smoked. Non-psychoactive effects include dilated pupils, flushed skin, confusion, blurred vision, increased heartbeat, and anxiety. In the fall, the plant produces thorny fruit pods that, if eaten, can lead to bizarre and violent behaviour. This behaviour may necessitate hospitalization until the effects subside. As little as a teaspoon of seeds can produce an overdose that results in circulatory collapse, coma, and, in severe cases, even death (McKim & Hancock, 2013).

Dissociative Anaesthetics
These hallucinogens belong to the arylcycloalkylamine family and possess stimulant and depressant properties along with their hallucinatory effects. They produce a wide spectrum of responses, making it difficult to predict experiences from one usage to the next. The term "dissociative anaesthetic" refers to the state in which a person is aware of physical sensations such as touch, pressure, and pain, but the brain does not interpret the messages.

Phencyclidine (PCP)
Slang: amoeba, angel dust, animal tranquilizer, beam me up Scotty (mixed with cocaine), black dust, busy bee, crystal, DOA (dead on arrival), hog, elephant tranquilizer, embalming fluid, mint leaf, mint weed, monkey tranquilizer, orange crystal, rocket fuel, soma, snorts, tic tac, wack

The pharmaceutical company Parke Davis originally developed PCP in the 1950s as an experimental general intravenous anaesthetic. It was called Sernyl to reflect the idea of the serenity it was hoped the drug would create. The company was preparing to market PCP for human use when it discovered, at the clinical experimentation stage, that the undesirable possible side effects included convulsions during surgery, delirium, confusion, visual disorientation, and hallucinations as the drug wore off. Not to experience a total economic loss, Parke Davis re-labelled PCP as Sernylan and marketed it as an anaesthetic for non-human primates. A decade later, PCP was available to street drug users in San Francisco, and during the 1970s, abuse became widespread throughout North America, primarily because the drug was extremely inexpensive and relatively easy to produce.

PCP is not chemically related to either LSD or mescaline. It produces its hallucinogenic effects by blocking a specific neurochemical receptor site, the NDMA (N-methyl-D-aspartate) subtype of glutamate, which plays a part in pain perception, learning, memory, and emotion. PCP is a difficult drug to classify accurately. Different doses produce different effects as it interacts with most neurotransmitter systems because it is an arylcyclohexlamine compound. This gives it not only hallucinogenic and CNS-depressant effects, but also weak stimulant properties. It is also known to control dopamine in the brain, causing a person to experience elation. These effects may resemble the action of a stimulant, an analgesic, an anaesthetic, or a hallucinogen (McKim & Hancock, 2013).

PCP at low doses will most often produce a feeling of euphoria, relaxation, and sedation. Perceptual distortions of time, space, body image, and visual or auditory stimuli are fairly common. There is often a feeling of dissociation from the environment so that the user feels totally isolated. Impairment of a number of higher cortical functions, such as attention, concentration, judgment, motor coordination, and speech, can also occur. Physiological effects include constriction of the pupils, blurred vision, an increase in body temperature, and mild stimulation of the cardiovascular system. Higher doses of PCP, which can be as little as 10 mg in a non-tolerant user, can induce an acute toxic psychosis, including paranoia, confusion, disorientation, restlessness, hallucinations, anxiety, agitation, personal alienation, delusions, and bizarre and sometimes violent behaviour. Muscular rigidity and spasm, twitching, or absent reflexes may appear at high doses. When given in large amounts, PCP also has an analgesic effect that prevents users from experiencing pain resulting from injuries. This factor tends to increase the severity of injuries, because the user fails to take any type of protective action. Other physiological effects experienced at high doses include irregularities in heartbeat, fluctuations in blood pressure, abnormally high body temperature, respiratory depression, severe nausea and vomiting, and hypersalivation. At very high doses (150–200 mg), seizures, coma, and respiratory arrest may result in death. Hypertensive crises, stroke, and renal failure have also been reported, as has stupor, catatonic rigidity, and accidental and/or violent death (Carroll, 1985, 1990).

Long-term effects of PCP include the possibility of flashbacks, prolonged anxiety, social withdrawal and isolation, severe depression, impairment of memory, and the inability to think abstractly. Impairment of thought, along with unpredictable and violent behaviour, has also been observed in chronic PCP users. These symptoms may take several months to abate once the user has stopped ingesting the substance. A toxic psychosis has also been observed in chronic users of PCP with no history of psychiatric disorder, though the exact role of PCP in the etiology of these symptoms is unclear. Tolerance does appear to develop to PCP use. Withdrawal symptoms have been reported in animals, but the development of physical dependence has yet to be confirmed in humans. Psychological dependence appears to occur in some users, but the prevalence is unknown (Domino & Luby, 2012).

Ketamine

Slang: big K, breakfast, cat killer, cat tranquilliser, cat valium, donkey, horsey, jet, K, ket, kitkat, kitty, special K, super acid, vitamin K

Ketamine is a white, powdery, short-acting synthetic dissociative anaesthetic developed in 1962 at the Parke-Davis laboratories in Michigan. Despite its hallucinogenic properties, it is still used in short surgical procedures where a patient needs to be unconscious for only 10–15 minutes as it does not suppress the respiratory system and after-effects last only 1–3 hours. However, it is has become much better known through its use as an animal tranquilliser for a wide range of mammals, including elephants, camels, gorillas, horses, pigs, sheep, goats, dogs, cats, rabbits, snakes, guinea pigs, birds, gerbils, and mice (Jansen, 2000).

Ketamine produces feelings of serenity, changes in perception, and dissociation between mind and body (termed the "K-hole" effect). However, when too much is consumed, feeling of confusion and loss of short-term memory occur, and, in severe cases, stupor or unconsciousness, which some have equated to an out-of-body or near-death experience. While it produces anaesthesia quickly, even low doses can produce delusions and mental confusion that can progress to hallucinations and degrees of dissociation bordering on a schizophrenic-like state. Violent dreams and flashbacks have been associated with both clinical and non-medical use of the drug. Ketamine was one of a number of drugs that gained popularity at raves and all-night dance clubs, and it has been associated with spiked drinks and used as a date-rape drug. Physical effects can include a loss of motor control, leading to difficulties in walking, standing, and talking; cardiovascular issues; temporary memory loss; numbness; nausea; loss of sensory perception; and respiratory depression. It is possible to overdose on ketamine, and deaths have been reported from its misuse. Chronic use may produce kidney damage, shrink the bladder irreversibly, impair memory and cognitive functions, and produce delusional, dissociative, and schizotypal symptoms (Curran & Morgan,

2000; Morgan, Muetzelfeldt, & Curran, 2008). However, clinical trials have indicated that, in small doses, it can reverse depression faster than traditional pharmaceuticals and rapidly reduce suicidal thoughts (Price, Nock, Charney, & Mathew, 2009).

Cannabis

Slang: A-bomb (mixed with heroin or opium), Acapulco gold, Acapulco red, ace, bazooka (mixed with cocaine), BC Bud, bhang, blunt, boom, B.T., chronic, Columbian, doobie, dope, gangster, ganja, grass, hemp, herb, home grown, jay, kiff, Mary Jane, Maui Wowie, Northern lights, pot, purple haze, ragweed, reefer, sinse, skunk, smoke, spliff, tea, Thai stick, weed

Cannabis is classified as a hallucinogen because of its ability to alter perception at low doses and produce hallucinations at high doses. The use of cannabis is widespread because the hemp plant is remarkably hardy and can grow easily and quickly in almost every climate zone. Cannabis preparations are obtained primarily from the female flowers of the plant *Cannabis sativa* and, to a smaller extent, from the leaves and shoots. Like opium, it is a biological product with many components. While the plant contains numerous cannabinoids, the constituent of cannabis mainly responsible for its psychoactive effects is delta-9-tetrahydrocannabinol (THC). The potency of a given preparation is largely determined by its concentration of THC, although the presence of other cannabinoids, notably cannabidiol (CBD) and cannabinol (CBN), may influence the effects to a small extent. In total, there are 72 distinct cannabinoids.

Marijuana varies in colour from greyish-green to greenish-brown. Hashish is the dried caked resin produced from the tops and leaves of the female plant and is sold in solid pieces. A cigarette is typically dipped into cannabis oil, a liquid, before lighting. Cannabis oil typically has the greatest average potency, though levels of marijuana potency have increased substantially with the development of hydroponics. Marijuana was first criminalized in Canada in 1923, in part because of the publication of activist Emily Murphy's (1922) book *The Black Candle*, which described marijuana as a drug menace. Cannabis was thus included, along with heroin and cocaine, as an illicit drug when Canada implemented its first drug laws.

When a person smokes cannabis, the active ingredient, THC, travels quickly to the brain. THC binds to THC receptors, anandamines, which are concentrated in the limbic system, areas within the reward system of the brain. Other parts of the brain with large amounts of anandamide receptors include those regulating the integration of sensory experiences with emotions, as well as those controlling functions of learning, motor coordination, and some autonomic nervous system functions. The action of THC in the hippocampus explains its ability to interfere with memory, and the action of

THC in the cerebellum is responsible for its ability to cause incoordination and loss of balance. However, while THC quickly penetrates the CNS, the proportion of a dose that crosses the blood-brain barrier is low because of the high proportion of THC that binds to plasma proteins. This means that after smoking, peak CNS levels occur within 10 minutes (European Monitoring Centre for Drugs and Drug Addiction, 2009a).

First cultivated in prehistoric Asia, virtually every part of the plant is usable, though it is only the leaves and flowers that have psychoactive properties. There has been increasing acceptance of cannabis's therapeutic qualities, including its ability to: produce relief from the nausea and vomiting often caused by cancer chemo- or radiation therapy; increase appetite among people with HIV; aid in the treatment of glaucoma, migraines, muscle spasms, seizures associated with spinal cord injury and disease, and some types of epilepsy; alleviate gastrointestinal disorders, depression, anxiety, and tension; and aid with sleep and severe pain associated with arthritis, multiple sclerosis, spinal cord disease, cancer, or other end-of-life diseases (Health Canada, 2013b). However, the therapeutic potential of the cannabinoids does not diminish the risks associated with excessive recreational use. Chronic use can produce side effects, and tolerance can develop to some of the beneficial effects.

At low to moderate doses, the effects of cannabis products are somewhat similar to those of alcohol: relaxation, disinhibition, euphoria, and the tendency to talk and laugh more than usual, though it can also cause unpleasant effects in some users. However, these seem to occur less frequently and generally with less intensity than with other hallucinogens. Using cannabis can increase the pulse and heart rate, as well as heighten appetite, while reddening the eyes and producing a quite reflective sleepy state in the user. Cannabis also impairs short-term memory, logical thinking, and the ability to drive or operate machinery because it impairs judgment and motor control. It also produces changes in the perception of time, distance, touch, sight, and hearing, and can affect balance. Risk of automobile collision begins at low levels of use and escalates with the dose, increasing even more so when alcohol is also consumed. After alcohol, cannabis is the second most common cause of impairment leading to traffic collisions for males in the 18–30 age range (Asbridge, Hayden, & Cartwright, 2012; Santamarina-Rubio et al., 2009). An examination of fatally injured drivers in Canada between 2000 and 2006 revealed that 14.9 percent of those tested were positive for cannabis. Since then, cannabis use across the country has increased (Beirness & Beasley, 2009).

At very large doses, the effects of cannabis are similar to those of LSD and other hallucinogenic substances. The user may experience anxiety, confusion, restlessness, depersonalization, excitement, anxiety reactions, and even acute psychosis. Panic reactions are occasionally produced by smaller doses in inexperienced users. Flashbacks have also been reported occasionally in cannabis users. These are defined as recurrences of cannabis-induced symptoms that appear spontaneously days to weeks after the acute drug effects have worn off. The underlying mechanism is not clear, but it is likely that the drug experience has triggered some change in thought patterns that can be evoked by environmental stimuli.

There is a strong association between cannabis use and a broad range of primary mental illness, particularly bipolar disorder and anti-social, dependent, and histrionic personality disorders. Cannabis can enhance or trigger a psychotic episode in persons with family histories of this type of mental health problem, manifesting earlier than with the disease alone (González-Pinto et al., 2008). Cannabis use has been confirmed to have a definitive adverse effect on mental health, with frequent current use having a larger effect than infrequent current use or past use. Factors that make individuals more susceptible to cannabis use also make them more susceptible to mental illness (van Ours & Williams, 2009). However, cannabis use has still to be shown to cause schizophrenia, yet for those who are genetically predisposed to schizophrenia, there seems to be a correlation between cannabis use, onset of psychotic symptoms, and relapses. Children with a mother with schizophrenia are at a five times greater risk of developing schizophrenia and a two and a half times greater risk of developing cannabis-induced psychosis. Thus, while it may not be psychologically dangerous for most people to use this drug, there is a distinct risk among a small proportion of the population (Arendt, Mortensen, Rosenberg, Pedersen & Waltoft, 2008). People with first-episode psychosis tend to have smoked higher potency cannabis, for a longer time and with greater frequency, than healthy controls. Among individuals with anxiety disorders, regular cannabis users report mental health–related functional problems more often than non-users. Regular cannabis users also report accomplishing less due to emotional problems and more commonly having emotional problems interfere with social activities than do non-using controls. This is of note, given the reported poorer mental quality of life among individuals with anxiety disorders when compared to the general population (Lev-Rana, Le Foll, McKenzie, George, & Rehme, 2013; Lev-Rana, Le Foll, McKenzie, & Rehme, 2012).

Cannabis is not water soluble, and thus it is retained in a user's body fat. Cannabinoids from one joint may be retained in the body for up to a week. Once a chronic user stops using cannabis, he or she could still test positive 45 days after the last administration. Long-term effects of cannabis include impaired cognitive function on several levels, from basic motor coordination to executive functioning, including the ability to plan, organize, solve problems, make decisions, remember, think abstractly, and control emotions and behaviour. Additional effects include emotional lability (flatness), apathy, learning deficits, decreased energy, increased risk of mood depression, increased risk of stroke, decreased ability to fight infections, greater risk of head, neck, and throat cancers than non-users, increased endocrine system difficulties, decreased testosterone production and sperm count, inhibition of ovulation, and decreased fertility, depending on the quantity, frequency, age of onset, and duration of marijuana use (Aldington et al., 2007; Crean, Crane, & Mason, 2011; Daling et al., 2009; Hubbard, Franco, & Onaivi, 1999; Messinis, Kyprianidou, Malefaki, & Papathanasopoulos, 2006).

Cannabinoids cross the placental barrier and may affect the expression of key genes. Though there is no evidence to suggest an association of cannabis use during pregnancy with an increased risk of premature birth, miscarriage, or major physical abnormalities, reduced birth weight and body length among babies born to heavy cannabis smokers has been noted. However, greater impacts arise as children grow into adulthood. By age 4, deficits in memory, verbal and perceptual skills, and verbal and visual reasoning can be noted. Impaired performance in verbal and quantitative reasoning and short-term memory has also been found in a study of 6-year-olds whose mothers reported smoking one or more marijuana joints per day while pregnant. Testing of children in Grade 3 has found that prenatal cannabis exposure can impair abstract reasoning, and reading and spelling achievement. Children of maternal cannabis users expressed significantly more depressive and anxious symptoms at age 10 compared to children of non-users, and increased risk of ADHD and other learning disabilities. Brain imaging studies of young adults ages 18–22 indicate that in utero cannabis exposure negatively impacts the neural circuitry involved in aspects of executive functioning, including working memory. There is clear evidence that while there is no fetal cannabis syndrome, prenatal exposure to cannabis has subtle adverse effects that are greater the more cannabis a mother smoked while pregnant (Porath-Waller, 2009; Psychoyos & Vinod, 2013).

Smoking a single joint of cannabis has the same impact on breathing capacity as up to five cigarettes. Cannabis smokers had lighter symptoms, such as wheezing, coughing, chest tightness and phlegm, compared with tobacco smokers. However, they suffer more fine damage to their lungs, impacting the ability to bring in oxygen and take away waste gases. As a result, lungs have to work harder. As well, smoking marijuana can cause changes in lung tissue that may promote cancer. Cannabis can harm the lungs' airways more than tobacco as its smoke contains twice the level of carcinogens (such as polyaromatic hydrocarbons) compared with cigarettes. Additional health risks arise as joints are typically smoked without a proper filter and almost to the very tip, which increases the amount of smoke inhaled. Cannabis smokers also tend to inhale more deeply and for a longer time, facilitating the deposit of carcinogens in the airways, than do tobacco smokers. This can mean that cannabis smokers end up with five times more carbon monoxide in their bloodstream compared to tobacco smokers (Aldington et al., 2007, 2008). Marijuana condensates have been found to be more toxic than those of tobacco, though tobacco condensates appeared to induce genetic damage in a concentration-dependent manner, whereas the matched marijuana condensates do not (Maertens et al., 2009).

Other problems associated with tobacco smoking, such as constriction of airways and development of emphysema, also appear to be more of an issue with cannabis smoke, as the intake of tar and other carcinogens is greater with cannabis than with tobacco smoke. Studies that examined lung cancer risk factors or premalignant changes in the lung found an association of marijuana smoking with increased tar exposure, decreased immune response, increased risk of tumours, increased oxidative stress, and bronchial abnormalities compared with tobacco smokers and with non-smokers (Mehra, Moore, Crothers, Tetrault, & Fiellin, 2006).

Considerable tolerance can develop within a week to most of the acute effects of cannabis if the drug is administered several times per day. Less frequent smokers report a loss of sensitivity to the desired effects of the drug over the course of several months of regular administration. Despite earlier beliefs to the contrary, both psychological and physical dependence to cannabis do occur. Physical dependence can occur with as little as two joints per day. Withdrawal symptoms occur 4–8 hours after abrupt termination of drug administration and can last three to four weeks. They can include anger, irritability, aggression, insomnia, anxiety, and sleep disturbances accompanied by vivid dreaming (Copeland, Frewen, & Elkins, 2009). Users have also been reported to "green out" after using cannabis, which is when a person feels particularly unwell after smoking cannabis. This unpleasant experience can make the user turn pale green and feel sweaty, dizzy, and nauseous. It is similar to an overdose, with some people even passing out. Combining cannabis with alcohol appears to increase the likelihood of a user "greening out" (Vandrey, Budney, Hughes, & Liguori, 2008). Increasing cannabis use in late adolescence and early adulthood is also associated with a range of adverse outcomes later in life, including poorer educational outcome, lower income, greater dependency on social assistance, unemployment, and lower relationship and life satisfaction (Ferguson & Boden, 2008).

Synthetic Cannabis
Slang: none known

Synthetic cannabis is produced by spraying analegic naphthoylindole chemicals (such as JWH-018, JWH-073, JWH-200, JWH-250, and JWH-398) on inert plants or those with minor hallucogenic properties (such as blue water lily, wild dagga, honeyweed, lion's tail, and rosehip), which are then smoked to replicate the effects of THC. Members of the JWH chemical family are unregulated, but do act as a partial agonist at CB_1 and CB_2 receptors and therefore produce cannabis-like effects. The most common forms of synthetic cannabis are Spice, K2, and Izms, the latter of which is manufactured in Canada. The substance resembles crushed marijuana except that it is brown in colour and typically smells fruit-like. However, unlike delta-9-

tetrahydrocannabinol, the synthetic cannabinoids present are high-potency, high-efficacy cannabinoid receptor agonists. This can lead to consistently greater effects, though there is variation from brand to brand (European Monitoring Centre for Drugs and Drug Addiction, 2009b).

There are currently no drug tests that can detect synthetic cannabis, making it a viable alternative for those who want the effects but are subject to school, workplace, or prison testing. Synthetic cannabis affects mood, attention, perception, and thinking. It can produce anxiety, agitation, rapid heart rate, nausea, hallucinations, seizures, panic, and a paranoid state that has lasted several days for some users. Fortunately, as with cannabis, most symptoms last only a few hours, though, as with cannabis, those with pre-existing mental health issues are at greater risk for the most significant and longer-lasting side effects, including psychosis. As well, long-term use has been linked to kidney damage and episodes of cyclic nausea and vomiting (Spaderna, Addy, & D'Souza, 2013). Preliminary studies with animals also indicate that there are potential adverse developmental consequences of in utero exposure to synthetic cannabis. Excessive use has been linked to pre-eclampsia and a high level of protein in the urine, which can lead to seizures in pregnant women (Psychoyos & Vinod, 2013).

3.5 PSYCHOTHERAPEUTIC AGENTS
Antidepressants
Antipsychotics
Mood-Stabilizing Drugs

Psychotherapeutic agents are psychoactive substances used to treat patients with specified forms of mental health problems. They modify thought processes, mood, and emotional reactions to the environment. Many substances within this family of drugs, particularly those developed during the 20th century, produce unpleasant side effects, including involuntary movements and tremors, a shuffling gait, nausea, dry mouth, insomnia, constipation, and excessive weight gain. As these psychoactive agents also tend to change mood slowly, over a period of four to five weeks, they are not generally subject to non-medical use, with compliance being more an issue than misuse. Tolerance does develop to most of these substances, as does physical and psychological dependency. Some classify anxiolytic drugs, including barbiturates, benzodiazepines, non-barbiturate sedative-hypnotics, and psychostimulants, such as amphetamines and caffeine, in this family. However, those psychoactive agents do not primarily provide the central nervous system with the balancing effect produced by true psychotherapeutic agents. These other psychoactive drugs have been discussed previously, as they fit better into other families. Table 3.11 lists the substances predominately considered to be psychotherapeutic agents.

Interestingly, a second surge of diagnosed mental illness occurred after 1987, when Prozac, the first of the new generation of antidepressants, became available for clinical use. All psychotherapeutic medications disrupt brain chemistry, creating a range of side effects such as delusions, hallucinations, disordered thinking, and mood swings—the symptoms of mental illness itself. However, the side effects of second-wave drugs are much less severe. It is important to realize that chronic use of psychotherapeutic drugs is a primary predictor of a person's mental illness becoming more severe over time, as the body often responds to being medicated by seeking its original point of equilibrium. As well, chronic use of many of these substances can lead to disability in distinct and even more severe ways than can infectious agents, tumours, or metabolic or toxic disorders (Whitaker, 2005).

Antidepressants

The two original types of antidepressants were tricyclic antidepressants and Monoamine Oxidase Inhibitors (MAOIs). To these have been added Selective Serotonin Reuptake Inhibitors (SSRIs), Norepinephrine Dopamine Reuptake Inhibitors (NDRIs), Selective Serotonin Norepinephrine Reuptake Inhibitors (SNRIs), and Serotonin-2 Antagonists/Reuptake Inhibitors (SARIs). The most popular antidepressants in Canada are currently citalopram (Celexa), venlafaxine (Effexor), trazodone (Desyrel), escitalopram (Lexipro), and amitriptyline (Elavil, Levate, Peram) (Morgan et al., 2013). Antidepressants are used to treat clinical depression, otherwise referred to as unipolar mood disorder, which consists of a variety of symptoms including, but not limited to, the following:

- persistent sadness
- a lack of interest in previously enjoyed activities
- thoughts of death or suicide
- difficulty sleeping
- feelings of worthlessness
- feelings of guilt
- difficulty concentrating
- change in appetite
- agitation
- irritability
- feeling tired and worn out (Virani, Bezchlibnyk-Butler, & Jeffies, 2009)

All psychotherapeutic agents actively alter neurotransmitter functions, forcing the brain into a series of compensatory adaptations. The sedative effects of some antidepressants can impair vigilance, significantly decrease reaction time, and impair a person's ability to operate machinery or motor vehicles. Tricyclic antidepressants work by preventing the reuptake of neu-rotransmitters in the brain, thus allowing more to remain in the synaptic cleft. However, this immediate stimulation is not enough to create a sig-nificant change in mood. This family of antidepressants brings the cell back to normal functioning by prolonging the exposure of the receptors to the neurotransmitters in the synaptic cleft over a number of weeks. MAOIs work by preventing monoamine oxidase, an enzyme that breaks down neurotrans-mitters, from being released. The end result is similar to that produced by tricyclics (McKim & Hancock, 2013).

The newer group of drugs in use targeting serotonin includes SSRIs (Cel-exa, Lexapro, Paxil, Prozac, Zoloft), SNRIs (Cymbalta, Effexor) and SARIs (Desyrel), along with NDRIs (Wellbutrin). This group works much more specifically than did its predecessors. Serotonin is a neurotransmitter that carries messages between brain cells. Serotonin is released into the space between nerve endings, the synapse, where it connects with the next nerve ending and passes along information. All neurotransmitters remain in the synapse for an exceedingly brief period of time. If they are not used, then they are destroyed or return to the original neuron. SSRIs block the reuptake of serotonin, and thus allow the chemical to remain in the synaptic space for a longer period of time. In theory, this leads to improved mental functioning. Among the best known, and thus most controversial, of these SSRIs, is Prozac (fluoxetine). Prozac has been studied since 1974, though it was not until 1988 that pharmaceutical company Eli Lilly began marketing it. Prozac has been clinically demonstrated to act as an antidepressant, anti-obsessional, and anti-bulimic agent, with good to excellent short-term outcomes. There is no doubt that Prozac and the psychoactive drugs related to it produce positive outcomes, and while there are distinct negative side effects in some users, most do not suffer from these (Kramer, 1993; Krogh, 1995). However, this group of drugs is also up to seven times more costly than older antidepressants and still produces some of the same side effects. It has also been documented that Prozac is Eli Lilly's bestselling drug and was behind the company's increase in share price during the 1990s. The initial trial of another SSRI, Paxil (paroxetine), demonstrated no greater benefit among adolescents than a placebo, and yet this was not included in the original information release (Garland, 2004). The questions that have arisen concern who should be using Prozac and other SSRIs, to what extent, and for what reasons. When SSRIs are administered, neurons both release less serotonin and also decrease the number of serotonin-specific receptors. The density of serotonin receptors in the brain may decrease by 50 percent or more. After a few weeks, the patient's brain is functioning in a manner that is qualitatively and quantitatively dif-ferent from its normal state (Whitaker, 2005).

Prozac, like many wonder drugs before it, was initially touted not to produce addiction, though rebound depression has been observed after such

188 Substance Use and Abuse

withdrawal effects as dizziness, fatigue, weakness, headache, muscle pain, and tingling sensations (Therrien & Markowitz, 1997). Conditions appear one to four days after discontinuation of a variety of SSRI inhibitors and last more than three to four weeks. From the reports that Therrien and Markowitz examined, withdrawal did not seem related to dose or length of treatment, though they did caution that some of the symptoms are similar to those reported by persons suffering from anxiety and depression. Kennedy and Cooke (2000) have also documented additional unintended consequences of SSRIs, including nervous system damage and sexual dysfunction. There is also a greater risk of miscarriage during the first trimester of pregnancy when this drug is regularly used. Further controversy was raised by Kirsch and Sapirstein, who contend that 75 percent of the beneficial effect of antidepressant medication can be ascribed to a placebo effect and only one-quarter to actual changes in brain chemistry (Cowen, 1998). In examining individuals with depression and co-morbid alcohol use, antidepressant therapy using first-generation antidepressants was found to be more effective than a placebo. However, that was not the case with SSRIs. In those trials, there was no significant difference in the relative efficacy of SSRIs versus a placebo for either major depressive disorder or dysthymia, with or without alcohol-use disorders (Iovieno, Tedeschini, Bentley, Evins, & Papakostas, 2011).

Another major caution with these drugs is their use with children and young adults. Youth receiving high therapeutic doses are at heightened risk of deliberate self-harm when the drug is first introduced, even greater than among those receiving a placebo. Thus, if a young person is prescribed an antidepressant for any reason, their affect should be monitored closely for several months (Miller, Swanson, Azrael, Pate, & Stürmer, 2014).

With chronic use, even the newest antidepressants can create more issues than they resolve. While SSRIs regulate mood and relieve the symptoms of depression by increasing the levels of serotonin in the brain, the vast majority of serotonin that the body produces is used for other purposes, including digestion, the formation of blood clots at wound sites, reproduction, and development. While regulating serotonin in the brain, SSRIs create developmental issues in infants, who should not receive the drug directly or indirectly through breastfeeding. In adults, they cause problems with sexual stimulation, function, and sperm development; digestive problems, such as diarrhea, constipation, indigestion, and bloating; and most seriously, abnormal bleeding and stroke in the elderly (Andrews, Thomson, Amstadter, & Neale, 2012).

Antipsychotics
Antipsychotics, or neuroleptics, are psychoactive drugs used to treat various psychoses by reducing behavioural and physiological responses to stimuli, producing drowsiness and quieting emotions. Psychosis is a condition in

which the individual is out of touch with reality and is unable to determine what is real and what is not; it is typically characterized by delusions and hallucinations. In one National Institute of Mental Health study, patients who received short-term treatment with an antipsychotic drug were much improved compared to a placebo group, 75 percent compared to 23 percent. However, the patients who received the placebo treatment were less likely to be re-hospitalized over the next three years than were those who received any of the three active antipsychotics. Relapse was found to be closely related to the dosage of the medication the client received—the higher the dose, the greater the probability of relapse. The irony is that, while these drugs work in the short term, the longer a person takes the drug, the greater the risk of relapse. When an antipsychotic drug is administered and dopamine receptors are blocked, over time the brain compensates by increasing the number of receptors. They then overwhelm the effect of the medication, at which time dosage levels are increased, and the brain continues to compensate. As well, these potent drugs can lead to atrophy of the cerebral cortex and an enlargement of the basal ganglia; in essence, causing structural changes in the brain. Drug-induced enlargement of the basal ganglia is associated with greater severity of schizophrenic symptoms—a worsening of the very symptoms the drugs are intended to alleviate. While counterintuitive, the best response is to allow the psychotic episode to end naturally (unless the person is a danger to themself or others) and then provide counselling and behavioural supports. While not an effective strategy with all clients, it is estimated that minimal or no use of antipsychotics would lead to a return to non-problematic behaviour for 40 percent of those who suffer a psychotic break and are diagnosed with schizophrenia. However, once first-episode patients are treated with neuroleptics, a different outcome arises, as their brains undergo drug-induced changes that increase both their long-term biological vulnerability to psychosis and the likelihood that they will become chronically ill and be re-hospitalized (Whitaker, 2005).

A 20-year study based in Chicago followed 139 early psychotic clients, 70 with schizophrenia and 69 with diagnosed mood disorders. Participants were assessed with standardized instruments for major symptoms, psychosocial functioning, personality, attitudinal variables, neurocognition, and treatment. Beginning at the 4.5-year follow-up period, those diagnosed as having schizophrenia but who did not take antipsychotics for prolonged periods were less likely to be psychotic and experienced more periods of recovery. Though still experiencing relapses, they did so less frequently than those regularly taking antipsychotic drugs. Those self-selecting not to use drugs developed better coping skills and were assessed as being more resilient, having lower anxiety scores, and having superior neurocognitive skills (Harrow, Jobe, & Faull, 2012).

Between 1996 and 2011 in British Columbia, there was an overall fourfold increase in the prescription of antipsychotic drugs. However, second-genera-tion drugs surged eighteenfold, from 0.3 to 6.0 per 1,000 people. The groups with the greatest increases were males ages 13–18, males ages 6–12, and females ages 13–18; in other words, children and adolescents (Ronsley et al., 2013). In Canada, second-generation antipsychotic drug prescriptions for children in-creased 114 percent between 2004 and 2009, compared to 36 percent for ADHD drugs and 44 percent for SSRIs. While a proportion was used to treat psychosis in children, the majority was prescribed for off-label mental health disorders, including aggression in ADHD, oppositional defiant disorder, and conduct disorder; irritability related to autism spectrum disorders; and other related mood disorders. The most commonly prescribed drug, Risperdal (risperidone), was used on average for 90 days in children ages 1–6, 180 days in children ages 7–12, and 200 days in children ages 13–18, despite concerns about metabolic side effects and the lack of formal sanction by Health Canada for their use with children. A similar trend has been reported both in the United Kingdom and the United States, raising the question of whether mental health assessment has truly improved or if more children are simply being medicated as a means of social control (Pringsheim, Lam, & Patten, 2011).

Mood-Stabilizing Drugs

Lithium carbonate, carbamazepine, and valproic acid may be used by persons suffering from bipolar mood disorder, formerly referred to as manic depres-sion syndrome. Mania is a specific diagnosis that relates to an episode of per-sistently elevated or irritable mood associated with a decreased need for sleep, excessive talkativeness, racing thoughts, easy distractibility, or grandiosity. Lithium carbonate is a naturally occurring salt whose antimaniac effects can be felt as soon as one week after administration. It also works in stabilizing symptoms of depression in those with bipolar disorder. However, the side effects can be unpleasant, and monitoring is essential as the substance can accumulate in the body. Effects of lithium intoxication include drowsiness, anorexia, muscle twitching, vomiting, and, at higher levels, convulsions, coma, and potentially death. Therefore, levels of the drug in the body must be regularly monitored through blood tests (Licht, 2011; Virani et al., 2009).

While lithium is highly regarded in the treatment of bipolar disorder and has recently been used in treating suicidality in PTSD, issues remain with its chronic use (Gupta & Knapp, 2013). High doses of lithium can cause chronic kidney inflammation and, eventually, kidney failure. It can also interfere with thyroid metabolism, increasing the incidence of hypothyroidism and hyperparathyroidism, which can produce significant medical conditions. In these circumstances, a person must choose whether to remain on lithium and become physically ill or taper off the drug and potentially return to a bipolar affect (Fuentes Salgado, Sutor, Albright, & Frye, 2014; Hundley, Woodrum, Saunders, Doherty, & Gauger, 2005).

The major distinction between psychotherapeutic agents and the other psychoactive substances discussed previously is that with appropriate use with specific populations, the long-term consequence, in a normative sense, is positive mood and behavioural change. These substances are not a cure for mental health problems. Rather, their effects on the central nervous system and thus on behaviour are balancing rather than destabilizing. As with benzodiazepines, women and seniors are the predominate users of these substances. Other alternatives may be appropriate for some potential users and should be considered rather than immediately medicating the situation. This is especially relevant since, for some clients, the side effects and chronic effects of the drugs can be more debilitating than the mental health problem they are supposed to alleviate (Valentine, Waring, & Giuffrida, 1992). General practitioners prescribe a majority of antidepressants and anti-anxiety agents, as well as a proportion of antipsychotic and antimania drugs. While this improves access to treatment, perhaps the best place for mental health care provision is within evidence-based guidelines (Moran, 2009).

TABLE 3.11: PSYCHOTHERAPEUTIC AGENTS

Type	Drug	Brand Name
Antidepressants		
Monoamine Oxidase Inhibitors	moclobemide	Manerix
	phenelzine	Nardi
	tranylcypromine	Parnate
Norepinephrine Dopamine Reuptake Inhibitors	bupropion	Zyban
Serotonin Antagonist and Reuptake Inhibitor	trazodone	Desyrel, Trazorel
Selective Serotonin Norepinephrine Reuptake Inhibitors	desvenlafaxine	Pristiq
	duloxetine	Cymbalta
	venlafaxine	Effexor
Selective Serotonin Reuptake Inhibitors	citalopram	Celexa
	escitalopram	Lexapro
	fluoxetine	Prozac
	fluvoxamine	Luvox
	paroxetine	Paxil

	sertraline	Zoloft
Serotonin-2 Antagonists/ Reuptake Inhibitors	trazodone	Deseryl
Tricyclic Antidepressants	amitriptyline	Elavil, Levate, Peram
	amoxapine	Asendin
	clomipramine	Anafranil, Clomicalm
	despramine	Norpramin, Pertofrane
	doxepin	Adapin, Sinequan, Zonalon
	imipramine	Tofranil
	nortriptyline	Aventyl, Norventyl
Antipsychotic Agents		
Butyrophenones	haloperidol	Haldol
Phenothiazines	chlorpromazine	Largactil, Thorzine
	trifluoperazine	Stelazine
	thioridazine	Mellaril
Rauwolfa Alkaloids	resperpine	Serpasil
Thioxanthenes	chlorprothixene	Tarasan
	thiothixene	Navane
	fluphenazine	Prolixin
New Antipsychotics	clozapine	Clozaril
	loxepine	Loxitane
	olanzapine	Zyprexa
	quetiapine	Ketipinor, Seroquel
	risperidone	Risperdal
Mood Stabilizers (Bipolar)		
	carbamazepine	Tegretol
	lithium carbonate	Carbolith, Duralith, Eskalith CR
	valproic acid	Depakene, Depakote

Note: Due to the lack of recreational use of these drugs, there is limited slang terminology associated with these psychoactive agents.
Source: Virani, Bezchlibnyk-Butler, & Jeffies (2009)

3.6 FINAL CONSIDERATIONS

The various effects of different drugs have been discussed throughout this chapter. However, the substance comprises only one-third of the equation in determining the actual effect an individual experiences when he or she uses a drug. Not surprisingly, the other two components are the environment and the user. Factors associated with these other two components of the equation are presented in Table 3.12.

TABLE 3.12: FACTORS INFLUENCING ADDICTION

Individual Factors: Short-Term	Individual Factors: Long-Term	Environmental Factors
Expectations	Emotional stability	Where you are
Build and weight	Self-esteem	Who you are with
Sex	Confidence	Comfort level
Fatigue	Role models	Cost
Illness	Coping skills	Availability
Medication	Other resources	Social Acceptance
Other drug use	Leisure skills	Legality of the drug
	Predisposition	

Table 3.13 provides a summary of the lethal dose level for drugs from the different families discussed in Chapter 3 for both a person weighing 54 kg and one weighing 77 kg. This allows for a comparative examination of the relative biological risk associated with various psychoactive agents. Likewise, Table 3.14 offers a comparative analysis, but in this case of reported costs of buying various drugs on the streets of Toronto, Ontario, in 2009.

TABLE 3.13: DRUG AND CHEMICAL INGESTION LETHALITY

Drug	Dose Level	Lethal Range for a 54 kg/ 120 lb. Person	Lethal Range for a 77 kg/ 170 lb. Person
Acetone (nail polish remover—inhalant)	liquid	1–6 oz.	1–8 oz.
Amobarbital (barbiturate)	65 mg capsules	18	25
Amoxapine (antidepressant)	100 mg tablets	27–270	39–390
Benadryl (antihistamine)	25 mg capsules	44–88	62–124
Caffeine (Diet Coke)	liquid	180 cans	260 cans
Caffeine (Nodoz)	100 mg capsules	100–136	141–193
Dexedrine (amphetamine)	10 mg capsules	10–20	10–20
Doriden (non-barbiturate sedative-hypnotic)	250 mg tablets	22–109	31–155
Dramamine (antihistamine)	50 mg tablets	27–270	39–390
Elavil (antidepressant)	100 mg tablets	19–27	27–39
Haloperidol (antipsychotic)	5 mg tablets	164–1,640	232–2,320
Fiorinal (opioid and barbiturate)	300 mg tablets	23–31	33–44
Lithium (bipolar medication)	300 mg tablets	15–20	15–20

Methadone (opioid)	5 mg tablets	16	22
Methyl alcohol (depressant)	liquid	2–6 oz	2–9 oz
Miltown (pre-benzodizaepine tranquillizer)	200 mg tablets	27–136	39–193
Nembutal (barbiturate)	50 mg capsules	16	22
Oxazepam (benzodiazepine)	10 mg capsules	273–2,730	387–3,870
Oxycodone (opioid)	4.5 mg tablets	78	110
Phenobarbital (barbiturate)	30 mg tablets	39	55
Placidyl (non-barbiturate sedative-hypnotic)	200 mg capsules	27–136	39–193
Quaalude (non-barbiturate sedative-hypnotic)	150 mg tablets	37–183	52–260
Ritalin (stimulant)	10 mg tablets	16	22
Seconal (barbiturate)	50 mg capsules	31	44
Sudafed (decongestant—stimulant)	30 mg tablets	26	36
Talwin (opioid)	50 mg tablets	5	7
Toluene (in nail polish—inhalant)	liquid	0.16–1 oz	.0.25–1.25 oz
Thioridazine (antipsychotic)	25 mg tablets	33–330	46–460
Trilafon (antipsychotic)	2– 25 mg tablets	76–100	108–142
Valium	5 mg tablets	545–5,450	773–7,730
Valproic acid (antipsychotic)	250 mg capsules	11–110	15–150
Xanax (benzodiazepine)	1 mg capsules	6,229	8,834

Source: Smith, Conroy, & Ehler (1984)

TABLE 3.14: TORONTO STREET DRUG PRICES, 2009

Drug	Family	Average Unit Cost		
		Gram	Ounce	Tablet/ Single Use
Cocaine powder	stimulant	$90.00	$1,200.00	
Codeine	opioid			$5.00
Crack cocaine	stimulant	$90.00	$1,200.00	
Demerol	opioid			$40.00
Diazepam	benzodiazepine			$3.00
Ecstacy (MDMA)	hallucinogen			$15.00
Hashish—solid resin	hallucinogen	$25.00	$350.00	

Hashish oil—liquid resin	hallucinogen	$35.00	$850.00	
Heroin	opioid	$300.00	$4,000.00	$40.00
Hydromorphone	opioid			$50.00
Ketamine (Special K)	hallucinogen	$70.00	$800.00	$10.00
Khat	stimulant	$0.50		
LSD	hallucinogen			$3.00
Marijuana	hallucinogen	$15.00	$225.00	
Methamphetamine	stimulant	$100.00	$1,500.00	
Opium	opioid	$20.00	$900.00	
Oxycodone	opioid			$5.00
OxyContin	opioid			$50.00
PCP	hallucinogen	$100.00		$20.00
Psilocybin	hallucinogen	$10.00	$175.00	$5.00
Ritalin	stimulant			$5.00
Rohypnol (roofies)	depressant	$80.00		$5.00
Seconal	depressant			$5.00
Talwin	opioid			$5.00

Source: Royal Canadian Mounted Police (2010)

DISCUSSION QUESTIONS

1. Discuss the implications of long-term alcohol use. How did your understanding of addiction influence your discussion?
2a. Which drug is more problematic in terms of short-term use and long-term use: nicotine or cannabis?
   b. After you have listed your points, reflect on how many of them are based on facts, how many on your beliefs, and how many on the media and what your peers think.
   c. Which of the two has more therapeutic utility?
3. Opioids are more hazardous than depressants. Do you agree or disagree with this statement? Discuss why.
4. Rank the CNS stimulants from most to least problematic. What factors do you need to consider in creating your ranking?
5. In what context would you recommend the use of psychotherapeutic drugs? What are the ethical implications of recommending for or against the use of these drugs?
6. What constitutes safe psychoactive drug use?
7. A new group of people has been discovered on a desert island. They have never been exposed to any psychoactive drugs. You are minister of the Drug Secretariat and must decide which psychoactive drugs (discussed in Chapter 3) you would allow to be brought to the island and which you would ban. Create two lists and explain your rationale.

Chapter 4

TREATMENT OPTIONS

Substance abusers are a heterogeneous group, necessitating different types of intervention methods. As a result, matching a client to the most appropriate program and counselling approach has taken on ever-increasing importance. Some treatment facilities favour a medical model featuring the principles of Alcoholics Anonymous, others take a social support approach, while still others still are more cognitive and behaviourally orientated. Many different methods have been proposed for how to best treat those addicted to psychoactive drugs, though some are slightly more enigmatic than others. Among the options that have been tried are:

- acupuncture (Cho & Wang, 2009; Janssen, Demorest, Kelly, Thiessen, & Abrahams, 2012)
- animal-assisted therapy (Martin, Minatrea, & Watson, 2009; Pugh, 2004)
- chiropractic care (Holder & Shriner, 2012; Nadler, Holder, & Talsky, 1998)
- horticultural therapy (Neuberger, 2012; Young, 2007)
- humour therapy (Arminen & Halonen, 2007; Ptaszik, 2007)
- hypnosis (Flammer & Bongartz, 2003; Green, Lynn, & Montgomery, 2006)
- laser therapy (Marovino, 1994; Zalewska-Kaszubska & Obzejta, 2004)
- logotherapy (Crumbaugh & Carr, 1979; Hart & Singh, 2009)
- meditation (Carlson & Larkin, 2009; Pruett, Nishimura, & Priest, 2007)
- mindfulness (Garland, Schwarz, Kelly, Whitt, & Howard, 2012; Zgierska et al., 2009)
- music therapy (Buino & Simon, 2011; Winkelman, 2003)
- neurofeedback (Dehghani-Arani, Rostami, & Nadali, 2013; Scott, Kaiser, Othmer, & Sideroff, 2005)

198 *Substance Use and Abuse*

- prayer and religious intervention (Holt, 2015; Kus, 1995; Womack, 1980)
- spontaneous remission (Fillmore, Hartka, Johnstone, Speiglman, & Temple, 1988; Walters, 2000)
- subliminal audio tapes (Merikle, 1988)
- traditional Chinese herbal remedies (Lu et al., 2009)
- transcranial magnetic stimulation (Barr et al., 2011)

The lack of any acknowledged best practice and the diversity of approaches may partially explain why addiction counselling is underutilized and characterized by high attrition rates (Gainsbury & Blaszcynski, 2011). It may also explain why one in six counsellors had clients whose substance use became worse after seeking counselling (Kraus, Castonguay, Boswell, Nordberg, & Hayes 2011), with observable clinical deterioration occurring in 7–15 percent (Ilgen & Moos, 2005; Moos, 2005).

Despite a distinct proportion of negative outcomes, that treatment works and that it has substantive economic benefits is no longer in question. Multiple studies have indicated positive cost returns, including reduced health care system use, reduced criminal justice costs, and increased workplace productivity (Asay & Lambert, 1999; McCollister & French, 2003; Popova, Mohapatra, Patra, Duhig, & Rehm, 2011). At the height of the cocaine scare in North America, it was determined that $1 allocated to treatment caused the same decrease in the flow of cocaine as $7 spent on enforcement (Rydell, Caulkins, & Everingham, 1996). The benefits of addiction treatment accrue not only to individuals but also to society as a whole. The question that still needs to be answered is what works best and with whom. There are three myths regarding addiction treatment: (1) that nothing works, (2) that everything works, and (3) that all modalities work about the same. Deciding if one approach tested under highly controlled conditions works better than another form of treatment is not the same as determining what works best for the next client. Taking a client-centred approach, a treatment plan and a definition of what constitutes success should be based on the client's needs and not the counsellor's or facility's, and especially not exclusively on the latest trend. In their meta-analysis, Callahan and Swift (2009) found that clients who were provided with their preferred treatment were 58 percent more likely to show greater outcome effects compared to clients who did not.

The matching hypothesis suggests that treatment will be more effective when clients are matched with optimal interventions. This suggestion is logical, having face validity, and also has the potential of providing substantial savings if unnecessarily intensive and expensive treatment can be averted through an appropriate matching process. What is most important is not what therapy is offered, but how it is delivered (Gottheil, Thornton, & Weinstein, 2002; Thornton, Gottheil, Weinstein, & Kerachsky, 1998), along with the attributes of the counsellor. However, there are some factors that should be considered in determining which treatment approach might offer the best likelihood of assisting a client:

1. Treatment Setting: Where is treatment done?
   - community-based outpatient program
   - court-ordered (driving while impaired programs)
   - day treatment
   - in-patient hospital
   - non-medical residential facility
   - workplace-based (employee assistance program counselling)
2. Treatment Regimen: What focus is taken in treatment?
   - behavioural—to control or change maladaptive behaviours and to increase or teach adaptive behaviours
   - cognitive—to correct maladaptive cognition
   - developmental—to remedy structural deficits in ego development
   - exploratory—to increase understanding/resolution of intrapsychic conflicts and problems
   - pharmacological—to use drugs to treat addiction
   - supportive—to help manage problems in daily living by supporting clients' existing coping skills
   - systemic—to structure patterns of interactions, communications, and roles in the family social system
3. Treatment Format: With whom is treatment done?
   - educational groups
   - families/couples
   - individual
   - therapeutic group
4. Treatment Frequency: How often is treatment done (which also relates to the treatment setting)?
   - less than once per week
   - once per week
   - twice per week
   - daily
5. Treatment Duration: How long does treatment last?
   - less than one month
   - 21 to 42 days
   - three to six months
   - six to twelve months
   - open-ended
6. Therapy Process: Is there a relationship between the client and therapist that promotes learning?
7. Treatment Readiness: Is the client ready and/or receptive to treatment now?

8. Treatment Quality: How does the client like the treatment process? How is it in terms of the following?
   - accessibility
   - availability
   - cost
   - counsellor characteristics
   - intensity
   - proximity to home and supports
9. Therapy Philosophy: Is the client responsible for either the problem or the solution?

		Client Responsibility for Solution	
Client Responsibility for Problem		High	Low
	High	Moral	Enlightenment
	Low	Compensatory	Medical

Treatment philosophy may be the most important of all the variables in that it provides insight into what being client-centred truly means in the addiction field. During the assessment and matching process, it is critical to determine the extent to which clients view the problem as being their responsibility and to what extent they believe it is due to circumstances beyond their immediate control. The counsellor also needs to assess how active a client wishes and/ or is able to be in the change process, and to what extent the client views the counsellor as needing to lead the change process. While we must always begin where the client is, the fact that psychoactive drugs alter clients' central nervous systems and thus their cognitions and behaviours means that, in some cases, being client-centred will actually mean being more directive. Non-directive counselling approaches better suit clients who are resistant to or upset about having to attend counselling, as these individuals do not think they have an addiction issue. Thus, clients who react against the directions of a counsellor will do best when the counsellor gives them little direction to react against. Clients that externalize problem responsibility and resolution, who have an external locus of control, tend to do better with symptom-focused counselling that utilizes skill development and targets symptom change. Clients that internalize these two factors tend to do better when counselling focuses on providing insights and awareness regarding their drug misuse (Beutler, Harwood, Kimpara, Verdirame, & Blau, 2011).

Additional factors that have been found to be important in matching clients to a treatment program include:

- *Conceptual level:* Clients with a low conceptual level prefer simpler constructs and rules and tend to do better in directive programs. Those with higher conceptual levels do better in non-directive intervention modalities.
- *Neuropsychological impairment:* It is believed that clients with greater neuropsychological impairments do poorer in treatment. These individuals would benefit from longer, more intensive treatment.
- *Severity of dependence:* The greater the dependency, the more intense therapy needs to be.
- *Family history:* Those with a family history of problematic alcohol or drug use appear to need a distinct method of intervention from those without such a history (De Leon, Melnick, & Cleland, 2008; Miller & Hester, 1986a; Minkoff, Zweben, Rosenthal, & Ries, 2004).

As a result of the matching hypothesis, regular use of client-treatment matching has arisen within the substance abuse field, which appears to provide better client outcomes while diminishing excessive or repetitive treatment. No one technique stands out as the panacea for substance dependency treatment or as better than any other treatment in every case, which demonstrates that using matching techniques prior to prescribing an intervention method can improve treatment. As well, much of what one believes is successful depends on how success is defined. Cade and O'Hanlon (1993) perhaps best summarized some of the differences we see in treatment in the following statement:

> Behaviourists see behaviour problems with clients, psychotherapists discover intrapsychic problems originating from childhood, while brief therapists discover self-reinforcing patterns of thought and action during the course of treatment. Thus, a good clinician in developing a treatment plan needs to work from a holistic stance and listen to the client. (p. 1)

4.1 PHARMACOLOGICAL THERAPIES (PHARMACOTHERAPY)
Anti-Alcohol Drugs (Antidipsotropics)
Antagonists
Drug Substitution
Underlying Disorder Treatment

Pharmacological treatments were among the first approaches to emerge to address addiction, though with limited success. Codeine and heroin were substituted for morphine while cocaine was prescribed as an alternative during the 19th century. The further conceptualization of alcoholism as a disease in conjunction with the biological nature of excessive consumption of any psychoactive substance has led to and fostered the investigation of a large number of drugs as potential treatment methods for drug addiction.

Anti-Alcohol Drugs (Antidipsotropics)

These drugs, also referred to as antidipsotropics, have traditionally been prescribed to create an adverse physical reaction when the individual consumes alcohol. The basic paradigm is that of conditioned avoidance and conditioned aversion. When taken before alcohol ingestion, these drugs produce a strong and unpleasant aversive reaction that is intended to deter further drinking. Treatment with the alcohol-sensitizing drugs assumes that

- an aversive reaction will occur after alcohol ingestion;
- the reaction will be sufficiently unpleasant to deter further drinking; and
- the ensuing reduction in alcohol use will result in overall improvement in the behavioural and medical problems that led to excessive drinking or resulted from it.

The two drugs that were commonly employed for this purpose were Antabuse (disulfiram [tetraethylthiuram disulphide]) and Temposil (citrated calcium carbimide), both of which interfere with the breakdown of alcohol, though neither is now readily available. The human body has a good process for removing alcohol, which is a poison to it. When an antidipsotropic interacts with alcohol, a person's face and neck may become quite warm and flushed, and the individual can experience dizziness, a pounding heart, a throbbing head, and nausea. In essence, it is an exaggerated hangover effect. The severity of the reaction varies from person to person, but the more one drinks, the worse the reaction will become. If a person continues to consume alcohol, he or she can lose consciousness. It may take several days or even up to two or three weeks after the last dose of disulfiram before the body will be able to handle alcohol without an unpleasant reaction. The effects of calcium carbimide may last up to two days after the last dose is administered (Smith, Mansfield, & Herrick, 1959).

The use of disulfiram and calcium carbimide seemed reasonable initially: the chemical effectively makes it impossible for anyone to drink any beverage with alcohol in it. Even the description of violent reaction can be enough to deter an individual from taking an alcoholic drink. Success, however, depends entirely on the drinker's willingness to take the drug consistently. The chemical provides a prop for a drinker who is already, for other reasons, strongly committed to abstention and to a schedule of doses. If a drinker does not have a desire to stop heavy drinking, he or she may resist a casual impulse to drink because of the drug already ingested, but could still skip several doses and then resume drinking. Studies have indicated that even small pharmacologically inactive doses of Antabuse produced abstinence rates as great as that of a full active dose. The finding confirmed that the belief one is taking Antabuse or Temposil is as effective as taking the chemical itself. The therapeutic effects of anti-alcohol drugs derive primarily from a placebo effect (Roth & Fonagy, 2005). Thus, it is not surprising that these drugs are now used sparingly as a treatment or even as an adjunct.

Acamprosate is the newest drug used to prevent relapse among alcohol-dependent patients. Taken orally three times a day, the drug ameliorates the symptoms of alcohol withdrawal and helps to limit reactions to drink-related cues. It makes drinking less pleasurable, thereby potentially stopping lapses from becoming relapses. Acamprosate also has fewer side effects than other antidipsotropics. It is thought to stabilize the chemical balance in the central nervous system that is disrupted by both alcohol and benzodiazepine withdrawal, though the exact mechanism of action remains uncertain. Acamprosate has a significant but modest ability to decrease relapse rates as compared to a placebo when combined in counselling at both three and twelve months after the conclusion of treatment. However, a proportion of those in clinical trials did relapse and return to their previous drinking patterns (Rösner et al., 2010).

Antagonists

Antagonists are drugs that block the effects of abused drugs by occupying receptor sites in the brain. When used, antagonists extinguish the behavioural aspects of drug abuse. A drug user receives no positive reinforcement if the drug of choice is administered after the antagonist. Antagonists have been found for opioids and benzodiazepines. More recently, carbamazepine, an anti-seizure medication, and buprenorphine, a pain-masking agent more commonly used with opioids, have been advocated for use with cocaine-dependent individuals, as have anti-schizophrenia drugs that block the release of dopamine. However, as with the anti-alcohol drugs, the effectiveness of this method of intervention rests solely on the dependent person's willingness to take the drug (Peachy, 1986). As well, there is always a risk of overdose when using these drugs as dependent persons attempt to overcome the antagonistic effect by increasing the amount of psychoactive drug they consume.

Naltrexone, initially developed as an opioid antagonist, has been shown to also have value as an adjunct therapy in treating alcoholism (Litten & Allen, 1998). When using naltrexone, which is marketed under the name ReVia, the pleasurable effects some people experience when they drink are diminished or do not occur. As well, there is no experience of nausea such as with the use of antidipsotropics. However, unlike its interaction with heroin, naltrexone does not prevent one from becoming impaired or intoxicated with the use of alcohol, as alcohol does not attach itself to only one type of receptor site in the brain as do opioids (Berg, Pettinati, & Volpicelli, 1996; O'Malley et al., 1992; Volpicelli, Alterman, Hayashida, & O'Brien, 1992). In a review of 29 studies where naltexone was provided in conjunction with psychosocial treatments, it was found that relapse rates were, on average, 36 percent lower than when clients received only counselling (Srisurapanont & Jarusuraisin, 2005), results similar to acamprosate in reducing heavy drinking (Kranzler & Van Kirk, 2006).

Drug Substitution

Drug substitution is simply the replacement of an abused drug with an alternative drug, or an alternative way of administering the psychoactive substance that has been deemed to be safer. The alternative drug is theoretically used to slowly withdraw the dependent person until a time when he or she neither craves the original drug nor requires the substitute. Drug substitution was typically offered in conjunction with other treatment methods, though this has changed, with a greater emphasis on methadone maintenance programs rather than methadone treatment. The most commonly used substitute drugs are methadone and buprenorphine, used with opioids; Valium, used with both alcohol and other benzodiazepines; and nicotine patches, gum, lozenges and now e-cigarettes as a substitute for smoking or chewing tobacco.

Opioids

Drug dependence that involves heroin and other opioid agents is a chronic, relapsing condition with a generally unfavourable prognosis. The outstanding characteristic elements include an overpowering drive or compulsion to continue to take the drug and to obtain it by any means for pleasure or to avoid the extreme discomfort of withdrawal. The basic premise for opioid substitution therapy is that a suitable oral opioid agent that is administered daily is effective in suppressing withdrawal symptoms and reducing the use of illicit opioids. Of the many opioid antagonist drugs that are available, methadone is currently the most widely used pharmacotherapeutic agent for maintenance treatment, with a history dating back to the Vietnam War–era (Dole & Nyswander, 1965). In 2007, Health Canada also approved Suboxone, a combination of buprenorphine and naloxone, for use with persons dependent on heroin, Dilaudid, and OxyContin. When Suboxone is administered sublingually, the naloxone remains inactive while the buprenorphine antagonizes the painful physical effects of opioid withdrawal. However, if the drug is injected, the naloxone blocks buprenorphine's effects and the person rapidly enters a very painful opioid withdrawal. This interactive mechanism greatly minimizes the improper use of the drug. When used as intended, Suboxone has fewer side effects, builds tolerance slower, and offers a lower chance of overdose than methadone. Its greater financial cost has limited its use where opioid antagonists are paid for through universal health care (Fareed, Vayalapalli, Casarella, & Drexler, 2012). However, as with all other opioids, users remain dependent on the drug and experience withdrawal if they stop using Suboxone.

Opium continues to be used in some countries, such as Thailand, while heroin is routinely made available, under medical supervision, to substance-dependent persons in several European nations. It is also available to a limited number in British Columbia, after successful clinical trials. Though the federal government strenuously attempted to stop the practice, the courts intervened on the side of those in need (also see section 4.7, "Heroin-Assisted Treatment").

No serious chronic side effects have been reported with the therapeutic use of methadone, though methadone itself is an addicting substance. As such, methadone should be used only with those who are unable to curtail their excessive opioid use and who are already physically dependent. While studies have indicated the use of methadone as a maintenance drug decreases the costs of criminal behaviour, health care, and employment (Zarkin, Dunlap, Hicks, & Mamo, 2005), a major question with the use of methadone maintenance rather than methadone treatment is in whose interests is it used: the client's or society's? The other pressing issue is at what point a person should be encouraged to move toward abstinence.

Nicotine

In a similar vein, nicotine patches have become popular as a method of weaning smokers from cigarettes along with the more traditional use of Nicorette chewing gum. However, Nicorette use tends not to gradually decrease as is the clinical intent. One form of nicotine is simply being replaced by another, though all the other harmful side effects of smoking are eliminated. Another alternative drug substitution method used by smokers is a transdermal therapeutic system or skin patch or simply "the patch." First approved in Ireland in 1990, two forms were sanctioned for use in Canada in 1992: Habitrol by Ciba Geigy Pharmaceuticals and Nicoderm by Marion Merrell Dow Pharmaceuticals. These became available without a physician's prescription in 1998.

Resembling a small adhesive bandage, the patch uses a rate-controlling membrane to deliver nicotine via the surface layers of the skin to the bloodstream. A fresh patch is applied once a day to a clean, dry, hair-free area of skin on the upper body or upper arms. For most users, the initial 21 mg per day dosage is used every day for six weeks. It is then replaced by a 14 mg per day patch for two weeks, which in turn is then replaced by a 7 mg per day patch for the final two weeks of the 10-week treatment program. Clinical studies have indicated greater success with nicotine patches than with placebo control groups, though participants in both groups had members who quit smoking while others continued to smoke. The continuation of smoking while using the patches remains a concern with this method of drug substitution as users can experience adverse health effects due to much higher peak levels of nicotine than those experienced from smoking alone. As well, because nicotine is a noxious agent, this method of drug substitution is not recommended for pregnant women as potential harm to the fetus may occur, including the risk of spontaneous abortion, though the risk for spontaneous abortion is also greater among smoking women, compared to non-smokers. This treatment option is also not recommended for use by persons with heart disease, hyperthyroidism, insulin-dependent diabetes, hypertension, and peptic ulcers (Tsilajara, Noda, & Saku, 2010).

If a patch, particularly the 21 mg per day one, is ingested or applied to a child, potentially fatal poisoning can occur quickly due to peripheral or central respiratory paralysis or even cardiac arrest. Another much less severe but much more frequently reported side effect with the patches has been redness, swelling, and irritation at the administration site because nicotine, along with all its other negative effects, is also an irritant to the skin. In 2003 the American Food and Drug Administration approved an over-the-counter lozenge produced by GlaxoSmithKline, called Commit. Smokers suck on a lozenge when they feel a craving, with the intent of gradually reducing use over a three-month period. A British study found lozenges more effective than either gum or patches, with a 25 percent smoke-free status six months after quitting (Alberta Tobacco Reduction Strategy, 2003).

The latest nicotine replacement alternative is e-cigarettes. Electronic cigarettes have the look and feel of cigarettes but do not burn tobacco. Instead, e-cigarettes use a battery and an electronic device to produce a warm vapour from a cartridge containing nicotine, often propylene glycol, and some flavouring additive. Cartridges can be refilled with different flavours and nicotine concentrations. E-cigarettes still contain some carcinogens (including nitrosamines), toxic chemicals (such as diethylene glycol), and tobacco-specific components that are harmful to humans, but they do deliver less nicotine per puff than tobacco cigarettes. E-cigarettes deliver nicotine to the blood more rapidly than nicotine inhalers, but less rapidly than cigarettes. As a result, the effect of the e-cigarette on nicotine craving is similar to that of the nicotine inhaler, but less than that of cigarettes. Short-term use of e-cigarettes produces issues with lung capacity and air flow, though not more than tobacco smoke. E-cigarettes contain fewer toxicants than cigarette smoke. However, studies evaluating whether e-cigarettes are less harmful than cigarettes are inconclusive. Some evidence suggests that e-cigarette use may facilitate smoking cessation, but definitive data are lacking. Since most e-cigarettes are manufactured in China and quality control still varies greatly, the products may contain pesticide-grade nicotine rather than pharmacological-grade nicotine. The long-term effects of second-hand vapour from e-cigarettes is unknown. As concerns have not yet been empirically substantiated, most jurisdictions are moving toward the same restrictions on their use as apply to tobacco cigarettes. Much research is needed on e-cigarettes, and their efficacy in nicotine replacement therapy is undetermined (Callahan-Lyon, 2014; Etter, 2010).

Benzodiazepines

Benzodiazepines with long half-lives are used to assist persons to withdraw from dependencies on benzodiazepines with short half-lives. A typical five-step intervention model incorporating benzodiazepine drug substitution with ongoing counselling would consist of the following:

1. For two weeks, clients monitor and record their daily drug consumption.
2. Eight one-on-one therapy sessions follow at a rate of one per week.
3. Gradual reduction of drug use begins by switching to drugs with longer half-lives.
4. Ongoing supportive care and reassurance continues until cessation of any drug use.
5. A one-year follow-up period commences, using a support group model.

Stimulants

No medications have yet been proven effective for cocaine and methamphetamine addiction. Ritalin is currently being used in an attempt to improve brain function among those addicted to cocaine (Konova, Moeller, Tomasi, Volkow, & Goldstein, 2013), while both D-amphetamine and methylphenidate are being used to treat heavy amphetamine users, with some limited success (Elkashef et al., 2008). When given disulfiram for the treatment of their alcoholism, individuals who abuse both cocaine and alcohol also reduced their cocaine use from 2.5 days per week to less than once per week (Whitten, 2005).

Underlying Disorder Treatment

Co-morbidity is the occurrence of two or more illnesses in the same person. Alcoholism and other forms of drug abuse are frequently found in association with a variety of mental health issues. Meyer (1989) reported that up to one-half of those receiving treatment for alcohol dependency had been diagnosed as having suffered from a major clinical depression or a major anxiety disorder in their lifetime. For these persons, drug use may be a form of self-medication. Alcohol or drug abuse may be secondary to the actual problem of anxiety, depression, neurosis, or psychosis. This belief system led to the unsuccessful trials of LSD with alcohol-dependent persons in the 1960s. The rationale for LSD use was that dependent individuals would have a psychedelic experience or would undergo an altered state of consciousness that would render them more amenable to personality change. Early uncontrolled studies enthusiastically reported positive results, with abstinence rates ranging as high as 94 percent (Smart et al., 1967). However, long-term studies repeatedly found no advantage in using LSD as a treatment method, and by the early 1970s, the use of LSD in alcoholism treatment had all but disappeared. Similarly, controlled research has provided no persuasive support for using benzodiazepines or other anti-anxiety agents to treat underlying disorders that possibly precipitate substance abuse. However, where psychopathology persists, particularly after initial sobriety has been achieved, a carefully chosen medication may be appropriate for treating these concurrent problems (Anton, 1994). While there had been some hope that certain antidepressants and lithium carbonate could reduce the desire for and consumption of alcohol, more recent studies have shown the limited effectiveness of antidepressants as a primary treatment for alcohol dependency (Miller, Book, & Stewart, 2011).

In the 1990s, with increasing knowledge of neurotransmitters, antidepressants began to be prescribed as smoking cessation aids. Among those was Zyban, the trade name for bupropion hydrochloride. Zyban was introduced in Canada in 1998 to aid tobacco users in dealing with their craving for nicotine once they stopped smoking. The drug was believed to work by stimulating the production of dopamine and noradrenaline, neurotransmitters associated with creating feelings of well-being. The drug's predominant side effects, dry mouth and insomnia, were deemed minor in comparison with the damage caused by nicotine and tobacco. Champix is another anti-depressant whose side effects aid tobacco smokers in quitting. Its introduction led to an increase in the number of persons attempting to quit smoking, as it had minimal side effects and positive results. However, as its primary use is for those with mental health issues, it has been associated with a number of deaths, primarily by suicide (Stapleton, 2009), and has been the subject of a Canadian class-action lawsuit due to its alleged psychiatric side effects. These outcomes yet again demonstrate that, despite extensive laboratory testing, there is no such thing as a totally safe psychoactive agent.

4.2 INDIVIDUAL COUNSELLING
Psychotherapy Overview
Brief Solution-Focused Therapies
Feminist Approach
Narrative Therapy
Confrontation

Individual counselling covers as much territory as almost all other forms of intervention combined. It ranges from neo-Freudian and Adlerian psychotherapeutic techniques to the breakthrough thinking of feminist therapy and the newer areas of narrative, brief, and solution-focused therapies. This brief overview cannot cover all of these topics adequately, especially as many were not developed to deal directly with addiction issues; rather, they have been adapted for use with this clinical population. Nevertheless, a brief synopsis of some key approaches is provided. Regardless of the specific technique utilized by a clinician, therapeutic individual counselling should always be purposeful and goal-centred, should occur only by mutual consent, and should have a specific beginning, middle, and end phase.

Psychotherapy Overview
Psychotherapy is a broad title that incorporates a host of talk therapies as opposed to physical or chemical treatments. At its root, which dates back to

Sigmund Freud's abandonment of hypnosis, is the belief that substance abuse is a function of some underlying psychopathology. Popular psychotherapy deals primarily with the aloneness of modern life, the absence of purpose or meaning in our lives, the difficulty of knowing who you are, how you should behave, and what your obligations are (Specht & Courtney, 1994). Treatment focuses on identifying underlying unconscious or intrapsychic problems, redirecting patients' defences, ego strengthening, self-criticism, and helping to establish stable relationships within the client's environment. Psychotherapy entails, by definition, an attempt to facilitate a major personality change through personal insights, relying on historic events, major life developmental stages, and traumas as a guide. At its core are the fundamentals of human personality and one's family position and role. Early psychotherapy saw oral dependency as being at the root of addiction. An addictive personality and the need to actively and aggressively confront addiction are ideas that contemporary counselling has countered with alternative approaches. Psychotherapy has evolved and now views addiction as a stress response. Drugs are used to maintain and protect an existing sense of self, and suffering is further perpetuated by their continued and escalating use (Weegman, 2002). The role and significance of trauma as an antecedent event has also taken on prominence (Kalsched, 2014).

Psychotherapists are expected to have certain personal qualities, such as warmth, expressiveness, genuineness, empathy, unconditional positive regard, and relative absence of emotional problems, but above all they must have professional training that will allow a consistently applied approach (Kolden, Klein, Wang, & Austin, 2011). They also need to be able to effectively develop alliances with their clients to support the change process (Friedlander, Escudero, Heatherington, & Diamond, 2011). The counsellors' training should be extensive, as they are the experts and the "knowers" in most modalities, though this has begun to change with postmodernist approaches, such as feminist and narrative therapies. Several studies report that psychodynamic factors create internal conflicts within an individual's psychic structure, which predisposes him or her to the development, maintenance, and relapse of drug use (Khantzian, 2003). Studies also assert that psychotherapeutic techniques addressing these internal conflicts can be successful in the cessation of substance use (Woody, 2003), but that positive regard toward the client is essential throughout the process (Farber & Doolin, 2011). Examples of traditional psychotherapy systems are presented in Table 4.1.

A contemporary focus in the addiction field is that of the strength-based approach. Originating in the United States in the 1980s, the strength-based approach was a radical departure from traditional addiction counselling. Its emphasis is on a client's abilities, competencies, and available social resources, rather than the pathology, deficits, and problems emphasized by the dominant view. The six principles of the model are as follows:

- clients with addiction issues can recover, reclaim, and transform their lives
- the focus is on individual strengths, not deficits
- the community is viewed as an oasis of resources
- the client is the director of the helping process
- the worker-client relationship is primary and essential
- the primary setting for work is the community, not a residential facility

The strength-based approach is more than a philosophy or perspective, although it is both of these things. In its essence it is a set of values and principles, a theory of practice, and the explicit practice methods and tools that, once employed, help clients achieve the goals they set for themselves (Rapp & Goscha, 2006).

TABLE 4.1: TRADITIONAL MODELS OF PSYCHOTHERAPY

System	Therapeutic Goals	Methodology
Psychoanalytic therapy (Freud & Jung)	To reconstruct the personality; to promote insight; to make the unconscious conscious; to resolve internal conflicts; to understand the effect of early experience on adult functioning	Free association; dream analysis; interpretation; reconstruction of early experience and analysis of its present influence; study of client's feelings toward therapist as revealer of current interpersonal difficulties
Client-centred therapy (Rogers)	To experience and accept aspects of self formerly denied or distorted; to encourage personal growth; to trust the self and remain open to experience; to maximize self-awareness and self-actualization	Creation of a safe climate in which client can explore self-functioning; communicate qualities of the therapist (warmth, respect, genuine regard for client) to the client to promote realistic self-appraisal and personal growth; communicate empathic understanding to client to promote self-awareness
Existential therapy (May, Frankl)	To accept responsibility for one's own life and choices; to discover meaning in life; to gain freedom by removing block to self-awareness and fulfilling potential; to clarify values	Elicit client's being-in-the-world; establish a genuine encounter between therapist and client; examine choices client has made; lead client to make independent choices and adopt own unique values

Transactional analysis (Berne)	To re-examine decisions and to make new decisions based on accurate perceptions; to recognize the influence on behaviour and attitudes of parts of the personality; to improve interpersonal relationships	Analyze social transactions between individuals, especially games people play; psychodrama and role playing; explore consequences of commitment to adopting a rigid life pattern (script)
Reality therapy (Glasser)	To learn to appraise the self and the world realistically; to develop the capacity to make and carry out plans for reaching realistic goals	Therapist requires client to face reality and to make value judgments about his own behaviour; determine specific desirable behaviour changes; commit client to follow through on behaviour changes; promote sense of personal responsibility

Source: Lewis, Dana, & Belevins (1988)

Brief Solution-Focused Therapies

Sigmund Freud practiced short-term therapy with a few of his clients as early as 1908. In the 1940s serious challenges began to be made to the psychotherapy community's stance that longer treatment was better treatment. To this was added the work of Virginia Satir and Milton Erickson who continued to evolve individual counselling to a briefer, more problem-solving, solution-focused, strength-enhancing orientation. Erickson stated that one must keenly watch what a client presents during the interview, and urged counsellors to use the information provided by their clients to help them realize their potential for change. At the end of the 20th century, several prominent practitioners came to the forefront in systems theory and social constructionism, including Scott Miller, Insoo Kim Berg, and Steve de Shazer (O'Hanlon & Weiner-Davis, 1989; Berg & Miller, 1992; Miller & Berg, 1995).

In this form of individual counselling, various strategies are used to ameliorate the drug use and disrupt the trajectory of more serious issues. Brief interventions are useful primarily as early interventions for individuals without substantive physical or psychological dependency (O'Hare, 2005; Nilsen, 2010). Sessions are directed by the counsellor, focusing on the drinking or drug problem and how it is maintained. It is postulated that the problem behaviour is perpetuated or maintained by ineffective or inappropriate solutions. There is no denial. Rather, the tactics clients know and use regularly worsen or escalate the situation relating to their drug use. Clients engage in behaviours that they believe will solve the problem but, in fact, do not. In the brief, problem-focused therapies, clients are helped or instructed to alter or reverse the way in which they have attempted to resolve problems thus far in their lives. The counsellors' language is positive and strength-based, and the client-centred approach provides clients with choice at all stages of the process (de Shazer & Dolan, 2007).

Parsimony is important in this approach. Counsellors are encouraged to take the most direct route to a solution, keeping focused on the present and the future, using the simplest and least invasive treatment option. The major distinction between this approach and competing therapeutic models is the belief that no matter how problematic the client's situation, small changes in behaviour can make profound differences with a clear focus on solutions and not problems. Emphasis is on mental health rather than on mental illness, on client strengths and not weaknesses, while always maintaining a present and future orientation. There is a collaborative relationship between the worker and the client. However, change remains the responsibility of the client. Goals are typically practical and concrete, and they are based on the client's description of the behaviours, thoughts, feelings, interactions, and relationships that will be present when the problem is resolved (de Shazer & Dolan, 2007).

There are several schools of brief therapy that share similar beliefs and processes. Obviously, client and counsellor meet for a limited time. While the counsellor initially tends to direct sessions, this approach works with client-determined views of the presenting situation and uses the client's strengths to build a solution. Regardless of how entrenched a situation may appear, the counsellor needs to look for ways in which the client is already building solutions, one of which is seeking formal help with the problem. The counsellor's role is to find ways to best engage the client to facilitate the change process (Lethem, 2002). Six common components of many brief interventions are known by the acronym FRAMES: Feedback of personal risk due to alcohol/drug use/drug use, emphasis on personal Responsibility of the patient, Advice to change drinking behaviour, a Menu of options to reduce drinking/drug use, Empathic counselling, and Self-efficacy for the client (Bien, Miller, & Tonigan, 1993).

Miller and Berg (1995) have developed a rudimentary five-step method employing solution-focused principles to work with problem drinkers:

1. Develop a co-operative client-therapist relationship in which the client is actively engaged in developing the solution.
2. Set small, concrete, specific, behavioural, client salient treatment goals that have a beginning rather than an end, and that are realistic and achievable.
3. Interview toward finding a solution using very specific questions, including the "Miracle Question":

> While you are sleeping a miracle happens and the problem that brought you here is solved—just like that. Since you were sleeping you didn't know that this miracle has happened. What do you suppose will be the first small thing that will indicate to you tomorrow

morning that there has been a miracle overnight and the problem that brought you here is solved?

With scaling questions, the client ranks the seriousness of the problem on a scale of one (worst) to ten (best). The counsellor then works at moving the client from one to two, two to three and upward, using the client's ideas on what steps could be taken to improve the situation.

4. All solution-focused interventions, including interviews and homework assignments, are designed to elicit, trigger, and repeat new successful strategies for problem resolution.
5. In maintaining goals do not focus on high-risk situations; rather, focus on high-success situations.

De Shazer and Dolan (2007) offer counsellors a three-step framework:

1. If it ain't broke, don't fix it. In other words, if the client does not present it as a problem do not spend time addressing the issue.
2. Once you know what works, do more of it.
3. If something is tried and it doesn't work, stop doing it and try something else.

Counsellors using this approach encourage clients to continue to engage in actions that were functional during their misuse of a substance, increase the number of new actions that are functional, and not engage in any action that leads to a regression or lapse.

Figure 4.1 illustrates a brief solution-focused approach. In this model, the counsellor begins by asking the client: "Why today? What specific event or incident was the direct cause of your coming for counselling at this point in time?" The situation is then discussed and one of three avenues is chosen. The first is to ask what the client would like to change about their situation (wishes and complaints). In addiction counselling, this typically focuses on the drug use, though it does not need to initially. This establishes some concrete goals for the client to work toward. The second option is to explore what the client does when the problem is not happening (exceptions frame). The counsellor then further explores the behaviours the client engages in when this occurs or what activities led away from the drug-using behaviours. This then gives the client some specific targets to work towards or to do more of and also gives the client actual examples of things he or she did rather than drink and/or do drugs to illustrate that the client can control the substance. The third option is the hypothetical frame. In this instance the counsellor has the client imagine what activities he or she would be engaged in when they were no longer using drugs. A plan is then developed to start working in small ways toward this goal.

FIGURE 4.1: PATHWAYS FOR CONSTRUCTING SOLUTIONS

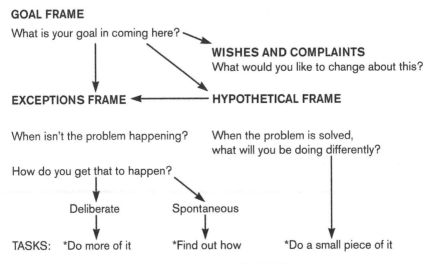

Source: Walter & Peller (1992)

Feminist Approach

What the feminist agenda brings to the addiction field is a new way to conceptualize the problem. It integrates the bio-psycho-social approach to addiction with the person-in-environment context, along with empowerment principles and practice (van den Berg, 1995). A feminist perspective on addiction necessitates a greater appreciation of the roles of social and cultural factors in the development of substance abuse (Bepko, 1991). The feminist approach refocuses how we define problems and how we identify what is important to examine. It takes the perspective of examining problems of those who have not dominated the culture or societal decision making. It challenges not only the questions that have been traditionally asked, but also those that have not been asked. The goal is to provide women's explanations of social phenomena, for the context of discovery is as important as the context of justification (Harding, 1987). The feminist perspective has a unique standpoint because of women's gender and their being part of a dominated class. At a basic level feminism is a recognition and critique of patriarchy and sexual politics, including historically within psychotherapeutic approaches. As opposed to pathologizing problems as individual deficiencies, the feminist approach broadens the scope, placing the onus upon the inherent structures of society. Applying a feminist perspective forces us to examine the larger societal constructs that divide our society rather than focusing on individual weaknesses. It is a model that questions existing societal hierarchies and their role in creating addiction. Feminism challenges the concept that biology alone creates destiny (Abbott, 1994).

There are three primary feminist values:

1. *The personal is political*: Each woman's personal experience and situation is a reflection of the position of women generally in our society.
2. *Choice*: Women have historically had limited choices as a result of their economic and social oppression and the internalized beliefs which stem from that oppression. Feminist therapy's goal is to help women become aware of their options and self-actualize by developing greater psychological and economic autonomy.
3. *Equalization of power*: There needs to be a greater equalization of power among persons, and the counsellor needs to take care not to add to a woman's oppression through his or her actions.

There are four major approaches that are specific to feminist therapy:

1. *Consciousness raising*: A small group process examines how oppression and socialization have contributed to the distress and dysfunction experienced by women.
2. *Social and gender-role analysis*: Implicit and explicit sex roles contribute to the development of the addiction. Labels such as co-dependency are re-examined and placed within a context where the question of why traditionally socialized female characteristics have been pathologized is examined.
3. *Resocialization*: The woman's belief system is reorganized based on new insights into the role of gender in creating excessive drug use. Women are taught to differentiate between what they have been taught and have accepted as socially appropriate, and what may be more appropriate for them. This approach combines both an inward and outward examination.
4. *Social activism*: Incorporating the notion of "the personal is political" into the recovery process, this approach addresses structural inequalities in society that apply both to psychoactive drugs and to larger societal issues that oppress women and make them vulnerable to addiction (Dutton-Douglas & Walker, 1988; Jones-Smith, 2012).

Women have not been well served by all forms of counselling. Traditional approaches often negatively perceived women's functioning and contributions (Russell, 1984). Counselling in a feminist framework has several goals:

- symptom removal
- increased self-esteem
- improved interpersonal relations
- competence in role performance
- resolution of target problems through problem solving
- increased comfort with body image and sensuality
- encouragement of political awareness and social action, emphasizing independence, autonomy, and personal effectiveness

Powerlessness and despair are central to understanding women's addiction as a position of oppression within society. As women experience greater stigma with drug use they tend to drink and do drugs alone more often than men. Many women substance abusers have a history of physical and sexual abuse, and this trauma is highly correlated to substance abuse (Collins, 2002; Hiebert-Murphy & Woytkiw, 2010). Female substance abusers also tend to have a family history of abuse and feelings of rejection stemming from childhood, depression, and a low degree of trust and self-esteem, along with high levels of anxiety. These characteristics are also often correlated with a history of trauma (Wilsnack & Beckman, 1984).

Another feminist perspective views substance abuse among women as a result of the suppressed anger and self-hate that occur among many women in our societal context. Substance abuse numbs this anger, and thus cessation is only the initial step in the treatment process, not the end goal. The next step is to help women identify, respect, and appropriately direct their anger. An important consideration is the use of alternative resources. As Alcoholics Anonymous is a white, middle-class, Protestant, male-created form of helping, it is important to help women in recovery find a women's support group that recognizes their unique problems in recovery (Dutton-Douglas & Walker, 1988; Ettore, 1992). However, with its base in oppression, and with a focus on the role of larger societal factors, the principles of feminist intervention may be transferred to any population that is marginalized and has turned to drug use to cope with their situation.

Narrative Therapy

Narrative therapy, developed by Australian postmodernists Michael White and David Epston (1990), was heavily influenced by the work of Michel Foucault (1965). It is very distinct from other forms of individual counselling pertaining to addiction issues. Postmodernists believe that there is no one reality but rather multiple interpretations of it, all of which have some legitimacy. What we take as truths are in fact social constructions. The underlying premise of narrative therapy moves counsellors away from pathologizing drug use. It is philosophically opposed to treatment ideas based on the disease model.

The goal of this form of individual counselling is to externalize the drug use. A client is discouraged from seeing him or himself as the problem and as an addict, an object with no other attributes. In narrative therapy, the client's story is the base unit of experience. Labels are considered part of the larger mental health discourse that maintains rather than resolves the problems of daily living (Carr, 1998). The use of the label "alcoholic" or "addict" increases the importance of the substance so that it becomes the central focus of a person's life story. No other aspects are considered, especially their existing strengths in other areas. This focus draws attention away from the times when the person is not using and minimizes his or her attempts to not use or delay use. In the process of narrative therapy, individuals begin to see themselves as other than simply an addict and as more than a problem. Their problem then ceases to represent the truth of who they are, which allows them to focus on other options and resolutions to their excessive use of drugs (White, 1995). Individuals examine what is occurring when they are not using and thus view themselves in another light. The process of "re-authoring the story" highlights the discrepancy between one's life story and one's actual lived experience in the development of an alternative, preferred story.

The role of the counsellor in narrative therapy is a collaborative one. The counsellor works with the client to discover alternative storylines. They work as a team to find exceptions to the problem, thicken the story's plot, and link the presenting problem to the past as well as to the future. Examples of internalized and externalized problems are presented in Table 4.2. The newly constructed life narrative then becomes more powerful than the problem, and the client becomes the author of a new identity. The counsellor addresses three areas during narrative therapy:

1. the meaning people make of their lives
2. the language used in creating meaning
3. the power relationships in which the client is involved

Also critical to this process is teaching the client to be mindful. The client must develop enhanced self-awareness, particularly of the thoughts and behaviours that lead to drug use as well as those that do not. Positive self-talk is stressed in this form of individual counselling, as is self-worth (Carr, 1998; White, 1995).

TABLE 4.2: COMPARING INTERNALIZED WITH EXTERNALIZED CLIENT ISSUES

Problem Internalized within Client	Problem Externalized from Client
The person is the problem.	The problem is the problem.
The problem is something wrong with the client.	The problem is external to the client's self-identity.
Experts are needed to explain the client's behaviour.	Clients can provide their own interpretation of self.
The counsellor is the expert.	Clients are the experts on their own lives.
Oppression is not a theme.	Counselling examines culture, race, gender, sex, class, ability, and sexual orientation.
The focus of counselling is the client's problem.	Counselling focuses on distinguishing the client from the problem.
Counsellor reorders the client's personality.	Clients re-author their own stories.

Source: Jones-Smith (2012)

Confrontation

There has been universal acclaim for confrontation and intervention and their role in addiction counselling, to the point where both fictional and reality-based television shows depict the process. Research studies, however, have not been as positive or as provocative. Therapeutic confrontation is the process by which a therapist provides direct, reality-oriented feedback to a client regarding the client's own thoughts, feelings, or behaviour. It was not only widely accepted but was often a formal component of many treatment programs, particularly residential, until the 1990s. The format can vary in its intent, timing, intensity, and emotional content. However, the common belief is that drug abusers as a group tend to deny or fail to recognize the reality of their problems, and that it is therapeutic to confront them with reality through the use of a dramatic intervention. The treatment literature includes dozens of descriptions of how to carry out a successful confrontation, and some of the employee assistance literature still refers to the idea of constructive confrontation for intervening in the workplace. In this approach, the person being confronted must accept the label of alcoholic or addict, that the disease of alcoholism is reducing their ability to control their life, and that their lack of insight into their situation is a result of denial (White & Miller, 2007).

Confrontation is also called the Johnson model of intervention by many after Vernon Johnson (1973) who believed that while alcoholics could have insight into their situation, this did not occur without formal active assistance. He believed that it was only through the creation of a crisis state that people would be adequately motivated to change and that by precipitating a crisis by a forceful confrontation this process could be enhanced.

Therapeutic confrontation was essentially founded on four interrelated assumptions. First, the core belief is that addiction is rooted in an immature, defective character encased within an armour-plated defence structure. Second, the passive methods of traditional psychotherapies are hopelessly ineffective in penetrating this defensive structure and altering this deformity of character. Third, the addict or alcoholic can only be reached by a "dynamite charge" that breaks through this protective shield. Finally, verbal confrontation is the most effective means of engaging and changing addictive behaviour (Bassin, 1975).

The usual procedure in confrontation includes a forceful and factual presentation of evidence that the individual has a drug dependency and the refuting of the client's protestations to the contrary. Yet confrontation need not be equated with strategies of coercion and extrinsic control. Alternatives include soft confrontation, which resembles a gentle persuasion and a feedback model in which the client is given information about his or her current health status. Minimal feedback procedures can have a substantial impact on behaviour and health if the emphasis remains on an honest and caring presentation. Yet confrontational approaches must be undertaken with care because of their potential to precipitate drop out from the process, negative emotional states, lowered self-esteem, and potentially relapse. The outcome literature indicates that there is little efficacy in this approach, with more long-term harm than benefit arising (White & Miller, 2007).

4.3 INTERVENTION

Intervention is based on similar principles as confrontation but is implemented to motivate an individual to seek treatment. It is intended to be a caring yet forceful process by which a concerned group presents reality to a family member or friend whose behaviour indicates a serious problem with an addiction. Historically, the belief was that individuals had to reach rock bottom before accepting that drugs had created a problem in their lives and that they needed treatment to become abstinent. Problematic drug use would thus continue unless significant negative consequences arose. However, because the effects of drugs, some people are unaware of the impact of their behaviour on themselves or others and genuinely believe that their drug use is under control. These individuals are candidates for an intervention, which, at its core, is a coercive practice.

Intervention in its simplest form is a direct conversation regarding another's inappropriate or excessive drug use. More typically, it is a formal, structured group of individuals who deliver rehearsed scripts in an orchestrated fashion. Practice is required so that those participating can control their emotions, as anger is a common response in an intervention. However, anger from those engaged in the process only creates additional defensiveness, and a defensive person has even greater difficulty in hearing what is being said about them during this trying activity (Lawson, 2005).

The intervention, which is best led by a trained professional, takes only 10–20 minutes. The counsellor, as the neutral party, chairs the process and begins by stating the reason for everyone being present. He or she ensures that everyone has the opportunity to speak before allowing the person who is the focus of the intervention the opportunity to respond. In a proper intervention, each person will prepare a written statement, beginning on a note of positive regard, followed by a factual, non-judgmental report of two or three incidents involving drug misuse, their consequences, and how they affected the speaker directly. After everyone has spoken, the counsellor will recommend that the person who is the focus of the intervention attend a residential treatment program. Typically a space has already been arranged. The counsellor will also clearly address the substantive consequence of non-compliance, which entails severing relations with those present until the person seeks treatment. It is important that the mood of the intervention be even, calm, and concerned, but with limited emotion. The normal response to an intervention by those who are its focus is anger, though some may try to bargain with the group or suggest that they can stop using drugs without formal help. It is important that those involved in the intervention be firm on what is and is not negotiable before beginning the process. Intervention is emotionally challenging and difficult, with significant treatment consequences. It should only be considered when all other methods of returning a person to health have been unsuccessful (Lawson, 2005).

4.4 GROUP COUNSELLING

Group work with clients has been a preferred intervention model in the alcohol dependency field since the inception of formalized treatment programs in the 1940s. This is partially due to the influence of Alcoholics Anonymous but also to the common experience of oppression of those with an addiction issue, despite the heterogeneity of this vast population (Csiernik & Rowe, 2010; Loughran, 2009). Group counselling is based on the recognition that, with proper guidance, substance abusers can help each other. Group counselling is also based on the universal human tendency to validate subjective experiences by comparing them with the experiences of others who are perceived as similar or share some common characteristic. In all forms of group counselling, clients and a clinician meet regularly to conduct specific structured activities within the framework of a mutually acknowledged group structure and code. Interactions with the leader and between members is the foundation for change. This interactive process allows for insight into behaviour and correction of maladaptive behaviours such as communication problems, leading to improved social and personal functioning. Groups for substance abusers are particularly helpful in assisting members to recognize, anticipate, and cope with drinking or drug-using triggers. They also help members move through the stages of change and work through the action phase of the Transtheoretical Model of Change (see section 4.8). The here-and-now orientation of groups is also an extremely valuable characteristic of this approach, as is a group's capacity to provide examples of drug avoidance and alternative coping methods. Groups are also safe havens for self-disclosure and provide opportunities for experimentation with new behaviours. The group process reduces social isolation and can provide wonderful opportunities for the development of insight into past and current behaviours (Flores, 1983; Hepworth & Larsen, 2012). All groups provide a level of mutual aid where individuals both receive and give help, and this mutuality is essential to the change process. While each group is a unique entity, its membership is representative of the range of issues persons with addictions face outside the group, and of the broader issues they experienced during the development of their drug use and will continue to encounter during their recovery. Finally, each group is a unique gestalt, which simply means that the group is greater than the sum of its individual members. What each person brings to the group makes it unique in its potential and outcome.

Many treatment programs utilize some form of small group experience with clients as a focus for change, especially given the flexibility of group formats and approaches. No single technique, type of group, or theoretical orientation succeeds for all group participants, and one cannot find a technique, type of group, or orientation that will not work with at least one person. However, no client should be expected to automatically be able to relate closely to whatever group he or she is asked to join. Consequently, a client's wish to switch groups may indicate resistance to treatment, but it may also signify a quite healthy judgment of feelings and needs. It is therefore incumbent on the group worker to foster a sense of psychosocial belonging between members in the beginning stages of group development (Loughran, 2009).

The composition of the group is a powerful determinant of what happens and what gains the participants ultimately achieve. Consequently, the process of selection is critical and, if carried out ineffectively, can lead to poor group dynamics, interactions, and outcomes. On the other hand, effective and sensitive selection can be the principle determinant of successful outcomes. The following are key in creating a small group whose purpose is to change behaviour:

- A high degree of group interaction is required, and exercises should keep group members interested in attending and facilitate development of the group.
- Group members need to be supported and protected to develop sufficient courage to speak about upsetting, problematic, and even traumatic aspects of their lives.
- Sufficient compatibility among group members is needed to increase personal attraction: "Can we actually like each other?"
- Adequate diversity and similarities among group members is necessary to provide examples to each other, so that the strengths and resources of each can be utilized. For example, some group members may be capable of expressing anger more easily than others, or be able to manage financial matters more adequately. The question is what each person can teach others in the room.
- The group facilitator needs to prepare clients to participate and provide them with clear and adequate information about the group treatment process. He or she must provide a safe environment, outline the group rules, and demonstrate the norms for appropriate participation. Special attention should be given to pre-counselling training and providing specific instructional materials about the nature, purpose, method, and goals of group exercises.

An important decision to make prior to beginning an addiction-specific treatment group is whether it should be open or closed. Open groups allow new participants to enter at any time during the group's life, while closed groups do not allow for the addition of new members. An open group format provides the opportunity for new members to bring new perspectives to the group and offers immediate support for those in need. However, open groups are more prone to instability, are more disruptive, and their members often do not develop the same level of trust that occurs within closed groups. Regardless of which option is selected, potential members should be informed prior to joining if the group is to be open or closed (Hepworth & Larsen, 2012).

Group counselling is a social experience with a focus on both the group and each individual member. As such, an optimum size is from six to eight members. Counselling groups are intended to allow a safe opportunity for clients to identify, express, and talk about their emotions. The group is a place where one is allowed and encouraged to search for and articulate feelings. The non-judgmental intent of groups also provides an ideal locale for practising newly acquired skills and behaviours. The here-and-now emphasis, the opportunity to gain insights from others' behaviours, and the opportunity for personal insights all speak to the value of including some type of group process in addiction treatment. However, while group and individual counselling and psychotherapy have become exceedingly popular elements in the standard treatment of drug users, there is now empirical evidence to demonstrate the long-term value of group versus individual interventions (Csiernik & Arundel, 2013; Csiernik & Troller, 2002). Current economic realities are also forcing more programs to use group interventions and the question must be asked as to whether this is in the client's or the facility's best interest.

Counselling groups can serve one of several purposes. They can assist with socialization, or, in the case of substance misusers, re-socialization, so that the behaviours associated with drug use are minimized if not eliminated. Group counselling can also focus on self-concept formation, where members grapple with being drug users or being outside societal norms or not feeling like citizens. Group work can also aim to directly change behaviours through role play that examines antecedent events leading to drug use, or learning avoidance or refusal skills. Group work may also function as a support to offer emotional and instrumental aid in becoming a non-user.

Educational groups tend to be larger than counselling groups as there is less one-to-one and counsellor-to-individual group member interaction. This type of group usually entails a series of lectures, films, readings, or discussions on a specific substance abuse–related topic. Members still share their experiences with the group and the group's facilitator, though there is a greater emphasis on how-to strategies. Specific how-to strategies include the following:

- how to problem solve
- how to self-monitor
- how to handle relapse
- how to decrease consumption
- how to abstain

Yalom (2005) discussed 12 curative factors in detail that are associated with group work:

1. provision of information
2. instillation of hope
3. universality—understanding that you alone are not affected by addiction
4. altruism—offering help to others
5. corrective emotional response to the primary group, one's family
6. development of socializing techniques
7. role modelling of alternative behaviours by other group members
8. interpersonal learning
9. group cohesion and the development of positive interpersonal bonds
10. catharsis
11. insight into existential factors of life, existence, and death
12. acceptance, safety, and support

Group workers should also be aware of the distinct stages of group evolution, from initiation to termination. Two fundamental models, the traditional Tuckman (Tuckman & Jensen, 1977) and the alternative, feminist-premised Schiller (1997), outline this development. Tuckman observed that there tend to be five distinct though overlapping stages in the life cycle of a group. The opening stage, "forming," is predicated on an approach-avoidance conflict. Members new to each other and to the group leader assess the group and decide whether to commit their time but also their affect to be part of the process. This is followed by the "storming" phase, where group position and status is determined. Group members are most likely to react negatively to the group leader rather than against each other in this phase, especially if the leader has no recovery history or is still using a substance in an integrated manner. If this conflict can be satisfactorily resolved, the group will enter the "norming" stage. Group members will move toward intimacy, where mutual trust and cohesion begin to develop and superficial support is replaced with earnest social and emotional interaction. The fourth stage is "performing," in which the group becomes less dependent on the group worker and relationships become more realistic. Members take more risks, and social support between members becomes more evident and more genuine. The termination stage in Tuckman's model is called "mourning." The function of the group leader in this stage is to lessen the members' need for the group while ensuring that they take what they have learned from the group, both about their drug use and about themselves, beyond the confines of the group.

Linda Schiller offers a different perspective from the Tuckman model. For her, the group dynamics among women differ from men, the only clients observed in Tuckman's and most other group development models. While Schiller's model also has five stages (see Table 4.3), the process varies in two key areas. After dealing with the discomfort of being in a new environment with unknown individuals, a stage she labels as "pre-affiliation," Schiller states that woman are not driven to establish social power and dominance. On the contrary, what women want is to form a "relational base" to work from, and to find common ground where trust and cohesion can develop. Once this is established, they can move to a state of greater openness, that of "mutuality and interpersonal empathy," when connections and similarities between group members become the overriding focus of the social exchange. At this point, women tend to become more comfortable in confronting each other to deal with the underlying issues that led them to a counselling group for addiction. Schiller calls this the stage of "challenge and change." Once a positive relationship is developed, it is easier, according to Schiller, for women to challenge each other regarding behaviours that led them to be part of the group.

TABLE 4.3: THE TUCKMAN AND SCHILLER MODELS OF GROUP DEVELOPMENT

Tuckman	Schiller	Major Characteristics
Forming	Pre-affiliation	Approach-avoidance
Storming	Establishing a relationship base	Interpersonal relationship focus
Norming	Mutuality and interpersonal empathy	Working stage
Performing	Challenge and change	Moving forward
Mourning	Termination	Consolidating changes

Group work has distinct advantages over individual counselling. It more closely resembles everyday life than does one-to-one work. And being part of a group reduces the social isolation many persons with addiction issues face, especially if their peer group continues to use. Group counselling offers greater feelings of support and caring for others through the dynamic of mutual aid, and as increases self-esteem through the giving and receiving of positive feedback. It also offers a safe environment in which to learn from others and the opportunity to imitate successes through social learning.

4.5 FAMILY COUNSELLING

Substance abuse treatment has traditionally focused on isolating the drug user from the family. By the time most substance abusers seek some form of treatment, their drug use has affected not only themselves but also their entire social and family structure, producing profound social, economic, legal, and health changes. Addiction affects the emotional and physical intimacy of family members, isolates the family and its individual members, and increases the risk of mental health issues, such as depression (Lander, Howsare,

& Byrne, 2013). Globally, it is estimated that more than 100 million adults are affected by their relatives' addiction problems. Affected family members experience multiple stresses, coping dilemmas, and a lack of information and support, making them vulnerable to their own health and social issues, both related and unrelated to the drug use (Orford, Velleman, Natera, Templeton, & Copello, 2013; Rojas, 2015). As well, when the substance abuse ceases, everyone within the family unit becomes vulnerable and disequilibrium may ensue. To remove this uneasiness, the family may attempt to return to the previous status quo, which can entail sabotaging treatment and the ongoing recovery process. Recognizing that problems both influence and are influenced by the family, clinicians and treatment programs have slowly begun to include the partner and other family members in the treatment process (Alaggia & Csiernik, 2010).

Family counselling, which emerged as a separate field in the 1950s, views the family as an organic whole. The treatment interview is usually conducted with the father, mother, and children, but can include other persons who have a functional participant role in the ongoing life of the family group, for example, grandparents, aunts, or uncles. In essence, the interview unit comprises all those persons who share the identity of a family and whose behaviour is influenced by the circular interchange of emotion within the group. The counsellor initiates the treatment process with the entire group, but may excuse the children and concentrate on the marital and parental pair or on a parent-child pair (Steinglass, 1992). There are four distinct options when working with a family:

1. *Family orientation*: This involves informing family members about the rehabilitation program on which the identified client is embarking. It is used to enlist family support in the client's treatment.
2. *Family education*: This approach is used to inform family members about family-relation issues and how they may be relevant to substance abuse and the substance abuser.
3. *Family counselling*: This is employed to bring about the resolution of problems identified by family members as related to the substance abuse.
4. *Family therapy*: This method is employed to bring about significant and permanent changes to intractable areas of systemic family dysfunction related to the substance abuse. (Boudreau, 1997)

The thrust of family work in addiction counselling evolves around several themes:

- All couples and families have problems, but psychoactive drug use prevents resolution of these problems and creates new and more complex ones.

- No individual can force another to change.
- Personal change comes through accepting responsibility for one's own behaviour.
- All members of the family are involved in the problem, and all have responsibility in finding some form of resolution.
- Removal of drugs from the family system represents a necessary beginning in the recovery process, yet is incomplete in itself.

The three prominent stages of family counselling are: (1) the attainment of sobriety and unbalancing of the system, (2) adjustment to sobriety and stabilizing the system, and (3) maintenance of sobriety and rebalancing the system (Todd, 1991).

A family system orientation provides a comprehensive and meaningful approach to addressing underlying issues related to drug use. It is an integrated approach that views drug abuse and family functioning as interrelated. One component that should not be overlooked in the process is the couple's sexuality, and sex therapy should be made available as one aspect of this type of intervention (Dowsling, 1980; Osmond & Kimberley, 2010). Family therapy, when incorporated with other treatment approaches, significantly increases the level of improvement observed at both short- and long-term follow-up intervals in interventions ranging from cognitive behavioural to pharmacological (Alaggia & Csiernik, 2010; Fals-Stewart & O'Farrell, 2003; McCrady, Epstein, Cook, Jensen, & Hildebrandt, 2009; Thomas, 1989).

While family counselling is an integral component for addiction intervention, there are certain instances when it should not be applied. If there is an alcohol-related crisis that is of greater urgency, family counselling needs to be delayed. Similarly, if there is great potential for violence in the relationship, safety concerns override the value of this type of intervention. Lastly, if family counselling leads to blaming or labelling of a partner, a re-examination of this intervention is required (Alaggia & Csiernik, 2010; Hester & Miller, 1995).

4.6 BEHAVIOURAL COUNSELLING
Operant Methods
Skills Training
Cognitive Behavioural Therapy
Dialectical Behavioural Therapy
Community Reinforcement Approach/Community
   Reinforcement Approach and Family Training
Aversion Therapy

While Freud's ideas and work were developing and promoting psychotherapy, the work of American John Watson was laying the foundation for behaviourism. Rather than looking at developmental stages and early psychological conflicts and trauma, Watson emphasized theories of learning and how the majority of behaviour originates through learning processes. Another early contributor to behaviour therapy was Edward Thorndike, whose law of effect stated that behaviour is shaped by the consequences it derives. To this was added Pavlov's ideas regarding classical conditioning, and Skinner's work on operant conditioning. Meichenbaum contributed the ideas of self-management, self-instructional learning, and stress inoculation (Jones-Smith, 2012; Wicks-Nelson & Israel, 1991).

Behavioural therapies apply to the full range of psychological events—attitudinal and emotional, as well as learned. These interventions are based on the belief that drug use is a socially learned behavioural pattern maintained by a wide variety of positive consequences and conditioned factors. Some forms of behavioural therapy bring about major changes in people's actions by modifying their emotional responses, while enduring changes in attitude can be most successfully effected through modifications in overt behaviour. Almost any learning outcome that results from direct experience can also come about on a vicarious basis through observation of other people's behaviours and their consequences. Providing an appropriate model may accelerate the learning process, and thus one prominent method of social-learning therapy is based on modelling desired behaviours.

Although differing in application, the behavioural component for treating drug problems is based on a common belief system:

- It is assumed that drug-using behaviour and behaviours affected by drugs, such as risk taking or aggression, are learned. Further, it is assumed that the learned characteristics of this behaviour can be modified.
- Drug use is usually dealt with directly, often by introducing the behaviour into the treatment strategy. Drug-use decisions are critical events; thus, the circumstances surrounding decisions to use a drug serve as a basis for determining their function.
- Emphasis is on operationally specifying treatment procedures and assessing treatment effectiveness by using empirical methods (Riley, Sobell, Leo, Sobell, & Klajner, 1985). In general, antecedent conditions (triggers) lead to behavioural responses (drug use). These lead to consequences in the form of initial positive reinforcement, which leads to continued drug use. A variety of behavioural approaches have been postulated to respond to this process.

Operant Methods

Operant conditioning techniques stress the relationship between behaviour and the environment, and attempt to alter the interaction through modification of behavioural consequences. First suggested as a treatment method in the mid-1960s (Ulmer, 1977), it is based on a community health approach that believes that mental health disorders result from forces operating in the community on the individual. This suggests that treatment occur through rearranging community influences on the client in the community, not in a hospital or other closed institution. With alcohol- and drug-dependent individuals, reinforcement and punishment contingencies are used to influence drug use and drug-related behaviours. A very large literature attests to the effectiveness of reinforcement contingencies in influencing drinking behaviour within laboratory settings (Miller & Hester, 1986a; National Institute on Drug Abuse, 1988; Pollack et al., 2002; Riley et al., 1985; Rychtarik, Foy, Scott, Lokey, & Prue, 1987). In this model, antecedent behaviours leading to drug use are punished while behaviours that substitute for drug taking are positively reinforced.

One specific type of operant conditioning is contingency management. This method involves arranging the individual's environment so that positive consequences follow desired behaviours, and either negative or neutral consequences follow undesired behaviours. These techniques require other persons, such as the partner and other family members, to enforce the contingencies, and are often used as part of a multimodal or family treatment program. The core tenets of this approach entail monitoring of target behaviour, quickly rewarding desired behaviour and withholding rewards in the absence of the desired behaviour (Petry, 2012).

A second form of operant conditioning is behavioural contracting. Behavioural contracting is similar to contingency management. Essentially, the process is one of explicitly defining a set of behaviours and their associated consequences. The contract is usually negotiated between two parties and stated in writing, as often it is only through explicit written agreements that the foundations for change can be established. Behavioural contracting ensures that all parties agree to expected behaviours, appropriate reactions, and how behaviour change will be recognized and rewarded. Behavioural contracting is very helpful in the initial stages of treatment as it can build in early recognition of behaviour changes and thereby motivate clients to make continued life changes.

Skills Training

Although most behavioural techniques involve the acquisition of skills, some focus on teaching specific adaptive behaviours that are presumed to be deficient prior to the individual's excessive drug use and may have been a major contributing factor to the alcohol or other drug problem. The main assumption underlying skills training techniques is that drug-dependent individuals have deficiencies in skills that are essential in achieving personal goals and solving interpersonal problems. If taught these skills, clients should be more successful in maintaining a drug-free lifestyle than those whose treatment focuses only on alcohol and other drug use.

Problem-Solving Skills

The problem-solving skills approach is a general behavioural treatment strategy that assures that a variety of highly specific and specialized behavioural procedures are considered by a client whenever a problem situation arises. It focuses strongly on identifying and evaluating multiple opportunities, categorized as behavioural options, for treatment intervention. The training typically incorporates a four-stage procedure:

1. problem identification
2. description of behavioural options or alternative responses
3. evaluation of each behavioural option for its possible outcome
4. employing the best behavioural option based on the best probable outcome

The behavioural technique of problem-solving skills training analyzes treatment operations on a continuing basis and directly involves the client in the treatment process. This approach involves the following:

1. Tailoring the treatment approach to the client rather than vice versa.
2. Removing the judgmental aspect of what is and is not appropriate by matching the model to the client. This is because behavioural consequences are specific to individuals and circumstances.
3. Precisely defining and evaluating behaviours and situations.
4. Avoiding the use of vague terminology or labels, such as dependency needs, alcoholic, or drug addict.
5. Increasing awareness of the powerful influence of the short-term consequences on perpetuating drinking and/or drug taking.
6. Increasing awareness that many appropriate behavioural options have long-term rewarding consequences.
7. Recognizing that as clients become better able to define, evaluate, and understand the influences on their behaviour, their personal problems correspondingly become less mysterious and more capable of positive resolution. This is predicated on clients being active participants in their own treatment and life planning.

Social Skills

The excessive use of some substance abusers can be traced to a deficit in social skills. Controlled research clearly supports skills training as a valuable component of alcohol and drug abuse treatment (Roth & Fonagy, 2005). Techniques useful in teaching social skills include role playing, modelling, social coaching, role reversal, and providing social rewards. Comparative findings suggest that focusing on assertiveness training and cognitive inhibitions is particularly helpful. Cognitive rehabilitation includes training in focusing, sustaining and dividing attention, discrimination between cues, inhibition, and differential responding to cues, along with problem solving (Fals-Stewart & Lam, 2010). The focus of cognitive self-change is to

- pay attention to thoughts and feelings;
- recognize that thoughts and feelings have risks leading to harmful behaviour;
- use new thinking to reduce the risk; and
- practice until proficient at the change (Barnett, 2009).

Interpersonal Skills

The evidence regarding deficits in interpersonal skills among drug abusers and alcohol-dependent persons is extensive (Longabaugh & Morgenstern, 1999; Nixon, Tivis, & Parsons, 1992; Roberts, Shaner, & Eckman, 1999; Sacks, Skinner, Sacks, & Peck, 2002). Some studies suggest that substance-dependent persons use drugs as a coping response to stressful interpersonal situations and relapse is often initiated by stressful situations. Therefore, it is possible that interpersonal skills training may increase the individual's real control over the stressor(s) by compensating for skill deficiencies, or increase the individual's perception of control over the stressor(s), leading, in either case, to control over the consequent drug use. One reason that training in coping skills may be useful is that it increases client self-efficacy, mobilizing skills they already possess but have not actively employed (Miller, Forcehimes, & Zweben, 2011).

Vocational Skills

Training in vocational skills is based on findings that many problem drinkers and abusers of psychoactive drugs have a poor employment history, and that employment status is a good predictor of treatment outcome. Vocational skills education usually involves assertiveness training and instruction in other skills for dealing with co-workers and employers. Generally, training in vocational skills has not been used alone but as one component of a multimodal treatment approach (Schottenfeld, Pascale, & Sokolowski, 1992; Wolkstein & Spiller, 1998).

Stress Management

Stress has been hypothesized as an antecedent of both drug use and of lapse and relapse after treatment. The theoretical rationale underlying the application of relaxation training techniques usually involves two assumptions: first, that the problem is caused or exacerbated by tension or anxiety and, second, that relaxation training can effectively deal with the problem either by reducing anxiety or by increasing the individual's sense of perceived control in stressful situations. Relaxation training can be particularly useful when it is used as part of a systematic desensitization treatment. Systematic desensitization is a well-defined procedure used to diminish specific fears. The client is gradually and repeatedly exposed to imagined or real aspects of the phobic situation. This is done under conditions that prevent or minimize the arousal of anxiety. Other popular relaxation training techniques include progressive muscle relaxation, meditation, and yoga (Back, Gentilin, & Brady, 2007; Noone, Dua, & Markham, 1999).

Cognitive Behavioural Therapy

Cognitive behavioural therapy (CBT) combines theories about how individuals learn behaviours with theories regarding how they think about and interpret a life event. CBT has an extensive history of empirical support in treating substance abuse, as the synthesis of cognitive and behavioural approaches was proposed in the 1980s (Carroll, 1996, Carroll & Onken, 2005; Marlatt, 1985; O'Hare, 2005; Pollack et al., 2002). The rationale behind using CBT is the assumption that the process of drug use, including lapse and relapse, can be controlled by making new cognitive and emotional and, therefore, behavioural choices. While the foundation was laid by John Watson, Aaron Beck also contributed extensively to the development of the therapy. CBT also draws from Albert Bandura's social learning theory, being premised on the belief that all thoughts and behaviours are learned through the results of direct experience as well as through vicarious observation (Wills & Sanders, 2013). It also assumes that cognitive processes lead to drug craving, though current research suggests that other neurobiological and physiological processes, which operate out of cognitively conscious awareness, may also influence behaviour (Waldron & Kaminer, 2004).

Cognitive behavioural therapy focuses on cognition as covert behaviour and holds the view that individuals' problems arise from their beliefs, evaluations, and interpretations regarding life events (Gabour & Ing, 1991). The first step in CBT is to take a functional analysis of the client's behaviours associated with drug use, focusing on patterns of use and frequency. CBT is based on several assumptions, including that drug use is often the result of maladaptive cognition, that drug and alcohol misuse is an attempt to solve such problems, and that adaptive cognition will decrease alcohol and drug use (National Institute on Drug Abuse, 1988).

Combining behaviour and cognitive therapies, CBT concentrates on the mental process mediating between stimuli and responses in the belief that a person's feelings and behaviours can be moderated by their thinking. Individuals have negative automatic thoughts (NATs), which are typically closely linked with their emotions and behaviours. As NATs develop, a person's interpretation of life can become skewed, creating a cycle of negative thought and self-doubt. Additional negative emotions and behaviours then reinforce the negative thoughts (Dryden & Branch, 2012). Skills training to break this cycle can be either intrapersonal (examining internal events) or interpersonal.

In either case, the counsellor draws on daily life examples to address both the cognitions and the behaviour. Self-efficacy is enhanced to the point where clients regain control over the active decision-making processes in their lives. This collaborative approach between client and counsellor places the client as active learner in the course of treatment, with the counsellor as teacher. Using positive reinforcement, the counsellor focuses on the assumptions that behaviour can change, based on how individuals think about themselves (Figure 4.2). If the thinking can become self-regulated, change can follow (Fisher, 1995).

FIGURE 4.2: INTERSECTION OF THOUGHT, BEHAVIOUR, AND EMOTION IN CBT

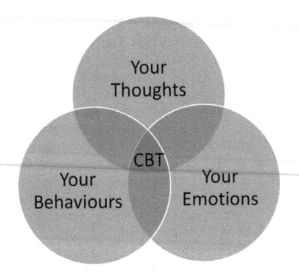

CBT seeks to bring about change during the therapeutic process by altering an individual's established cognitions, errors, and schemas. However, rather than addressing only distressing thoughts and feelings, contemporary CBT has evolved to promote an attitude of non-judgmental acceptance as part of the process (Herbert & Foreman, 2011). Waldron and Kaminer (2004) add that, within CBT, substance use issues must be conceptualized as learned behaviours that are initiated and maintained in the context of environmental factors. Recovery is a learning process, and time must be spent examining, explaining, and discussing high-risk situations that trigger drug use to build client self-efficacy in responding to them. Outcome studies indicate that becoming aware of these high-risk situations increases client confidence and provides them with an element of control over their lives (Vedel, Emmelkamp, & Schippers, 2008). However, this approach may appear to be more effective than others simply because it is used and evaluated more often. Overall, the advantage conferred by cognitive behavioural therapies over other counselling options is minor (Magill & Ray, 2009).

One of the most substantive addiction models premised on cognitive behavioural therapy was Marlatt and Gordon's (1985) relapse prevention approach (Figure 4.3). Historically, relapse had been attributed to factors such as cravings or withdrawal symptoms arising due to the disease of addiction. In contrast, the cognitive behavioural approach examines environmental factors and the context of drug use as leading to relapse. The approach also rejects the idea of a person being either successfully abstinent or failing and being a drug user. Rather, the transition is viewed as a process where lapses are not end points but learning opportunities. If a lapse becomes a relapse, it is still only a temporary setback, which is not unique to the individual but a common part of the process toward the end goal of abstinence. It is simply another learning opportunity, which, when resolved, becomes part of the person's behavioural repertoire. Primary goals of treatment are functional analysis, determining triggers and consequences of use, and skill building.

FIGURE 4.3: COGNITIVE BEHAVIOURAL MODEL OF RELAPSE

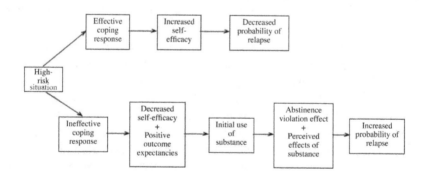

Source: Marlatt & Gordon (1985)

In Marlatt and Gordon's model, the basic belief is that relapse events are immediately preceded by a high-risk situation, defined as any context that places a person at risk of engaging in unwanted drug-using behaviour. These high-risk situations can be emotional or cognitive, such as negative feelings or a decrease in self-efficacy. An example is being back in a club where the person used to buy drugs. Whether the person uses in this situation will depend on his or her ability to enact an effective coping response, either cognitive or behavioural, to counteract the trigger that led to the psychological desire to use again. These are areas that cognitive behavioural counselling looks to develop and bolster. Clients need to learn techniques to help them to anticipate and cope with high-risk situations while reducing the risks by promoting positive lifestyle changes. Thus the foundation of CBT in relapse prevention is assessment of the client's substance use patterns, high-risk situations, and coping skills while enhancing the client's self-efficacy, outcome expectancies, and readiness to change. The process begins with a client identifying high-risk situations and then working in conjunction with the counsellor to develop both cognitive and behavioural coping responses to counter each situation (Hendershot, Witkiewitz, George, & Marlatt, 2011).

Dialectical Behavioural Therapy

Dialectical behavioural therapy (DBT) is an evidence-based form of skills training. It is often referred to, along with acceptance and commitment therapy or functional analytic psychotherapy, as part of a new wave of behavioural therapies (Hayes, Masuda, Bissett, Luoma, & Guerrero, 2004). Developed by Marsha Linehan (1993), DBT involves the synthesis of both change and acceptance. Linehan found that clients with suicidal ideation tend not to have the skills to solve their problems, which exacerbates their suffering. As well, due to high levels of frustration, these clients are extremely sensitive to criticism. When tasked with behavioural change options they could not successfully complete, their emotional state led many to either shut down or respond physically. Such clients would dramatically exit from counselling sessions or even forcefully confront their counsellors. Their distraught emotional state simply did not allow them to accept their circumstances. Linehan worked to bring about change in these clients using persuasion and by asking what had not been considered in prior work with them.

DBT was initially developed to treat the suicidal and parasuicidal behaviours of clients diagnosed with borderline personality disorder (Linehan, 1993). Borderline personality disorder (BPD) is a complex mental illness characterized by fear of abandonment, impulsivity, self-harm behaviours, and emotional dysregulation (American Psychiatric Association, 2013). DBT is best characterized as a combination of cognitive behavioural therapy (CBT) and mindfulness principles derived from Buddhist meditative practices. Its intent is to improve client motivation to change, enhance client capability, and generalize new behaviours through structuring the client's environment in a more positive manner. As with other behavioural approaches, the behaviours to be changed are placed in a hierarchy. Life-threatening behaviours are a priority for change, followed by those that interfere with the counselling process, and then by those that degrade the quality of life. In several studies, DBT has demonstrated that it may be the first effective treatment for borderline personality disorder (Kliem, Kröger, & Kossfelder, 2010; Linehan, Armstrong, Suarez, Allmon, & Heard, 1991; Linehan, Heard, & Armstrong, 1993).

The overlap between borderline personality disorder and co-morbid conditions precipitated the use of DBT with other clinical issues. In the BPD population, this often included substance abuse issues as well as homelessness, unemployment, and eating disorders (Hayes et al., 2004). In stage one of DBT, the focus is on the client obtaining basic information and skills to decrease counterproductive behaviours. This begins with decreasing substance use among clients presenting with this issue, followed by alleviating the physical pain of withdrawal, decreasing urges and temptations, and avoiding cues that could trigger a return to drug use (Dimeff & Linehan, 2008).

It has now been well established that a range of addiction treatment approaches work but that the greatest impediment remains client drop out (Csiernik & Arundel, 2013), with evaluation studies regularly being compromised as drop-out rates range close to 80 percent (Bornovalova & Daughters, 2007). In contrast, a major strength of DBT is its retention-enhancing strategies. DBT strategies that explicitly aim to increase treatment compliance may do so by

- increasing motivation to attend treatment;
- emphasizing the importance of the therapeutic alliance; and
- emphasizing therapist availability through frequent contact or case management approaches (Bornovalova & Daughters, 2007).

Similarly, many of the mindfulness-based practices in DBT have been previously demonstrated as useful in substance-use treatment (Brautigam, 1977; Monahan, 1977; Alexander, Robinson, & Rainforth, 1994). While the exact mechanism is unknown (Bowen et al., 2006), it is likely that the focus on behaviour change combined with validation is responsible for improved compliance. One of the primary reasons that people drop out of treatment is because the traditional treatment paradigm views their actions as only dysfunctional and pathological (Linehan, 1993). However, DBT views their actions as problems to solve and not as indicators of treatment failure, personal inadequacy, lack of desire to change, or moral failing (Dimeff & Linehan, 2008).

DBT's goals are to balance thoughts, emotions, and actions while restoring emotional regulation to interpersonal situations. The counsellor observes, describes, and participates in the process without judging to manage the substance use with strategies that are not self-punishing. The goal is to allow clients to become more patient and accepting of themselves, and thus the counsellor must accept the clients as they are while working to teach them the skills necessary for change. DBT is a modality of acceptance and gentle persuasion for vulnerable clients with one or more emotional, behavioural, interpersonal, cognitive, or self-dysregulation. In DBT, tolerance of distress, emotional regulation, core mindfulness, and interpersonal skills are taught (Dimeff & Linehan, 2008).

Community Reinforcement Approach/Community Reinforcement Approach and Family Training

According to Miller and Hester's (1986a) detailed analysis of treatment effectiveness, the community reinforcement approach (CRA) model is among the strongest interventions possible, though also one of the most labour-intensive. It is based on the belief that environmental contingencies can play a powerful role in drinking or drug use, and that substance abuse is heavily influenced by social and occupational environmental stressors. The CRA is designed to restructure family, social, and vocational factors in a manner that reinforces a drug-free lifestyle while discouraging future drug use. In CRA, a group of behaviourally based procedures designed to alter the contingencies for drug use are implemented so that sobriety is rewarded and drinking or drug use results in a "time out" from positive reinforcement. The intent is to increase satisfaction in major life areas, such as relationships, work, and recreation, so that the need to obtain positive reinforcement through alcohol or drugs is minimized (Azrin, 1976; Hunt & Azrin, 1973).

The first step in the process is a comprehensive functional analysis to determine when drug misuse occurs, and outline the chain of events that leads from non-drug use to a state of dysfunctional impairment. This entails identifying external antecedents, including with whom, where, and when the drug is used, as well as the physical and psychological triggers. The quantity and frequency of drug use, positive and negative outcomes, and legal, occupational, educational, and relationship factors are all part of the functional analysis. Understanding positive reinforcement is essential if a full range of interventions, to alter both psychological and environmental factors reinforcing drug use, are to be used. Otherwise, the behaviour will not be fully addressed, and the likelihood of a lapse or relapse increases. The CRA treatment plan is itself framed during a period of sobriety. However, while abstinence may be the ultimate goal, the client is initially asked to remain sober only during this planning phase and not indefinitely. The "Happiness Scale," which examines 10 areas of a person's life, is the foundation of the treatment plan. The client and counsellor identify areas that need focus. Strategies for goal development and a feasible time frame are then determined. The counsellor uses a positive reinforcement framework to establish reasonable goals that a client can achieve, which underscores how the treatment process aids the client in obtaining rewards important to her or him (Myers, Villanueva, & Smith, 2005).

A key initial focus in the assessment is behavioural skill deficits. The three main training components of CRA are problem solving, communication skills, and refusal skills that emphasize assertiveness in uncomfortable and difficult settings. These are supplemented with social and recreational counselling and job skills, given that many clients are either unemployed or their existing employment is a substantive drug-using trigger. Mood monitoring and cognitive restructuring are important components of the counselling process, as is relationship counselling. CRA was among the first treatments to recognize the importance of family members in maintaining ongoing sobriety, and to stress the inclusion of other significant people in the client counselling process. Interestingly, the CRA process begins by anticipating relapse, and thus the functional analysis immediately begins by identifying future risks for use. Homework is an ongoing part of the treatment process. A major caveat is to not create a plan that is so complex or has so many goals initially that it cannot successfully be carried out. Along with avoiding high-risk situations, every step in the plan should be one over which the client has control (Myers, Villanueva, & Smith, 2005).

The focus on family involvement has led to an enhanced version of CRA, known as CRAFT (community reinforcement approach and family training). CRAFT more actively engages non-using family members, typically partners and children, to affect the behaviour of substance abusers (Sisson & Azrin, 1986). Both CRA and CRAFT stress the importance of relationships in the treatment process. Focusing only on using behaviours and not including interpersonal problems will decrease the likelihood of success with the approach model. What is key is reciprocity, with both partners being allowed to express themselves, avoiding blaming, and speaking in a positive, reinforcing manner. Issues need to be clearly stated by both partners, including the overt discussion of their feelings. In both CRA and CRAFT, supportiveness, empathy, and a genuine caring attitude are critical to establishing the client-counsellor relationship. These treatment models are action-orientated approaches involving modelling, role playing, and shaping. They require the counsellor to be directive, energetic, and engaging, actively encouraging the client and pointing out all the successes in the client change process, regardless of how small they may initially seem (Myers & Miller, 2001; Roozen, Waart, & Van Der Kroft, 2010).

Aversion Therapy

Aversion therapy, the least favoured form of behavioural therapy, was among the earliest approaches to treating addiction. Aversion therapy induces a state of mind in which attention to an object is coupled with repugnance and a desire to turn away from it. Historically, it has been produced by drugs or electric shock, though the most recent format uses verbal conditioning, forming a new relationship between an aversive stimulus and an undesirable response through the use of words. On presentation of the stimuli—either alcohol or another drug—the response is punished. When the response becomes infrequent or disappears, the repugnant stimuli are reduced or terminated.

The common goal of aversion therapies is to alter the individual's attraction to a drug. Through counter-conditioning procedures, the abused substance is paired with any of a variety of unpleasant experiences. If the conditioning is successful, the individual shows an automatic negative response when later exposed to the drug alone, much like the protagonist in Stanley Kubrick's *Clockwork Orange*. Aversion therapies should not be confused with pharmacological interventions where the intended effects rest not on conditioning by repeated aversive pairings but rather on suppression of fear of immediate aversive consequences. Aversion therapy is a form of classical (Pavlovian) conditioning procedure.

Four variants of aversion therapy appear in the literature. The oldest form of aversion is a procedure that typically paired either alcohol or heroin with the experience of nausea. With alcohol, several sessions are typically held where nausea is induced, usually through injection or oral consumption of a noxious substance while the individual drinks his or her favourite alcoholic beverage. The nausea effects may linger for several hours after the "intervention." Apnea was a short-lived experiment in aversion therapy during the 1960s. In the procedure the aversive stimulus was an injection of succinylcholine, which induced total paralysis of movement and breathing for an interval of up to 60 seconds. During this interval, alcohol was placed on the lips of the paralyzed patient. If the patient did not begin breathing after 60 seconds, he or she was ventilated. Not surprisingly, clients reacted quite negatively to the bottle containing alcohol after the trial. However, in one reported study, 17 of 23 males were again drinking regularly less than eight months after their last apnea session. Ethical factors, the severe nature of this treatment, and the lack of positive results quickly discouraged its application (Elkins, 1975).

Electric shock was also first employed in attempting to treat alcohol-dependent persons during the late 1960s. In one common procedure, clients received several sessions of electric shock, usually applied to the forearm, paired with the smelling or tasting of alcoholic beverages. At the direction of the therapist, clients poured themselves a drink and then tasted it without swallowing. Shocks were applied randomly throughout the process. Sessions ran over a 10-day period and lasted from 20 to 45 minutes, depending on the client's level of alcohol abuse (Jackson & Smith, 1978). Outcome studies painted a confusing picture, as some noted strong and significant effects, while others found virtually no long-term benefit of this technique. The apparent lack of long-term success with this procedure led a young researcher named G. Alan Marlatt to one of the most important addictions insights of the late 20th century—the need for relapse prevention training as integral to maintaining sobriety (Marlatt, 1973; Marlatt & George, 1984).

The newest addition to the repertoire of aversion techniques was covert sensitization. This technique occurred entirely in the patient's imagination and entailed pairing aversive scenes with drug-use imagery. Covert sensitization using nausea scenes operates by establishing a conditioned aversion response. The procedure is related to that used in hypnosis.

The fact that aversion techniques, especially chemical aversion, produce substantially superior outcomes with older subjects who are of higher socioeconomic status suggests that the principal benefits of these techniques may relate to factors other than classical aversive conditioning, including motivation, social stability, and a stable support system. In general, aversive conditioning procedures appear to be effective largely with those individuals who have a relatively good prognosis at the outset. Because of the relatively poor long-term effectiveness of aversion techniques, it is difficult to justify their use, especially in light of their highly invasive nature. Reduction of consumption rather than total abstinence is a common observation following aversion therapies, and thus the success of these approaches would not be well reflected if complete abstinence were used as the primary criterion of success (Miller & Hester, 1986a).

4.7 HARM REDUCTION
Needle-Exchange Programs
Methadone Treatment and Methadone Maintenance
Heroin-Assisted Treatment (HAT)
Safe Injection Sites
Controlled Drinking

Harm reduction is a form of treatment that has multiple possible successful outcomes, one of which is the drug user becoming abstinent. It is officially one of the four pillars of Canada's drug plan and involves any strategy or behaviour that an individual uses to reduce the potential harm that may exist for him or her. In the field of addiction, this translates into a range of options, from safer drug use techniques, to using licit rather than illicit drugs where the quality and purity of the product is better known, to decreasing either the amount of drugs administered or the frequency of administrations or both, to moving toward abstinence. While initiatives such as controlled drinking, designated drivers, contracts for life, and methadone treatment have been available for decades, it was the emergence of AIDS and HIV that brought harm-reduction initiatives to the forefront of the addiction field and shifted the focus more toward strategies relating to decreasing injection drug use (Collin, 2006; Thomas, 2005).

A 2001 meeting of Canadian provincial and federal health ministers formally established a new drug strategy for Canada. It was recognized that harm reduction was an important component of the addiction intervention continuum (Health Canada, 2001). However, harm reduction is more than just intervention, as it relates to "any policy directed toward reducing or containing adverse health, social and economic consequences of alcohol, other drug use and gambling without necessarily requiring a reduction in consumption or abstinence from substance use or gambling strategy or behaviour that an individual uses in their life to reduce the drug related harm which may exist for them in their life" (Alberta Alcohol and Drug Abuse Commission, 2001, p. 3). By adopting a harm-reduction perspective, we are obligated to also adopt a new philosophy toward users of drugs, including those who primarily use illicit drugs. While historically they have been judged through a moral model lens, and intervened with primarily using the criminal justice system, harm reduction offers a much different perspective. It rejects the belief that increasing law enforcement is the optimal approach to decreasing drug use. Instead, this philosophy embraces the following beliefs:

- All humans have intrinsic value.
- All humans have the right to comprehensive non-judgmental medical and social services.
- Licit and illicit drugs are neither good nor bad.
- Psychoactive drug users are sufficiently competent to make choices regarding their use of drugs.
- Outcomes are in the hands of the client.
- Options are provided in a non-judgmental, non-coercive manner. Harm reduction practitioners acknowledge the significance of any positive change that individuals make in their lives (Hagan, 1999).

Harm-reduction interventions are facilitative rather than coercive, and are grounded in the needs of individuals. Small gains are viewed as success, just as abstinence is, for in the process of change, individuals are much more likely to take many small steps rather than one or two huge leaps. Harm reduction begins with the most feasible changes to keep people healthy as they slowly move toward abstinence, knowing that many will never reach that end goal. However, keeping people alive and preventing irreparable damage is regarded as the most urgent priority. International health bodies, including the World Health Organization and the Joint United Nations Programme on HIV/AIDS (UNAIDS), recommend harm-reduction programs as best practices and as crucial for reducing HIV infection among those who inject drugs.

Needle-Exchange Programs

Needle-exchange programs allow injection drug users (IDUs) to trade used syringes for new, sterile syringes and related injection works. In recent years, though, many of these fixed and mobile outreach programs have also begun to offer crack pipes and straws for cocaine use. Needle exchange is a harm-reduction strategy that arose as a direct result of the blood-borne infections of HIV, hepatitis C (HCV), and hepatitis B (HBV), which were unintended outcomes of injection drug use. However, this is not only a form of intervention for IDUs but is also part of a broader public health model. Funding for these initiatives is intended to limit the transfer of these diseases into the general population. Needle-exchange programs have been empirically demonstrated to reduce the spread of blood-borne infections and also to create supportive relationships between IDUs and the health and social services systems, often for the first time in their lives (Hankins, 1998; Hyshka, Strathdee, Wood, & Kerr, 2012; Stimson, 1995, Vertefeuille et al., 2000).

Methadone Treatment and Methadone Maintenance

Both subjective and health-related quality of life are relatively poor among opioid-dependent individuals compared with the general population, and also when compared to people with other medical illnesses (De Maeyer, Vanderplasschen, & Broekaert, 2010). Methadone, a synthetic opioid analgesic with a long half-life, was first widely used as a drug for those dependent on heroin in the 1960s. Most programs were of limited duration, and it was discovered that once users were weaned off methadone, many returned to heroin use. Methadone produces morphine-like actions and cross-tolerance but does not produce significant euphoria. As it is administered orally, its use as a drug substitute eliminates the associated risks IDUs have when injecting heroin and other opioids. However, methadone is not without its limits, as tolerance and withdrawal do occur, and, with extended use, addiction does arise to this psychoactive drug. Both methadone maintenance (MM) and methadone treatment (MT) consist of an individual drinking a sufficient dose of methadone on a daily basis to eliminate withdrawal symptoms from other opioids. The basic premise for opioid substitution therapy is that methadone administered daily by mouth is effective in the suppression of withdrawal symptoms and in the reduction of the use of illicit opioids. MM involves determining a correct dose for each individual and providing regular health care and treatment for other addiction issues. MT programs also entail the provision of counselling and support, mental health services, health promotion, and disease prevention and education, along with advocacy and linkages to community-based supports and services, such as housing. Unfortunately, for many individuals living with opioid addiction, the damage that has occurred to their bodies as a result of prolonged drug use may not allow them to ever withdraw completely from methadone (Watkin, Rowe, & Csiernik, 2010).

Opioid-dependent individuals who receive treatment with methadone or who enter an MM program do use fewer illicit drugs (not only heroin), have better health than IDUs not in a program, access health care more readily, develop a greater sense of wellness, have higher rates of employment and less use of social assistance, report better interpersonal relationships (including improved parenting and child rearing), and have overall better social functioning. As with needle-exchange programs, the benefits of both MM and MT extend to the general community by reducing the spread of infectious diseases (Methadone Strategy Working Group, 2001; Sun et al., 2015). Methadone substitution programs also have a positive effect on quality of life, especially during the first months of treatment, as the crisis or symptoms that precipitated it recede. Initial gains tend to be maintained over time, though they do typically fall back unless the underlying reasons for drug use are addressed. Drug use is not always the reason that people seek treatment, but rather problems in other life domains (De Maeyer et al., 2010). Recent developments have seen some methadone maintenance programs no longer target only individuals dependent on heroin but also those addicted to non-injected opioids, such as Dilaudid, Percocet, and OxyContin, and even opioids with a lesser dependency liability than methadone itself, including codeine.

This evolution and growing prominence of MM rather than MT raises the troubling question of who is being helped the most: the user who remains addicted to a psychoactive drug, the general public, or those manufacturing, prescribing, and distributing this socially acceptable licit opioid drug. It is acknowledged that longer treatment periods are associated with improved outcomes, including reduced use of other opioids and reduced criminal activity. Grella and Lovinger (2011) reported that 40 percent of methadone users achieved stable remission after five to eight years, with one year being considered the minimum to achieve better and sustained benefits. A 2010 economic study completed in Ontario found that the average daily cost of treatment was only Can$15.48 per day, which consisted of physician billing (9.8 percent), pharmacy costs (39.8 percent), and urine toxicology screens (46.7 percent), with the methadone itself costing $0.59 per day. On average, the annual cost is $5,651 or the equivalent of an annual three-week hospital stay (Zaric, Brennan, Varenbut, & Daiter, 2012). This is eight times less than the average health, social, and criminal costs associated with an untreated person using illicit opioids, which was estimated to be $44,600 per year (Health Canada, 2008). However, over the course of the next 35 years, with inflation factored in, the cost of keeping each person legally addicted in a methadone maintenance program will total over $250,000. This long-term cost could be substantially offset if counselling were incorporated throughout the process to help individuals move towards abstinence. Even though the process of MT often takes two to four years, it is of much shorter duration and is much less costly (both economically and personally) than the 3.5 decades currently spent regularly ingesting an addictive substance.

Heroin-Assisted Treatment (HAT)

Some individuals do not respond well to methadone. It may not ease the physical or psychological pain of withdrawal, or negate the craving, or an individual may have a negative reaction to its synthetic nature. Historically, these individuals either endured a cold turkey withdrawal or more typically went back to using street heroin. By returning to use, they again put themselves at risk for life-threatening health issues, including drug overdose, blood-borne viral infections, and endocarditis, as well as the violence that accompanies illicit drug transactions. One controversial alternative is heroin-assisted treatment (HAT). Under a HAT protocol, street heroin users are prescribed pharmaceutical quality heroin, which is injected in safe, clean, specialized medical clinics. In 2005, a randomized controlled trial was conducted in Vancouver and Montreal to evaluate the feasibility and effectiveness of HAT in Canada. The results showed that participants were less likely to use street drugs than those in a MM program, and they were also less likely to engage in criminal activity, increasing the likelihood of an eventual move toward abstinence (Nosyk et al., 2010). A follow-up study compared prescription heroin with hydromorphone. It too reported superior outcomes among those using the prescription heroin, which further reinforced earlier findings from studies in the United Kingdom, Germany, the Netherlands, and Switzerland (Ferri, Davoli, & Perucci, 2011).

The results of the two Canadian studies led to a recommendation by Health Canada to allow prescription heroin use among individuals who could not successfully use methadone. However, Conservative Health Minister Rona Ambrose objected to Health Canada's approval and introduced regulations to make prescribing the drug outside of clinical trials illegal. In turn, Supreme Court Chief Justice Christopher Hinkson ruled against the Minister of Health, stating that risks associated with the severe heroin addiction of the 202 follow-up study participants would be reduced under this specialized medical program. However, the court ruling at this time allows only for the study's initial participants to continue to receive the pharmaceutical-grade drug and sterilized supplies with which to inject it (Woo, 2014). Despite decades of national and international research indicating the economic and health utility of various harm-reduction initiatives, the Stephen Harper government continued to oppose programs that offer choices to Canadian citizens with addiction issues.

Safe Injection Sites

Safe injection sites (SIS) are clinics designed to provide IDUs with clean needles and sterilized works to inject their drugs in a safer manner. The goal of an SIS is to provide individuals with a healthier environment in which to inject drugs while also providing related health and social services, all in one location. Switzerland, Germany, and the Netherlands adopted the concept of safe injection rooms during the 1970s, again as a general public health initiative. However, since then, the strategy has been demonstrated to decrease new HIV and HCV infections and reduce the number of overdose-related deaths while providing access to primary and emergency health care for a traditionally oppressed population. After the opening of a safe injection site, there is generally a decrease in public nuisance issues related to drug use, including public injecting, discarded syringes, and injection-related litter (Rowe & Gonzalez, 2010).

Supervised injection sites offer a safe place that drug-dependent individuals can access to inject drugs under the supervision of trained multidisciplinary health and social services staff who can provide education regarding safer injection practices, as well as respond appropriately in the event of an overdose. Each SIS varies in the way it operates; however, in general, injection drug users bring pre-obtained drugs to the site, are provided with sterile equipment to use, and inject their drugs with nurses and other trained staff nearby. Typically, needles, syringes, candles, sterile water, paper towels, cotton balls, cookers/spoons, ties, alcohol swabs, filters, ascorbic acid, and bandages are available in the injection areas. SIS allow IDUs to have their privacy while also offering the comfort of knowing that trained medical staff are available to respond in case of an emergency. SIS do not allow the sharing of drugs or equipment and prohibit assisted injection. Supervised injection site use by IDUs leads to a reduction in syringe sharing among users, which also reduces the spread of diseases and infections. It is critical to note how SIS differ markedly from illegal shooting galleries operating in many cities, where drug users pay a small fee for a few minutes in a private or semi-private room. The latter are profit-motivated, may be littered with trash and/or needles, violent, and controlled by drug dealers, may allow participants to share dirty needles, and show little regard for the user's health and safety. In contrast, SIS attempt to protect and promote the health of injection drug users by employing a non-judgmental, client-centred approach rooted in a harm-reduction philosophy (Rowe & Gonzalez, 2010).

A major social and community issue regarding SIS is the misconception that these sites bring with them an increase in drug dealing, using, and other crimes to the neighbourhood in which they are located. Interestingly, the risk of crime in a neighbourhood is more causally linked to the location of a convenience store than an SIS or any other type of harm-reduction program. The benefits of SIS on public drug use and HIV risk behaviour have not come at the cost of increases in criminal activity (Boyd, Fang, Medoff, Dixon, & Gorelick, 2012). In addition, SIS can actually enhance public order through a decrease in public drug use, and the introduction of SIS has led to an increase in addiction treatment and detoxification service use in most communities where they have been established. There is also no evidence to suggest that the presence of SIS leads to more individuals initiating injection drug use or that using SIS increases the relapse rate of injection drug use or decreases quitting injection drug use. Initial concerns of residents primarily stem from a fear of the unknown, a feeling of uncertainty, and a lack of knowledge regarding SIS, such as what they are and how they operate, rather than actual events or evidence. As with other forms of harm reduction, SIS benefit a hard-to-reach population of IDUs by offering services with minimal barriers to access and avoidance of interactions with the criminal justice system. Contact with these hard-to-reach persons can lead to important social and health referrals and treatment opportunities, which ultimately result in positive social and community opportunities. Client contact with SIS has contributed to individual improvements in health, social functioning, and stabilization. Clients generally cease to use the sites on attaining stable living arrangements. In this way, injection sites can improve the likelihood that IDUs can reintegrate into the mainstream (Wood, Kerr, Montaner et al., 2004; Wood, Kerr, Small et al., 2004; Wood, Tyndall, Lai, Montaner, & Kerr, 2006).

Controlled Drinking

In 1973, Sobell and Sobell introduced a highly controversial concept to the addiction field: controlled drinking. Seventy male alcoholics in an in-patient program were assigned either to experimental or control groups. Two experimental groups received individual counselling and behaviour therapy, with one group having abstinence as their outcome goal and the second, a goal of controlling their alcohol consumption. The two control groups received standard treatment, with one group having an outcome goal of abstinence while the goal of the second group was to control their drinking. At both six-month and one-year follow-ups, the treatment groups were doing better than the control groups but there was no significant difference on the outcomes measures between the two experimental groups. This led to the idea that controlled drinking was as effective as abstinence, which in turn brought waves of protest from Alcoholics Anonymous proponents, who believed it sent a message to its members that it was permissible to drink again. In 1974, Sobell and Sobell followed up their initial contentious study with an article claiming that "more than 600 total studies ... have reported that some alcoholic individuals have successfully resumed some type of non-problematic moderate drinking" (p. 10).

This furor was intensified when a study by Armor, Polich, and Stambul (1978) indicated equivalent relapse rates between those following a program of abstinence compared with those following a regiment of controlled drinking. Pendery, Maltzman, and West (1982) further heightened the controversy with a retrospective review of Sobell and Sobell's clients. They found that many members of the original controlled drinking group had relapsed into heavy drinking, with four having died due to alcohol-related causes. These authors, proponents of the abstinence approach, used their study to claim controlled drinking had no merit. However, what Pendery, Maltzman, and West failed to do was conduct a follow-up with the control groups to determine if in fact controlled drinking provided better outcomes than the traditional treatment.

Controlled drinking is an adapted behavioural technique with a specific defined goal. When the view of alcoholism broadened to incorporate the concepts of alcohol dependence, alcohol abuse, and alcohol-related disabilities, a wider range of treatment goals had to be considered. For those persons experiencing low levels of alcohol abuse, a treatment goal of controlled drinking can potentially be recommended. The assessment of the client's level of alcohol dependence is necessary to assist in the selection of a goal of either controlled drinking or total abstinence. As controlled drinking is a component of the behaviourist school of treatment, it follows that training in drinking skills is viewed as a learned response that has short-term effectiveness for the drinker in specific situations, particularly when the individual lacks effective non-drinking responses. Thus, drinking skills training is used with alcohol misusers to teach them to drink in a non-abusive manner as an alternative to abstinence, and usually forms part of a more broad-based treatment program. Matching for controlled drinking is targeted at individuals with a lack of control rather than a loss of control (Donovan & O'Leary, 1979; Glatt, 1980; Miller & Hester, 1986a).

The first step in controlled drinking is determining whether a client is a problem drinker or an alcohol-dependent individual. This is accomplished by first imposing a two- to three-week period of abstinence on a potential client. If the person can go without drinking, he or she is moved into the next phase. Those who cannot abstain during this baseline period generally do not qualify for a controlled drinking treatment program. In the program itself, clients are provided with a set of goals and rules to help them to control their alcohol intake. A common drinking goal of a set number of standard drinks per week is established, with numerous limitations. For a young healthy male approximately 1.8 m tall and 81 kg, the following regimen might be applied:

- no more than two standard drinks per day (one for women)
- no more than one drink per hour
- sip drinks and avoid carbonated beverages
- drink only on a full stomach
- two days per week must be set aside where no alcohol is consumed
- limit weekly intake to 14 standard drinks per week for men (7 for women)

Self-management or behavioural self-control training procedures, such as controlled drinking, require clients to implement their own treatment. The primary advantage of these procedures is that they can maximize the generalization of treatment effects during and after treatment. The main problem with such techniques, however, is that they are likely to be feasible with only highly motivated individuals. Self-management programs generally consist of behavioural strategies, such as the following:

- self-monitoring
- goal setting
- specific changes in drug-using behaviour
- rewards for goal attainment
- functional analysis of drug-using situations
- learning alternative coping skills (Hester, Nirenberg, & Begin, 1990)

Reduced drinking may be a viable alternative for those problem drinkers who do not exhibit levels of alcohol dependence, do not have alcohol-related physical damage, and have not experienced any serious personal, financial, legal, or employment problems as a result of their drinking. If they do not have a history of unsuccessful attempts to curb their drinking behaviour, and if they will not accept abstinence as a lifelong goal, they can attempt to become controlled drinkers. Obviously, systematic assessment is critical in establishing the severity of a person's alcohol problem and in deciding on the most appropriate long-term goal. It is also crucial in this scenario to monitor the problem drinker's progress to ensure that treatment goals are achieved.

The literature attests to the fact that controlled drinking is an attainable and successful goal for problem drinkers who have not established significant degrees of dependence. Abstinence does not have to be the only treatment goal (Miller, 1983a). However, controlled drinking training is not an alternative for those who are physically and psychologically dependent on alcohol or any other psychoactive substance.

Several groups have also advocated a "warm turkey" approach, a middle-ground tactic of moving toward abstinence using a controlled drinking philosophy. The 1996 National Institute on Alcohol Abuse and Alcoholism (NIAAA) program is simply called "How to Cut Down on Your Drinking." It is a basic three-step approach, accompanied by alternatives to drinking. The NIAAA's first step is to have someone considering reducing their alcohol intake to write down the reasons to cut down or stop. The second step is to set the drinking goal: one standard drink per day for women and a maximum of two for men. It is recommended that the person write down the goal and place it in a conspicuous spot so that he or she is reminded of the goal on a regular basis. The third step is to keep a weekly drinking diary that lists the day, the number of drinks consumed, the type of drink, and where it was consumed. In closing, advocates of this method of intervention advise those considering modifying their drinking pattern to not keep much alcohol at home, drink slowly when they choose to drink, try to abstain for a week or two, learn to say no to a drink, stay otherwise active, and seek additional social supports to stay focused.

4.8 THE TRANSTHEORETICAL MODEL OF CHANGE
Pre-contemplation
Contemplation
Preparation
Action
Maintenance/Adaptation
Evaluation/Termination
Techniques

Prochaska and DiClemente (1982) revolutionized thinking about addiction treatment with their integrative model of intentional change based on their work with tobacco smokers who stopped without any formal or self-help assistance. They took the idea of motivation as being a characteristic exclusively of clients and made it into an active counselling skill. Rather than being located exclusively within the client, they expressed the idea that motivation was an interpersonal, interactional process within which the probability existed for behaviours to occur that led to positive outcomes. Numerous studies have identified client motivation as having a substantial positive effect on program retention and client outcome (Heather, Hönekopp, & Smailes, 2009; Nidecker, DiClemente, Bennett, & Bellack, 2008; Prochaska, 2008). Prochaska and DiClemente identified six specific steps necessary for any type of radical change to occur, which represented a natural process of change that could be adapted by counsellors to assist any client to move forward (Figure 4.4).

The idea that drug use was a steady downward track that, with abstinence, became a steady upward track was replaced with the spiral model of change (Figure 4.5). This represents a more realistic representation of the change process, not only for drug use but for any behaviour. The spiral model of change demonstrates that there can be spurts of dramatic positive change interspersed with setbacks, not necessarily lapses or relapses but rather periods of time when the change process becomes more difficult and counselling for the client becomes tedious. However, if the counsellor continues to support and work with the client, further advances are possible if both partners in the process are patient and diligent.

Pre-contemplation

In the first stage of the model, it is recognized that an individual will resist change and typically has no intention of altering behaviour in the near future; the client does not recognize that any problem exists. This idea had historically been called denial. Critical to the entire premise of the Transtheoretical Model (TTM) of Change was the replacement of the longstanding idea that clients were in denial regarding their addiction with the concept of pre-contemplation. Prochaska and DiClemente (1982) reconceptualized the idea of denial, framing it so that clients are not viewed as wilfully deceiving themselves and, in the process, destroying themselves or their families; rather, these individuals were truly unaware of the impact of their behaviour on those around them. People with substance use disorders are often ambivalent about changing their harmful behaviour. They may continue their drug use because they are attracted to a particular lifestyle, want to be included in a peer group, or simply to cope with life's daily stresses. When the destructive effects of their behaviour become obvious, they are faced with giving up many of the people, places, and things they have come to enjoy and with which they may strongly identify. Without a clear view of the future, these individuals may be reluctant to change. A considerable effort is thus required not only by the individual with a substance use disorder, but also by his or her family members, friends, and helping professionals, to become willing to make a commitment to change.

In the pre-contemplation stage, clients are not searching for solutions or looking to change as they typically do not recognize the nature or severity of their substance misuse or abuse. Their drug use has become so normalized, so much a part of their everyday lives, that it is not viewed as a problem. Rather, it is a part of who they are. In this model, individuals who may well be demoralized and ill are assisted in gaining insight into their behaviour or situation by the provision of facts and information. The counsellor's role is to move a person to a point where she or he will consider change. Readiness to change is not a client trait, but a fluctuating product of interpersonal interaction. Pre-contemplation does not entail confrontation or advice. Rather, alliance building is critical, as is the use of cognitive dissonance. Counsellors assist clients in distinguishing between how they see their circumstances and the reality of their situation from an outside perspective. This is accomplished by providing information about the physical consequences of substance use and discussing the history of drug use and its consequences (DiClemente, 2007).

FIGURE 4.4: THE STAGES OF THE TRANSTHEORETICAL MODEL OF CHANGE

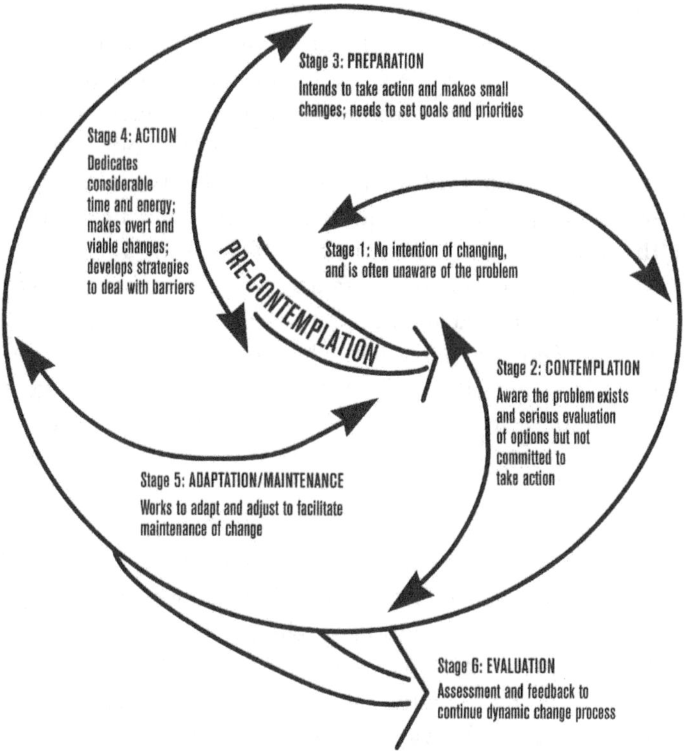

Source: Addiction Studies Institute (2010)

FIGURE 4.5: THE SPIRAL PROCESS OF CHANGE

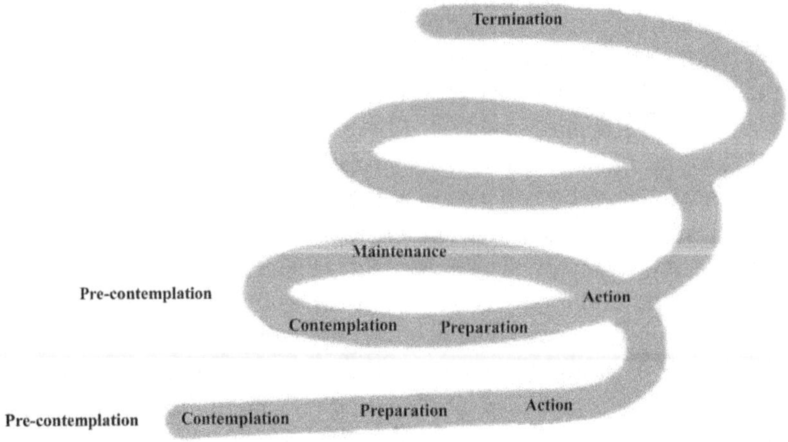

Termination

Maintenance

Pre-contemplation

Action

Contemplation   Preparation

Pre-contemplation   Contemplation   Preparation   Action

Source: Lalazaryan & Zare-Farashbandi (2014)

Contemplation

In the second stage of the model, clients become aware that they are stuck in a situation and must decide whether they wish to change or remain where they are. They are supported in gaining understanding of the consequences of their alcohol or drug use, but the counsellor does not force them to make a commitment to change. This is the stage where the counsellor must help balance in the client's mind the delicate equilibrium between the desire to change and the fear of changing and the associated unknown consequences. Counsellors need to reflect this ambivalence to help clients move forward to the next stage while recognizing and ac-knowledging the fear associated with change. Counsellors also need to be aware that some clients will drop out at this highly stressful stage, so there must be a willingness to work with the client in the future when he or she is ready and able to move forward again.

Preparation

The third stage, preparation, which is also known as the determination stage, is when clients consider changing their drug-using behaviour and anticipate what this future action might be. However, the counsellor needs to be aware that there may be much ambivalence to the idea and process of actual change. During the preparation phase, probing, review-ing consequences, and self-evaluation are areas of work with the client. A specific time frame (with a maximum target of one month) is established when the client agrees to begin changing existing practices and actions. The counsellor needs to support clients as they develop ways to replace what they are about to give up and begin to acquire new skills—such as assertiveness, relaxation, anger control, and problem solving—if they are to make the successful transition to changed behaviour during the next stage (the action phase). The main task of the preparation stage is to identify and resolve barriers to success, including friends and family who may still benefit from the client's drug-using behaviour, along with activities associated with their drug use. Areas to explore in preparing for success are the consequences for the client and those around him or her when change occurs, and what the reactions to the change process will be.

Action

In this stage, the work and behavioural change begins, with a heavy emphasis on problem-solving and problem-solving skills. However, action also entails changing awareness, emotions, self-image, and thinking. Support of positive decisions and positive reinforcement dominate this stage of moving forward by the client, which can last as little as one day or as long as six months. Emphasis is on the positive—what the client is doing, rather than what the client is *not* doing, which is using drugs. Clients need to be reminded that they have reached the mid-point when they are in the action stage, with two steps remaining. Planning for lapse and relapse is also a critical aspect of the action stage. This involves identifying and exploring times that may lead to use, such as when faced with unpleasant emotions, physical discomfort, pleasant emotions, urges, cravings, social pressure, or pleasant times socializing with friends, colleagues, or family.

Maintenance/Adaptation

Stage five focuses on supporting and consolidating the gains made during the action stage and avoiding lapse or the more significant relapse. Social skills training underscores this stage of continued change. This is the skills practice phase of the stages of change model.

Evaluation/Termination

The final stage of the Transtheoretical Model of Change sees the client move beyond problem solving, with a focus on relapse prevention and dealing with the reality of sobriety. During this phase, clients assess their strengths and areas that may be problematic in the future as they develop a relapse-prevention plan that can be undertaken on their own.

Techniques

A variety of techniques are used in the TTM. Consciousness raising, dramatic relief, and environmental re-evaluation are all critical during both the pre-contemplation and contemplation stages. Consciousness raising involves increasing information to clients about themselves and their problem by using observations, interpretations, feedback, education, reading materials, and challenges to what clients believe they are doing and what they are actually doing. Dramatic relief entails experiencing and expressing feelings about one's problems and solutions, grieving losses, and partaking in role play to appreciate the impact of the changed behaviour. The intent of this technique it to produce increased emotional experiences followed by reduced affect if appropriate action can be taken. Psychodrama and personal testimonies can also move people forward emotionally. Environmental re-evaluation assesses how the presence or absence of a personal habit affects one's social and physical environment and entails empathy training. It can also increase awareness that one can serve as a positive or negative role model for others. Empathy training is a critical component of this technique.

As a client moves from contemplation to preparation, self re-evaluation becomes important. Clients need to assess how they feel and think about themselves with respect to their use of substances and clarify their values, often engaging in corrective emotional experiences. Self re-evaluation combines both cognitive and affective assessments of one's self-image. Value clarification, healthy role models, and imagery are techniques that are used with this technique. Self-liberation is the step that moves a client from preparation through to the action phase. Clients choose and commit to change through both their beliefs and actions. It is both the belief that one can change and the enduring commitment to act on that belief. Motivation research indicates that people with two options have a greater commitment to change than those with only one option; those with three have an even greater commitment, though beyond this there is no further enhancement.

The following five tactics are used through both the action and maintenance steps:

1. *Reinforcement management*: Providing consequences for taking steps in a particular direction. While reinforcement management can include the use of punishments, rewarding oneself or being rewarded by others for making changes is far more powerful. Contingency contracts, overt and covert reinforcements, positive self-statements, and group recognition are procedures for increasing reinforcement and the probability that healthier responses will be repeated and maintained.

2. *Helping relationships*: Combining caring, trust, openness, and acceptance, as well as support for the healthy behaviour change. Rapport building, a therapeutic alliance, counsellor calls, and buddy systems can be sources of social support, though regardless of the technique employed, being open and trusting about problems with someone who

cares will help maintain the change. Therapeutic alliance is key during this process.

3. *Counter-conditioning*: Substituting healthier alternatives for problem drug-using behaviours. Relaxation can counter stress; assertion can counter peer pressure; nicotine replacement can be a substitute for cigarettes. With this technique, the focus is on substituting alternatives for problem behaviours with an emphasis on self-care.

4. *Stimulus control*: Removing cues for drug use and replacing them with prompts for healthier alternatives. Avoidance, changing one's environment, and actively participating in self-help groups can provide stimuli that support change and reduce risks for lapse and relapse.

5. *Social liberation*: Increasing engagement in non-drug-related behaviours, progressing emotionally so that the client considers the needs of others. This late-stage technique requires an increase in social opportunities or alternatives, especially for those who are relatively deprived or oppressed. Advocacy, empowerment procedures, and appropriate policies can produce increased opportunities for marginalized individuals and groups (Prochaska, DiClemente, & Norcross, 1992; Prochaska & Velicer, 1997).

Throughout all stages of the TTM, clients are continually asked to weigh the pros and cons of change. This is referred to as decisional balance. Decision making on the part of the client is not always fully conscious or rational, but by openly discussing options, unrecognized thoughts and feelings can be more judiciously examined and assessed. Critical issues that arise during the change process and techniques to counter them are presented in Table 4.4.

TABLE 4.4: CLIENT ISSUES AND COUNSELLOR STRATEGIES TO EMPLOY IN THE TRANSTHEORETICAL MODEL OF CHANGE

Stage	Client Issue	Counsellor Strategy
Pre-contemplation	Nothing needs to change.	Build rapport and trust; increase problem awareness; raise the sense of the importance of the change
Contemplation	I am considering change.	Acknowledge ambivalence regarding the difficulties associated with change; explore the discrepancy between present behaviour and the client's personal values and goals; discuss pros and cons of change; talk about ways to experiment with changing behaviour

Preparation	I am figuring out how to change.	Build client confidence; talk about timing of change; provide information, options, and advice; don't rush—work at the client's pace
Action	I am working on reaching my goals.	Offer planning assistance; provide support around the change process; develop attainable goals; monitor progress and assist the client in self-monitoring; help develop plans in co-operation with the client to maintain the changes over time
Maintenance	I've made my changes. I need to keep up my changes.	Support and encourage new behaviour; talk about possible trouble spots and develop plans to address triggers that can lead to lapse or relapse
Relapse	I've stumbled—how do I get back up? Have I lost everything?	Openly address lapse/relapse; negate shame; discuss and assess what led to the return to drug use; raise confidence; address that the client can begin again and be successful

Source: Waiters, Clark, Gingerich, & Meitzer (2007)

4.9 MOTIVATIONAL INTERVIEWING

"What do you make of all of this?"
"Where does this leave you?"
"What do you want to do next?"

Motivational Interviewing (MI) is closely associated with the Transtheoretical Model of Change and is integral to its success. Developed by William Miller (1983b), MI also draws from the work of Carl Rogers. MI is a brief, client-centred, directive method for enhancing intrinsic motivation to change. It explores and resolves client ambivalence using the ideas of empathy, attribution, cognitive dissonance, and self-efficacy. In MI, motivation is conceptualized not as a personality trait, but as an interpersonal process. The model de-emphasizes labelling, replaces confrontation with empathy, and places a much greater emphasis on individual responsibility and internal attribution for change. Cognitive dissonance is created by contrasting the client's ongoing problem behaviour with salient awareness of the behaviour's negative consequences. Empathic processes, motivation, and objective assessment feedback are used to channel this dissonance toward a behaviour change, being cognizant of and avoiding the typical client barriers of low self-esteem, low self-efficacy, and pre-contemplation. MI is a strength-based counselling style in which the counsellor works with the client, rather than doing things for or to the client. The focus is on locating natural motivating issues within a client's life or the client's system (Box 4.1). The counsellor needs to anticipate and respond to a client's genuine hesitation and insecurity to engage in a fundamentally life-altering change in behaviour. Simply giving clients advice to change is typically unrewarding and ineffective. Motivational interviewing is non-confrontational in nature and acknowledges that creating conflict, rather than ambivalence, in the therapeutic relationship is counterproductive and is more likely to create client resistance than client change. MI seeks to increase a client's awareness of their problematic behaviour, along with unrecognized strengths and opportunities for change (Miller, 1983b; Rosengren & Wagner, 2001).

Often when a client is asked or commanded to stop drinking or using drugs, the client is being told to give up his or her best friend. As a result, the counsellor should not be surprised by and, in fact, should expect hesitancy from a client who is being asked to give up what can be her or his one great love (and perhaps longest and only love). This ambivalence is the key barrier to change and the counsellor needs to respond by believing that change is possible and by actively and supportively conveying this belief to the client. It is the task of clients rather than counsellors to express and resolve their ambivalence to change. At its core, ambivalence is the basic conflict between the value of continuing to use versus cessation of use, each of which has distinct benefits and costs. The counselling process allows clients to openly articulate this confusion in a non-judgmental environment. The counsellor facilitates an examination of both sides of the ambivalence to guide the client toward action that will lead to positive change (Rollnick & Miller, 1995). During this process, the counsellor must assess the importance of change to the client, the reason behind their planned future actions, and how confident the client is in his or her ability to change. Clients who are uncertain of the importance of change are unlikely to benefit from a counselling process whose emphasis is on how to change. A focus on the reasons to change is irrelevant if the client is not motivated to work toward achieving an outcome (Rollnick, Miller, & Butler, 2008).

Four attributes are specifically stressed in motivational interviewing:

1. *Expression of empathy*: To be successful in motivational interviewing, a counsellor must be able to readily express empathy. This is a critical helping skill, regardless of which counselling approach is employed, entailing the ability to feel what a client feels and see the situation from his or her perspective. Even more importantly, empathy underscores the counsellor's understanding of the client's motives so that new motivational strategies can be utilized in the future. Empathy with a client also sets the stage for a client's acceptance of efforts to facilitate change. Carl Rogers (1959) hypothesized that accurate empathy, congruence, and positive regard are critical therapeutic conditions that create an atmosphere of safety and acceptance in which clients are freed to explore and change. These relational

factors were predicted in and of themselves to provide the foundation to promote and maintain positive change (Miller, 1983a).

2. *Develop discrepancies*: The client always needs to take responsibility for finding reasons to change. However, it is crucial for the counsellor to support this process, particularly early on in counselling. A list of the perceived values of drinking or using drugs in the client's life needs to be contrasted with the behaviours and outcomes of the drug use as compared to what the client wishes for himself or herself. This process, if successful, will unveil some negative insights that the client has not considered or fully recognized previously, and counsellors need to be in a position to support clients as they discuss who the drug use has led them to become. The change process is predicated on clients' ability to perceive the discrepancy between their present behaviour and the important personal goals and values they hold for themselves. A safe environment is a necessity for clients to be able to openly express the discrepancies and often the shortcomings of their lives. It is critical for the counsellor to distinguish for the client between the client and the client's behaviour. Thus, being a person addicted to drugs or a drug user, rather than a drug addict, may appear to be simply semantics, yet it can be critical in helping clients distinguish between themselves and their use of drugs, which is only one component of who they are.

3. *Roll with resistance*: Ambivalence, the hesitancy to change a well-established behaviour, is a normal state for client to experience when they are on the verge of giving up the most important thing in their lives for some uncertain outcome, such as abstinence or a decreased or altered pattern of drug use. Pushing or arguing against resistance is usually quite counterproductive counsellor behaviour, and rather than enhancing the therapeutic alliance a counsellor is attempting to create, it can instead evoke further defensiveness in a client. This, is turn, can further strengthen the client's existing pattern of behaviour. Thus, a guiding principle of MI is to have the client, rather than the counsellor, voice the arguments for change. The counsellor needs to avoid arguing with the client and understand that any new perspectives that the counsellor has to offer need to be invited by the client and not imposed by the clinician. A client's resistance to change is simply an indicator that the counsellor has to switch tactics or the approach and respond in a different manner. If it is not working, the counsellor should try something else; if it is working, the counsellor should do more of the same.

4. *Support self-efficacy*: Belief in the possibility of change is an incredibly important motivator. Thus, not only must the client believe that he or she can change, but so must the counsellor (Figure 4.6, p. 274). Hope, but not false hope, is another critical aspect of this process. The counsellor's belief in the individual's ability to change can become a self-fulfilling prophesy. However, it is always the client and not the counsellor who is responsible for choosing and carrying

out change. Counsellors are responsible for finding factors that motivate a client to change, but it is the client who is ultimately responsible for the change process and the speed of that process (Miller & Rollnick, 1991).

Behaviour change through the use of MI is promoted by supporting clients in verbalizing arguments for change; this is the very simple cognitive concept of "change talk." Encouraging change talk allows clients to openly discuss the new idea and thus think in a new way that is different from how they thought while misusing or abusing drugs. In contrast, "sustain talk," which is typically the conversation that active drug users and drug seekers engage in, favours the status quo and not changing. Proficient use of the techniques of MI will increase clients' in-session change talk and decrease sustain talk, which, in turn, is correlated with the likelihood of changing drug-using behaviours. One of the most important themes of positive self-talk in terms of predicting positive behaviour change is the strength and frequency of commitment language. The strength of expressed desire, ability, reasons, and need for change all positively relate the degree of commitment to change and the ability to move into a stage of contemplation and action within the TTM. Increasing commitment language during counselling sessions is also associated with moving toward abstinence or less frequent use of drugs. However, commitment language that begins high and then decreases or plateaus early in the counselling process is not as strong an indicator of a client's commitment to change as is a slow build-up over time (Miller & Rose, 2009).

As well, when using MI, it is important to whenever possible catch clients doing something right and positively reinforce it, shamelessly if need be. Counsellors should: look for strengths at all times and recognize even small steps that illustrate their ability to change; affirm their hard work and perseverance through the process, ask them to recount their most successful efforts and also their most difficult, and genuinely praise their success; and summarize their progress and look for further evidence that change is possible while still acknowledging, but not dwelling on, difficulties that clients have with the new learning they are experiencing (Miller, 1983b; Miller & Rollnick, 2002, 2009; Moyers, Martin, Manuel, Hendrickson, & Miller, 2005).

What motivational interviewing is not is merely a series of techniques or micro-behaviours linked together. Rather, it is a different philosophy of how clients are viewed and how the process of change is conceptualized. It entails both a relational component, focused on empathy and interpersonal interaction, and a technical component, centred on developing client change talk and implementing the client-generated ideas. This aligns with the knowledge that how counsellors practice is critical to successful client outcomes (Miller & Rose, 2009). Clinicians who were the most successful in producing change in clients were those who captured the spirit of the intent of motivational interviewing, and were adept at the various specific skills. This includes being collaborative rather than authoritarian in their counselling approach, evoking the client's own motivation and motivators rather than applying their own, and respecting the client's autonomy to make his or her own decisions even if the counsellor did not fully agree with them. Decreased use of alcohol as a result of MI has occurred when counsellors demonstrate acceptance with a motivational approach, and elaborated and expanded on the client's comments rather than simply reflecting them back or merely asking more questions (Jensen et al., 2011). Thus, MI involves an active engagement with the client and closely listening and responding to his or her story. All counsellors studied using MI were found to be able to assist already motivated clients to decrease their psychoactive drug use, while those who applied the principles in a consistent manner were also able to assist those who were much more ambivalent about their drug use, who were initially much less motivated to change, and who openly expressed more doubts. A counsellor's belief in the client's ability to change is crucial to the success of MI, as is the ability to engage the client in the change process (Gaume, Gmel, Faouzi, & Daeppen, 2009). Outcome evaluations have consistently demonstrated that motivational interviewing is an effective approach that positively contributes to counselling efforts, though its utility is still dependent on the counsellor's ability to engage the client (Britt, Hudson, & Blampied, 2004; Lundahl, Kunz, Brownell, Tollefson, & Burke, 2010; Vasilaki, Hosier, & Cox, 2006).

BOX 4.1: TOP 10 USEFUL QUESTIONS IN MOTIVATIONAL INTERVIEWING

What changes would you most like to talk about?
What have you noticed about...?
How important is it for you to change...?
How confident do you feel about changing...?
How do you see the benefits of...?
How do you see the drawbacks of...?
What will make the most sense to you?
How might things be different if you...?
In what way....?
Where does this leave you now?

Source: Rollnick, Miller, & Butler (2008)

4.10 MUTUAL AID/SELF-HELP
Overview
Alcoholics Anonymous
Alternatives to 12-Step Groups

> Self-help groups are informal, voluntary, small group structures for mutual aid and the accomplishment of a special purpose. They are usually formed by peers who have come together for mutual assistance in satisfying a common need, overcoming a common life-disruption and bringing about a desired social and/or personal change. The initiators and members of such groups perceive that their needs are not or cannot be met by or through existing societal institutions. Self-help groups emphasize face-to-face social interactions and the assumption of personal responsibility by members. They often provide material assistance, as well as emotional support. (Katz & Bender, 1976, p. 9)

> Self-help may be defined as a process, group or organization comprising people coming together or sharing an experience or problem with a view to individual and/or mutual benefit. As empowerment commonly means "becoming powerful," self-help may thus be viewed as one form of empowerment. (Adams, 1990, p. 1)

Overview
Self-help is an informal method of social support providing informational, effective, and instrumental support. Self-help groups give their members an anchorage, a reference point, companionship, and even a sense of belonging. These groups employ three major ingredients of social learning: (1) instruction, (2) reinforcers, and (3) models (Kurtz & Powell, 1987). Mutual aid is a process in which people who share common experiences, situations, or problems can offer each other a unique perspective that is not available from those who have not shared these incidents (Self-Help Clearinghouse of Toronto, 1991).

The one thing that self-help is not is a unitary phenomenon. It is a professional practice in which the role of consumer is that of producer of service. Self-help is based on the principle of reciprocity—of both giving and taking. A central axiom of self-help is the helper-helpee principle. The foundation of this principle is that the more one helps others, the more the person is helped, and thus those who help most are helped most. Great value is placed on shared experience, with minimal social distance between the helper and helpee. Social support is paramount, as help is not a privilege; rather, it is a right to be shared with others.

Initially new members receive support from other group members. As they discover their own capacity for helping they develop a feeling of equality with other members. By participating in the group they are able to play the role of helper-helpee, a person who, being conscious of his/her own capacities and needs and those of others knows how to give and receive help at the same time. It is through the practice of mutual aid that the self-helper in his helper role is able to accept the person receiving help as a true equal; there is no place for feelings of superiority or inferiority. (Romeder, 1990, p. 32)

Other characteristics commonly associated with mutual aid/self-help groups include the following:

- free membership and participation
- the voluntary nature of all activities
- a not-for-profit approach, with members controlling all resources
- the lack of financial support from external sources
- a membership based on individual circumstances and situations
- the structuring of meetings for mutual benefit of those participating
- a constructive action toward shared goals
- an egalitarian philosophy, including a belief in participatory and not just representative democracy
- equality of status and power within the group
- shared leadership and co-operation in decision making
- groups are member-led and organized
- a lack of reliance on professional helpers
- individual decision making by each member, with the group as a whole responsible for its own decisions
- the confidential nature of groups' proceedings
- participants move toward improving control over their own circumstances, and giving themselves more control over their own lives
- a general avoidance of hierarchical and bureaucratic patterns of organization
- a lack of importance of outside societal status within group proceedings; instead status is conferred by personal involvement in the group (Adams, 1990; Gartner & Riessman, 1977; Katz & Bender, 1976; Pape, 1990; Silverman, 1980)

Self-help has become a recognized process to deal with all types of problems in a setting where members are treated as equals. It entails openness, informality, friendliness, and getting involved as the norm (Hill, 1983). Professional service providers may participate in the self-help process at the request and sanction of the group but usually remain in an ancillary or consultative role. Self-help has no pre-appointed hours. Many groups operate so that if there is no formal meeting, there is a contact person or personal buddy or sponsor to call. Self-helpers are not separated by education, class, or experience (Robinson & Henry, 1977). Typically, persons join self-help groups to overcome feelings of rejection, isolation, and powerlessness and to break free of societal stereotypes. However, in many groups, members must identify themselves as having a specific problem, with many of these problems being compulsive behaviours (Katz & Bender 1976). Gartner and Riessman (1977) claim that one of the most significant characteristics of mutual-aid groups is that they are empowering and thus potentially de-alienating. They are empowering as they allow members to feel that they have greater control over their lives. To move from an external to internal locus of control is a significant achievement, but whether this affects the distribution of power in the community or society remains in question.

Katz and Bender (1976) proposed a variety of typologies in attempting to classify the myriad of self-help groups:

1. (a) self-fulfilment or personal growth (Recovery Inc.)
   (b) social advocacy (National Welfare Rights Organization)
   (c) alternative patterns of living or solidarity (women's groups)
   (d) outcast havens (X-Kalay)
2. (a) groups conforming to society's norms; also know as self-reforming (Alcoholics Anonymous)
   (b) groups wishing to reform society (gay and lesbian rights groups)
3. (a) inner-focused (Parents Without Partners)
   (b) outer-focused (wishing to change public policies) (Fortune Society)
4. (a) anonymous groups (Alcoholics, Gamblers, Overeaters)
   (b) living with groups (Cystic Fibrosis, Cerebral Palsy)
   (c) life transition groups (widows' support groups)
5. (a) rehabilitative (Stroke Club, United Ostomy Association)
   (b) behaviour change (Narcotics Anonymous)
   (c) primary care (disease where there is no cure but care is required) (Arthritis Association, Diabetes Association)

What becomes evident from the creation of this typology is that a myriad of self-help programs exist for a variety of different purposes.

Adams (1990) discussed four perspectives that attempted to explain the growth of self-help/mutual aid:

1. *Traditionalist*: A conservative view of history that claims that self-help has existed since humans first lived together. All that the 20th century introduced was a focus away from economic issues and toward deviance and problem-solving groups.

2. *Functionalist*: This viewpoint regards self-help as an automatic response to a changing society. It arises naturally between gaps left by existing services and complements other types of helping and social support. It is an inevitable consequence of the inability or unwillingness of the state, professionals, and agencies to meet needs.
3. *Liberal*: The liberal perspective claims that self-help is an alternative to existing forms of professional helping and grows because need is inadequately or incorrectly met, rather than because it is unmet.
4. *Radical*: Self-help is a response to widespread alienation in society and acts by fulfilling many of people's affiliation and identity needs. Negative consequences of industrialization and urbanization that are associated with the decline in the extended family have led to the rapid growth of self-help groups. Mutual aid has also grown because of rapid technological development, depersonalized and dehumanized institutions and the alienation of people from communities, institutions, and each other.

Hoehne (1988) attempted to explain the growth of self-help in North America as the consequence of four critical factors:

1. the fiscal crisis of the state leading to cutbacks in volume and quality of the services provided by governments at a time when demographic trends are leading to an increase of sectors of the population that are the most dependent on government services (unemployed, working poor, homeless, single-parent families)
2. a rise in the proportion of chronic diseases due to increasing life spans
3. the erosion of the traditional extended family network
4. health care and social service systems that are still rooted in 19th century models

Hoehne (1988) claimed that increasing self-help use equates to deficiencies in existing health care and social service systems. While health problems are seen as individual problems, social problems are individual only in their consequences; in their causes, they are collective. However, the state still tends to equate social problems with each individual's shortcomings. Social self-help groups pose a greater threat to the legitimization efforts of governments than do health-focused self-help groups. By becoming organized, those involved in social self-help groups take the first step in countering the "blaming the victim" strategy of the ruling ideology. Thus, government funding is primarily targeted to groups that have cost-cutting goals and seek to legitimize the status quo, rather than to those advocating for system change.

While having great potential, self-help groups are no panacea. Their proliferation needs to be examined in context. The availability of self-help can be used to justify the curtailing of services, with the risk of poorer clients being shunted off to self-help groups while more affluent individuals receive professional services. Self-help groups can also become the dumping grounds of professionals whose clients' problems are hard to resolve, or for cases where insurance and/or employer-financed counselling conclude yet more assistance is required. Self-help can thus become an inappropriate referral, replacing required professional interventions. Self-help groups focused solely on client-centred approaches tend to de-emphasize larger societal issues and take pressure off the need for societal changes. The issue of hitting rock bottom before becoming better, associated with anonymous groups, can create even poorer self-esteem and self-image in some participants. An overemphasis on self can lead to escapism and narcissism, with the potential to foster dependence and the need for a life-long commitment instead of a focus on getting better, or moving forward, for some. Those attending meetings may be able to participate but not necessarily obtain assistance. Self-help groups have also been called limiting because they only examine issues at the symptom level, looking at small-scale solutions and providing only marginal alternatives to existing systems (Gartner & Riessman, 1977). Nonetheless, in the United States alone, more than 5 million people attend addiction-related self-help groups (SAMHSA, 2008).

Alcoholics Anonymous

The initial and most prominent form of mutual aid/self-help in the addiction field has been, and remains, Alcoholics Anonymous (AA). Alcoholics Anonymous is not a treatment modality, though it remains an excellent relapse-prevention resource (Clark, 1995). When AA arose, the moral model was the prevalent attitude toward persons who were misusing and abusing alcohol. Thus, during the initial development of the AA model, alcohol-dependent persons concealed their problem because of the stigma and oppression associated with alcohol abuse.

AA consists of men and women who are recovering from alcohol abuse, and who provide help to other active users as one of the key steps in maintaining their own sobriety and contentment. This informal banding together rests on a cornerstone of common experience. The members seek to promote, through continuing support, the hope and determination of each other to achieve and maintain the sobriety on which they believe their recovery depends. Non-political, non-sectarian, and non-reformist in any way, AA neither espouses nor opposes any cause or movement. It exacts no dues and imposes no assessments. Each group supports itself by means of voluntary contributions within its own community and is loosely associated with other similar groups (Alcoholics Anonymous, 1976).

The AA program is based on the 12 suggested steps and on the 12 traditions. They embody the thinking and beliefs regarding the functioning of an individual in the program, and the functioning of AA as a unique fellowship and method of mutual aid. The following are the 12 suggested steps of Alcoholics Anonymous:

1. We admitted we were powerless over alcohol—that our lives had become unmanageable.
2. Came to believe that a Power greater than ourselves could restore us to sanity.
3. Made a decision to turn our will and our lives over to the care of God as we understood Him.
4. Made a searching and fearless moral inventory of ourselves.
5. Admitted to God, to ourselves and to another human being the exact nature of our wrongs.
6. Were entirely ready to have God remove all these defects of character.
7. Humbly asked Him to remove our shortcomings.
8. Made a list of all persons we had harmed and became willing to make amends to them all.
9. Made direct amends to such people wherever possible, except when to do so would injure them or others.
10. Continued to take personal inventory and when we were wrong, promptly admitted it.
11. Sought through prayer and meditation to improve our conscious contact with God as we understood Him, praying only for knowledge of His will for us and the power to carry that out.
12. Having had a spiritual awakening as the result of these steps, we tried to carry this message to alcoholics and to practice these principles in all our affairs.

The 12 AA traditions are:

1. Our common welfare should come first; personal recovery depends upon AA unity.
2. For our group purpose there is but one ultimate authority—a loving God as He may express Himself in our group conscience. Our leaders are but trusted servants; they do not govern.
3. The only requirement for AA membership is a desire to stop drinking.
4. Each group should be autonomous except in matters affecting other groups or AA as a whole.
5. Each group has but one primary purpose—to carry its message to the alcoholic who still suffers.
6. An AA group ought never endorse, finance or lend the AA name to any related facility or outside enterprise lest problems of money, property and prestige divert us from our primary purpose.
7. Every AA group ought to be fully self-supporting, declining outside contributions.
8. Alcoholics Anonymous should remain forever non-professional, but our service centers may employ special workers.
9. AA, as such, ought never be organized; but we may create service boards or committees directly responsible to those they serve.

10. Alcoholics Anonymous has no opinion on outside issues; hence the AA name ought never be drawn into public controversy.
11. Our public relations policy is based on attraction rather than promotion; we need always maintain personal anonymity at the level of press, radio and films.
12. Anonymity is the spiritual foundation of all our Traditions, ever reminding us to place principles before personalities (Alcoholics Anonymous, 1976).

Underpinning AA's 12 steps and 12 traditions is a strong spiritual dimension. For many members, this is a mechanism that allows them to think about and envision a future that does not involve alcohol use (Timmons, 2010). Attending AA meetings is also intended to address core issues in the emotional growth of the alcohol-dependent person. Telling and understanding one's life story, repairing past misdeeds, recognizing and correcting false beliefs and cognitive distortions, and shifting focus from unhealthy rumination to a consideration of appropriate actions are fundamental issues that participation is intended to address. The emphasis on humbling oneself is premised on the belief that alcohol-dependent persons are, at their core, narcissists and that their self-absorption does not allow them to earnestly address their alcohol misuse. Narcissists so love themselves that they cannot love others. Thus, in addressing this character flaw, AA allows individuals to open themselves up emotionally to others (Sachs, 2009).

Though it inspires worldwide acclaim and great enthusiasm among many North American alcoholism treatment personnel, AA lacks universal support for its efficacy and is viewed as rigid by some. Responses to this rigidity can be found in specific adaptions of the 12 steps and traditions, such as a First Nations adaption, the 12 Steps of Walking the Red Road (White Bison, 2002):

1. We admitted we were powerless over alcohol—that we had lost control of our lives.
2. We came to believe that a power greater than ourselves could help us gain control.
3. We made a decision to ask for help from a higher power and others who understand.
4. We stopped and thought about our strengths and our weaknesses and thought about ourselves.
5. We admitted to the Great Spirit, to ourselves and to another person the things we thought were wrong about ourselves.
6. We are ready, with the help of the Great Spirit, to change.
7. We humbly ask a Higher Power and our friends to help us change.
8. We made a list of people who were hurt by our drinking and want to make up for these hurts.
9. We are making up to those people whenever we can, except when to do so would hurt them more.

10. We continue to think about our strengths and weaknesses when we are wrong and we say so.
11. We pray and think about ourselves, praying only for strength to do what is right.
12. We try to help other alcoholics and to practise these principles in everything we do.

Likewise, a Millati Islami version of the 12 steps has emerged, based on Islamic principles:

1. We admitted that we were neglectful of our higher selves and that our lives have become unmanageable.
2. We came to believe that Allah could and would restore us to sanity.
3. We made a decision to submit our will to the will of Allah.
4. We made a searching and fearless moral inventory of ourselves.
5. We admitted to Allah and to ourselves the exact nature of our wrongs.
6. Asking Allah for right guidance, we became willing and open for change, ready to have Allah remove our defects of character.
7. We humbly ask Allah to remove our shortcomings.
8. We made a list of persons we have harmed and became willing to make amends to them all.
9. We made direct amends to such people wherever possible, except when to do so would injure them or others.
10. We continued to take personal inventory and when we were wrong promptly admitted it.
11. We sought through Salaat (a prayer service) and Iqraa (reading and studying) to improve our understanding of Taqwa (proper love and respect for Allah) and Ihsan ("though we cannot see Allah, He does see us").
12. Having increased our level of Iman (faith) and Taqwa, as a result of applying these steps, we carried this message to humanity and began practising these principles in all our affairs (Millati Islami World Services, 2010a).

The 12 traditions of Millati Islami are:

1. Shahadah—We bear witness that there is no God but Allah, and Muhammed is the last messenger of Allah.
2. Personal recovery depends upon Millati Islami unity. Believers are friends and protectors of one another.
3. For our individual and Jamaat (group) purpose there is but one ultimate authority which is Allah (God, the source from which all originates).
4. Requirements for participation are a desire to stop using and willingness to learn a better way of life.

5. Each Jamaat (group) should be autonomous except in their adherence to these traditions.
6. Our primary Jamaat (group) purpose is carrying out Al-Islam as the message of recovery to those who still suffer (Dawah).
7. Problems of money, property, and prestige must never divert us from our primary purpose.
8. Every Millati Islami Jamaat (group) should be self supporting but may accept sadaqa (voluntary charity) without attached obligations or promises to donating parties.
9. We may create service boards and committees directly responsible to those we serve.
10. The Millati Islami name aught never be drawn into public controversy.
11. Our public relations policy is based upon attraction before promotion. The criterion for both are decided by Jamaat (group), Taqwa, and Ihsan.
12. Iman (faith) is the spiritual foundation of all our traditions, reminding us to place principles before personalities (Millati Islami World Services, 2010b).

AA has grown from an organization of two in the 1930s to one that boasts millions of members globally. It has been incorporated into many treatment programs in both the United States and Canada (MacMaster, 2004). Despite its shortcomings, it remains a widely used resource because it is well known, inexpensive to join, accepting and tolerant of new members, open to everyone, and teaches by example. AA appears to be most effective for a specific subpopulation, though recent research has shown that it benefits non-traditional members as well (Csiernik, 2002). However, it should not be considered a remedy for all issues pertaining to alcohol misuse and abuse, nor for all issues persons in recovery face.

Alternatives to 12-Step Groups

As a response to concerns with the structure and message of 12-step groups, such as Alcoholics Anonymous, Narcotics Anonymous, Cocaine Anonymous, and even Nicotine Anonymous, other forms of addiction-specific mutual aid/self-help groups have arisen.

Women For Sobriety (WFS)

Women For Sobriety is an organization comprised of self-help support groups for women with a dependency on alcohol. It was founded to meet the recovery needs specific to women drinkers and may be viewed as both an alternative to AA and as a complement to it, depending on the comfort level a woman has with the original 12-step program. Women For Sobriety was founded in 1975 by Jean Kirkpatrick and was influenced by a mix of the medical model with feminist principles. WFS encourages women to take charge of their alcoholism and embark on a path of self-awareness, as alcohol-dependent women have fundamentally different needs in recovery than men. Interestingly, Men For Sobriety (MFS) groups have emerged due to the success of WFS and in response to the limits of AA.

Four central themes form the foundation of Women For Sobriety:

1. No drinking
2. Positive thinking
3. Believing one is competent
4. Growing spiritually and emotionally

While still premised on the overly rudimentary disease model, WFS differs from Alcoholics Anonymous. Rather than moving toward God for help in overcoming the compulsive use of alcohol, women are asked to discover why they initially became so dependent. Participants are helped to become self-empowered and to change their thinking. Lapses are more tolerated in WFS, with no need to begin again at day one of sobriety. Openly talking to other members during meetings is allowed, unlike in 12-step groups that have "no crosstalk" rules. Another significant difference is in the greeting. Rather than announcing and labelling oneself as an alcoholic, members introduce themselves by stating, "Hi, I'm ———, and I'm a competent woman." There is no emphasis on reducing ego or on being humble. For most women with an alcohol problem, there is a need for empowerment and increasing their self-worth (Kaskutas, 1989). The 13 affirmations of WFS are:

1. I have a life-threatening problem that once had me.
2. Negative emotions destroy only myself.
3. Happiness is a habit I will develop.
4. Problems bother me only to the degree I permit them to.
5. I am what I think.
6. Life can be ordinary or it can be great.
7. Love can change the course of my world.
8. The fundamental object of life is emotional and spiritual growth.
9. The past is gone forever.
10. All love given returns.
11. Enthusiasm is my daily exercise.
12. I am a competent woman and have much to give others.
13. I am responsible for myself and for my sisters.

SMART Recovery: Self Management and Recovery Training
SMART Recovery, which began in 1994, consists of facilitator-led, structured peer discussion groups that are premised on CBT counselling techniques. SMART Recovery was founded by Joe Gerstein, an American clinical professor

of medicine, to counter the myth that addiction is a disease that leaves its victims powerless and needing to stay in permanent recovery. Instead, Gerstein used rational emotive behaviour therapy (REBT) as the foundation for this form of mutual aid. Rather than steps, SMART Recovery is premised on a four-point program and a tool box that supports the framework:

1. Building and Maintaining Motivation
2. Coping with Urges
3. Managing Thoughts, Feelings and Behaviors
4. Living a Balanced Life (SMART Recovery, 2015)

All meetings are open, welcome both men and women, and last approximately 90 minutes. Participation is voluntary, and any member may choose not to contribute on the topic being discussed. Unlike Alcoholics Anonymous, SMART Recovery focuses on self-empowerment rather than surrendering to a higher power, believing that human beings have the capacity within themselves to overcome even severe addiction. SMART teaches participants how to disrupt their irrational belief system by helping them understand why they act as they do and then challenge that thinking. Unlike 12-step groups, cross-talk is permitted after the initial group check-in. Members are also encouraged to openly discuss lapses and relapses to help both the individual and the group understand what triggered the event and how to better respond in the future. Individuals who have been using may attend meetings but are asked to observe rather than actively participate. Members are invited to stay involved with the group after gaining independence but are not expected to attend indefinitely—in SMART Recovery, the end goal is to become recovered. In a pilot project in England, results from six SMART groups indicated that this mutual aid group addressed service gaps. It serves as a valuable alternative to AA while also being extremely cost-effective (MacGregor & Herring, 2010).

Secular Organization for Sobriety (SOS)

The Secular Organization for Sobriety was founded by Jim Christopher in 1985 in Hollywood, California, as an alternative recovery method for either alcohol- or drug-dependent persons who were uncomfortable with the spiritual component of 12-step self-help groups. SOS, which is also called "Save Our Selves" by participants, takes a secular approach to recovery and maintains that sobriety is a distinct issue from either spirituality or religion. The credit for recovery, as in WFS and SMART Recovery, belongs to the individual, without reliance on a higher power. SOS supports healthy skepticism and encourages the use of the scientific method to understand alcoholism. SOS also attracts members who wish to separate their recovery from their religious affiliation. Members are welcome to attend both SOS and traditional AA- or NA-type meetings, however, if it assists in their recovery (White, 2012).

SOS groups, whose members now number over 100,000 in North America, encourage those who attend meetings to acknowledge that they are alcohol- or drug-dependent and that abstinence is their only solution. SOS maintains that members have the ability to obtain a better quality of life only by abstaining, and they are asked to resolve not to drink or drug regardless of circumstances, feelings, or conflicts. Groups tend to consist of 20 members who take turns acting as the moderator, with new members being asked to attend once per week for six months and as needed after that for booster meetings (Secular Organization for Sobriety, 2014).

The following are the SOS Suggested Guidelines for Sobriety:

- To break the cycle of denial and achieve sobriety, we first acknowledge that we are alcoholics or addicts.
- We affirm this truth daily and accept without reservation—one day at a time—that as clean and sober individuals, we cannot and do not drink or use, no matter what.
- Since drinking or using is not an option for us, we take whatever steps are necessary to continue our Sobriety Priority lifelong.
- A quality of life, "the good life," can be achieved. However, life is also filled with uncertainties. Therefore, we do not drink or use regardless of feelings, circumstances, or conflicts.
- We share in confidence with each other our thoughts and feelings as sober, clean individuals.
- Sobriety is our Priority, and we are each responsible for our lives and our sobriety.

Rational Recovery (RR)

Rational Recovery describes itself as a mutual aid group for self-empowered recovery from substance dependency. RR, founded in 1986, views addiction as primarily a behavioural problem. It is affiliated with the American Humanist Association and also with the principles of Albert Ellis's rational emotive behaviour therapy (REBT). It has its own guidebook, written by Jack Trimpey, entitled *The Small Book*. In RR members learn that their use of alcohol and other drugs is an irrational choice. They also learn to listen, hear, and resist their internal irrational "Beast," a voice that urges them to drink and use. Rational Recovery believes in self-mastery rather than self-surrender, and is popular with those who have trouble or no interest in grasping the intent of a higher power, which is the foundation of the 12-step philosophy. Rational Recovery is described as a task-centred self-help group where one can totally recover (Self-Help Canada, 1992). RR believes in empowering members and Trimpey (1992) stated that Rational Recovery does not believe in the one-day-at-a-time philosophy, as this keeps the idea of drinking constantly before oneself, which reinforces one's lack of power. In Rational Recovery, to be successful is to be powerful, and in creating a state of mind for success, in creating motivation, guilt is the least effective of all mechanisms.

Moderation Management (MM)

Moderation Management is a support group for problem drinkers who wish to reduce their drinking and make other positive lifestyle changes. The group advocates a minimum 30 days of abstinence, followed by a personal assessment that assists the person to select either an abstinence or harm-reduction approach. Among proponents of this model are Frederick Glasser and Stanton Peele (Kishline, 1994).

Moderation Management (2014) provides a professionally reviewed nine-step program with information about moderate drinking guidelines and limits, exercises to monitor one's drinking, goal-setting techniques, and related self-management strategies. The goal of MM is to assist members in finding balance in their lives. This self-help group is not intended for those who have a significant physical or psychological dependency on alcohol, but rather for moderate drinkers who feel that alcohol is becoming too prominent in their lives. MM believes that people can change their behaviours and that a moderation-training program is effective for problem drinkers. Moderation Management is a non-disease model that believes in empowering participants and having members take personal responsibility for their own behaviour.

The nine steps toward moderation and balance are as follows:

1. Attend meetings and learn about the program of Moderation Management. For those who do not want to go to a support group, the program can be followed without attending meetings.
2. Abstain from alcoholic beverages for 30 days and complete steps three through six during this time.
3. Examine how drinking has affected your life.
4. Write down your priorities.
5. Take a look at how much, how often, and under what circumstances you used to drink.
6. Learn the MM guidelines and limits for moderate drinking. This information is provided at meetings and in MM literature.
7. Set moderate drinking limits and start weekly small steps toward positive lifestyle changes.
8. Review your progress and update your goals.
9. Continue to make positive lifestyle changes, attend meetings for ongoing encouragement and support, and help newcomers to the group.

4.11 INTERNET COUNSELLING

The emergence of Internet-based counselling and treatment modalities did not occur because existing treatment options have not been effective. Rather, Internet counselling offers another entry point, allowing counsellors to overcome some of the challenges associated with access and availability. It may be preferred by clients who are geographically isolated and cannot readily meet with an addiction specialist; who are experiencing the stigma and shame that is still associated with accessing addiction services; or who seek to benefit from the increased confidentiality and flexibility associated with Web-based modalities (Campbell et al., 2014; Moore, Fazzino, Garnet, Cutter, & Barry, 2011). The majority of Internet-based programs that have emerged over the past decade were tailored for alcohol abuse (Bewick et al., 2008; Campbell et al., 2014). However, as a treatment category, there is great heterogeneity in what Internet counselling entails, with substantial variation among the types of programs provided online. The quality of information, length, number of sessions or modules, and type of professional involvement, if any, all vary significantly (Moore et al., 2011). There is also variation in the amount of psycho-education versus direct counsellor interactivity, as well as in counsellor qualifications. Prior to the proliferation of digital media, interactive voice response systems via regular telephone were commonly used (Hall & Huber, 2000). These systems were gradually replaced with preprogrammed Web-based modules, but there was concern about how compatible these were with the fluctuating nature of addiction symptom severity (McKay, 2005). The alternative method provides real-time therapist involvement, and, indeed, this was demonstrated to be the superior approach (Spek et al., 2007). However, as with in-person counselling, drop out still remains an issue (King, Brooner, Peirce, Kolodner, & Kidorf, 2014).

Internet-based counselling is popular in addiction practice because of the cost of, and often time-limited resources for, individual counselling. This is also why group counselling is offered in place of individual treatment. Though additional counselling hours or more intensive services are required to encourage success (McLellan, Arndt, Metzger, Woody, & O'Brien, 1993), many clients may also be deterred by the increased frequency and perceived intrusiveness of attending in person (King et al., 2009). The first published evaluation of Internet-based counselling compared intensive, real-time therapy using video conferencing with traditional face-to-face counselling and found similar, if not superior, satisfaction by participants using the Internet option (King et al., 2009). Similarly, a randomized controlled trial found that problem drinkers engaged with a counsellor using text and chat formats had better outcomes than those who used a purely automated response, decreasing their alcohol intake by two-thirds more (Blankers, Koeter, & Scippers, 2011).

The use of Internet-based counselling, especially programs with direct therapist involvement, continues to gain legitimacy through positive outcome evaluations, client satisfaction reports, and lower costs, particularly when treating uncomplicated substance use and related problems (Gainsbury & Blaszcynski, 2011). As well, individuals can find a multitude of mutual aid groups online. The same issues regarding quality, however, pertain to self-help groups as to professional counselling. It is important to note that adopting purely Internet-based modalities would not support individuals of lower socio-economic status who may not have access to high-quality, if any, Internet service. This would also extend to clients with learning difficulties, who may be deterred by the technical skill required to operate a computer (King et al., 2009).

4.12 CONCLUSION

While there is no one perfect treatment approach, and controversy remains among treatment professionals regarding which method is "best," addiction treatment in general does produce positive outcomes, both for individuals and society (Babor & Del Boca, 2002). Studies from the United States (Ettner et al., 2006; Lipton, 1995; McCarty, 2008) and the United Kingdom (Davies, Jones, Vamvakas, Dubourg, & Donmall, 2009; UKATT Research Team, 2005) have indicated that individuals receiving treatment not only get better, but also that the economic returns are five to seven times greater than the cost of providing treatment (McCollister & French, 2003). As well, the average cost of treatment, even in the United States (with its private health care model) and now in Canada (with its drift away from universal health care for addiction treatment toward more privatized care providers), is less costly than acute hospital care, incarceration of users, and placing children in foster care (National Treatment Agency, 2012).

No single counselling method has been found to be universally successful in the treatment of those misusing or abusing psychoactive substances, though in each study, counselling was superior to no treatment. For many, a combination of several types of counselling will be more successful than recourse to any one alone. Two things are certain: that the therapy employed must be tailored to meet the specific needs of each individual, and that no client should be forced into a particular type of therapy simply because of the counsellor's convenience or prejudicial choice. The following critical factors should always be considered:

- the client choosing to enter treatment with an expectation of being helped to change his or her behaviour, thus having the motivation to change
- the credibility of the technique being used to both the therapist and the client
- consistent application of an empirically proven technique
- the ability to create optimism for a successful outcome
- the ability to create a foundation so that change may occur
- clinician discretion, flexibility, and emotional support
- the ability of the counsellor to create a supportive environment

Regardless of which approach one uses, it should always be consistently applied and client-centred so that the focus is on the individual in relation to her or his needs and wants, both perceived and actual (Imel, Wampold, Miller, & Fleming, 2008; Magill & Ray, 2009; Wampold et al., 1997).

Decades of research indicate that the actual intervention employed, while important, is far less vital than the process (Smedslund et al., 2011). In reviewing established alcohol treatment approaches, it was discovered that the therapeutic intervention alone was not solely critical, rather, so were the process and attributes associated with any empirically supported initiative. The counsellor-client relationship, client expectation, model employed, and other extra-therapeutic variables (or factors), such as the client's attributes, social system and social environment, and the treatment environment, all contributed (Figure 4.6). The therapist's personality, background, and understanding and patience all play significant roles in the success of the treatment, as the better the reported relationship at all stages of therapy, the better the outcome for the client and the client system. As well, rather than the type of treatment, the therapist's capacity to structure the treatment matters more. Regardless of the method or model used, if the client feels heard and supported, the treatment outcome is more likely to be positive for hope, and bringing hope is a critical part of the counselling process (Koehn, O'Neill, & Sherry, 2012). What the client expects, believes, and wants to happen in treatment contributes to its final outcome. Research indicates that what motivates people to change is positive, not negative, thoughts. The more one focuses on problems, the more stuck one feels. It is hope that causes people to change, not the pain of addiction or the losses it brings to them. Most critical, and reinforcing of the need to view addiction through a bio-psycho-social lens, is that other extra-therapeutic factors account for the greatest proportion of change. This includes all aspects of the client and his or her environment that facilitate recovery, including social support and social capital. Thus, to provide the best client-centred care, environmental factors must be considered and responded to in the counselling process. Effective addiction counselling can no longer consider only the individual but must always look at the person-in-environment (Hubble, Duncan, Miller, & Wampold, 2010; Magill, 2015), for you cannot treat an empty chair.

FIGURE 4.6: CONTRIBUTING FACTORS TO POSITIVE COUNSELLING OUTCOME

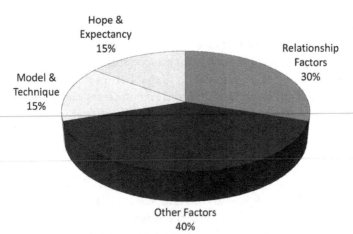

Source: Adapted from Hubble, Duncan, Miller, & Wampold (2010)

DISCUSSION QUESTIONS

1. Compare and contrast harm reduction with self-help. What are the major differences and similarities between these two approaches?
2. (a) As an addiction counsellor, which of the different treatment approaches do you think would be most effective in your practice?
   (b) What attracts you to those approaches?
   (c) What evidence informs your decision of the usefulness of these approaches?
3. Of the various treatment options listed, which do you think is the single strongest and the single weakest? What leads you to those choices? What factors did you consider? How much emphasis did you place on outcome studies versus your own experience?
4. What are the advantages of using the Transtheoretical Model of Change as the foundation for your counselling practice?
5. How does Motivational Interviewing differ from other counselling approaches that did not originate in the addiction field?
6. What role do you see Internet counselling having in the addiction field?
7. How will you use self-help groups as part of your practice as a counsellor?
8. What are the implications of Hubble, Duncan, Miller, and Wampold's (2010) findings on the way we should conduct counselling in the addiction field?

Chapter 5
TREATMENT RESOURCES

The implications are glaringly obvious; we do not provide adequate services for individuals with addiction issues. As a community we need to begin by identifying the individuals needing treatment in our schools, churches, workplace, hospitals, and families, we need to lobby the government for increased funding for addiction related programming, and shore up gaps in services and reduce wait times.
—2008 Annual Report of the Office of the
Auditor General of Ontario

Alcohol and other psychoactive drug abuse treatment is delivered by a diverse network of programs with administrative and fiscal linkages to government ministries, public institutions, private organizations, and lay groups. The Canadian federal government is responsible for dealing with addiction on two fronts. First, it has a direct responsibility for specific groups of Canadians: military personnel and veterans, federal penitentiaries inmates, the RCMP, and Canadian First Nations and Innu. Second, it is responsible for providing a national strategy for dealing with addiction, including transferring funds to provincial governments for data collection, research, and treatment (Kirby, 2004). The actual treatment of addiction in North America was initially organized and governed by groups of lay persons in recovery who were responding to the blatant neglect by helping professionals to this area of practice. By 1955, only 20 alcoholism treatment centres existed in all of Canada (Green, 1980). Prior to then, treatment was dominated by the moral model, with only a few psychiatric facilities or prison-based opioid-related programs in existence. Physicians were often forced to admit alcohol-dependent persons under false pretenses to get them any type of hospital care. The middle of the 20th century was dominated by the influence of Alcoholics Anonymous, with federal and provincial efforts leading to the development of treatment systems loosely connected to the health care system (Room, Stoduto, Demers, Ogborne, & Giesbrecht, 2006). This began to change during the 1970s, when both public agencies and private insurance companies began to recognize the need for formal treatment programming based on humanitarian and fiscal grounds. In Canada, nearly 300 specialized addiction services were established during the first half of the 1970s, with expenditure on treatment services growing from $14 million to $70 million. In 1978 the government of British Columbia legislated the first mandatory treatment in Canada with Bill 18, the Heroin Treatment Act, stating that compulsory treatment for heroin abusers was justified on economic grounds. This initial professionalization of the addiction field partially replaced the dominant role played by those using AA recovery principles as their foundation for helping. Tension grew between those with more formal post-secondary education and those with personal recovery histories who had been the primary helping resource in Canada for decades (Kirby, 2004; Rush & Ogborne, 1992)

The 1980s were marked by the specialization and diversification of services, and the beginning of a research-informed approach. The War on Drugs mentality of the era, though, stymied some of the empirically based ideas regarding treatment system development. With the emergence of AIDS and the fear that first accompanied HIV, another struggle arose between those supporting an abstinence-only approach and the often vocal advocates of nascent harm-reduction-focused organizations to deliver services to those with addiction issues (Roberts, Ogborne, Leigh, & Adam, 1999).

The economic downturn of the 1990s saw the consolidation and integration of programs and the slow emergence of two-tier addiction care. For-profit agencies were established and existing residential programs were no longer being fully funded, allowing those who could pay the full cost of care to no longer wait to receive treatment. A greater emphasis on neurobiological research in this century has contributed to a renewed interested in the pharmacological treatment of drug use. By 2002, an estimated $1.2 billion of funding was being allocated to specialized addiction treatment programs across Canada, with another $3.5 billion being directed toward medical and social issues arising from addiction (National Treatment Strategy Working Group, 2008; O'Connell, 2002).

Research and experience have shown that a continuum of care (Figure 5.1) is needed to serve the spectrum of drug-dependency-related problems (Csiernik, 2002, 2010; Csiernik & Troller, 2002). Both community- and institutional-based programs are needed, as are programs that serve specific groups such as women, youth, minority populations, and persons with concurrent disorders, though cost restraints continue to impede the growth of programs. Despite a demonstrated need, funding for new addiction facilities is slow to come, particularly for residential programming. In 2012 the Canadian Community Health Survey reported that 4.4 percent of Canadians met the criteria for a substance-use disorder. However, data collected by the National Treatment Indicators (NTI) project found that just over 150,000 Canadians accessed publicly funded treatment services. This number represents approximately 0.4 percent of Canadians ages 15 and older. Thus, a substantive gap exists between the number of Canadians with substance-use problems and those actually receiving treatment.

Table 5.1 presents an overview of the various government-funded components of the continuum of care. By far, non-residential treatment is the most prominent location for receiving assistance. However, there are no estimates of the number of individuals seeking assistance independently in fee-for-services programs, some of which remain totally unregulated. The 2008, the Office of the Auditor General of Ontario reported that adults seeking treatment could wait from a low of one day to a high of 189 days for an initial assessment, with the average being 24 days. Youths seeking help for substance abuse could wait from a low of one day to a high of 210 days for an initial assessment; their average wait time was 26 days. Adults seeking residential treatment could wait from seven to 340 days, with an average wait of 62 days.

FIGURE 5.1: ADDICTION TREATMENT CONTINUUM OF CARE

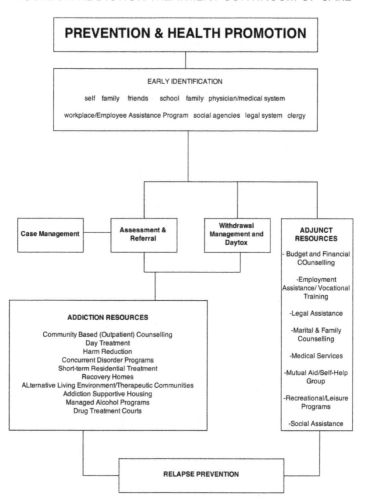

TABLE 5.1: OVERVIEW OF TREATMENT IN CANADA PROVIDED THROUGH GOVERNMENT-FUNDED PROGRAMS, 2011–2012

Jurisdiction	Population	Individuals Seeking Treatment	Issue					
			Residential Withdrawal Management (Detox)	Non-Residential Withdrawal Management (Daytox)	Non-Residential Treatment	Residential Treatment	Impaired Driving Program	Episodes where individuals were seeking treatment for family
Newfoundland & Labrador	526,900	1,223	334	n/a	1,789	209	79	93
Prince Edward Island	145,300	3,110	609	550	1,076	132	nr	180
Nova Scotia	944,800	7,400	1,116	287	5,408	147	1,309	459
New Brunswick	756,800	5,780	2,032	n/a	4,528	322	1,220	nr
Ontario	13,410,100	70,319	16,799	1,550	55,868	8,763	nr	5,555
Manitoba	1,250,500	10,900	1,027	n/a	7,998	2,444	1,588	1,337
Saskatchewan	1,087,300	15,240	3	297	11,755	1,666	3,755	1,316
Alberta	3,888,600	34,213	5,318	n/a	26,839	2,077	nr	4,861
Yukon	36,200	891	323	n/a	1,517	133	nr	nr

n/a = service not available

nr = not reported

Source: Canadian Centre on Substance Abuse (2014a)

5.1 ENTRY INTO THE ADDICTION CONTINUUM OF CARE
Assessment and Referral
Case Management
Withdrawal Management Services: Daytox and Detox

Assessment and Referral

Once an individual has been identified as having a substance abuse problem, the depth and breadth of the situation needs to be determined. Assessment and referral agencies provide services that use specific instruments and processes to determine the major issues, as well as the strengths and supports of the person with a substance issue. These agencies develop individualized plans for assistance, involving referral to other organizations for more intensive or residential treatment. A standardized assessment procedure can take anywhere from 2 to 3 hours to complete. While there is no national consensus on what constitutes comprehensive assessment, the Province of Ontario has developed a standardized assessment package for use by all assessment services. The package consists of seven core valid and reliable instruments: Drug History Questionnaire (DHQ), Adverse Consequences (AC), Stages of Change Readiness and Treatment Eagerness Scale (SOCRATES), Treatment Entry Questionnaire (TEQ), Drug Taking Confidence Questionnaire (DTCQ-8), Behavior and Symptom Identification Scale (BASIS-32), and Perceived Social Support. An assessment typically includes a history of the use of alcohol and other drugs, including age of onset, duration, patterns, consequences of use, and use of alcohol and drugs by family members, along with types of and responses to previous treatment initiatives. It is also recommended that assessments determine a client's physical health, environmental supports (including partner and family), accommodation, employment and/or school status, leisure activities, legal problems, sexual orientation, and any history of sexual or other physical abuse or trauma. It is also essential to initially assess the level and intensity of withdrawal management and stabilization services required. This systematic process must also identify the client's strengths and take into consideration what the client actually wants.

The principal function of assessment is to act as the entry point into the treatment system and to provide a comprehensive portrait of the client and her or his current situation. The assessment should culminate in an individualized treatment plan, including referral into the community's treatment service network when required. Some models for community-based assessment programs also include a case management role for assessment workers, thereby providing continuity to the client from assessment to treatment to aftercare, highlighted by a relapse-prevention plan.

Specialized assessment services have been promoted as an integral part of a comprehensive local treatment system and have become a vital resource in many communities. Staff at assessment centres should possess the following:

- in-depth knowledge of effects of alcohol and/or other psychoactive drugs on physical and mental health, employment, financial, and legal difficulties; marital and family relationships; and social, religious, and cultural identity
- in-depth knowledge of treatment resources available to deal with clients' problems, including resources specific to treating alcohol and drug problems
- knowledge of assessment tools specific to identifying drinking and/or drug-using activities
- access to psychological testing to determine the extent of damage from alcohol and/or drugs and thus the ability of clients to respond to treatment and interact in a treatment community
- ability to assess strengths and resources that would be a base for clients to begin to resolve their situation
- ability to identify environmental factors that might adversely effect treatment
- ability to prioritize clients' treatment needs
- ability to work co-operatively with clients and other stakeholders in the treatment system to design an appropriate treatment plan
- attitudes and specialized knowledge regarding needs of particular groups, such as youth, women, elderly, First Nations, and minority and newcomer groups
- specialized knowledge of resources directed specifically to the above groups

Case Management

Case management is a client-focused strategy to improve coordination and continuity of care. In many instances, the client will have to be linked to several different agencies to deal with the range of issues that have arisen due to an addiction. The case management role involves the counsellor serving as a referral agent, facilitator, and advocate for the client, ensuring that the client's assessment is accurate and up to date. The purpose of case management is to expedite the use of resources available in the community, consistent with an overall treatment plan, through a single, consistent point of contact. Without case management, the potential for inefficient use of limited resources increases. There may be misunderstandings among agencies as to who will deal with what problems, especially if the client begins to develop additional issues after the initial assessment has been completed. Some issues can be addressed by more than one organization, leading to duplication of services, while other problems may be missed altogether by all agencies unless there is one person responsible for coordinating the overall treatment plan in conjunction with the client. In Canada, when case management does occur, it is often taken on by staff at assessment agencies or by counsellors within opioid-treatment programs. The tasks of a case manager can include:

- providing continuity of care for the alcohol/drug-dependent person
- facilitating contact with appropriate treatment resources
- assisting the client in entering the appropriate treatment centre
- monitoring clients' changing needs and problems
- periodic assessment of clients' progress in terms of the agreed-upon treatment plan
- providing crisis intervention and ongoing support to clients and their families in solving immediate problems
- encouraging clients who leave treatment prematurely to return for further appropriate assistance
- facilitating, within the bounds of confidentiality, information sharing with all concerned parties, including other agencies, family, the employee assistance program, and/or family physician
- providing aftercare or follow-up care after discharge from treatment to ensure that clients receive continuing encouragement and, where necessary, additional services
- assessing the risk of lapse or relapse

Case managers can also become involved in helping clients learn social and domestic skills, develop constructive coping skills, and develop constructive leisure activities. Active case management increases treatment participation, decreases relapse rates, and is a cost-effective use of a counsellor's time (Saleh et al., 2006; Vanderplassscheen, Rapp, Wolf, & Broekaeert, 2004).

Withdrawal Management Services: Daytox and Detox

Withdrawal management, or detoxification services, is often a first step in the treatment process. It entails total abstinence from not only the drug of misuse, but often all other drugs, including, in some facilities, tobacco. This strict rule created an issue for decades in Canada, as potential clients who also had a mental health issue (concurrent disorder clients) could attend a detox program only if they discontinued use of their other psychotherapeutic medications, which would, in turn, place them at risk for other often serious behavioural issues. The detoxification process should be of sufficient length to allow all psychoactive drugs to be eliminated by the body. A client's safety is the first priority of all withdrawal management staff, though once an individual becomes more stable, staff also typically offer social and environmental support during the stay.

The effects of withdrawal can range from mild to severe and can, on occasion, be life-threatening. It is the function of a detoxification program to manage this withdrawal process in a safe, caring, non-threatening, and empathetic atmosphere. Initially detoxification occurred exclusively in hospital emergency settings if it was a severe case; otherwise a drunken or otherwise impaired individual was usually incarcerated. In Ontario in 1965, the Addiction Research Foundation was commissioned to undertake an examination of chronic drunken offenders. There was at this time a growing belief that alcohol abuse was more of a public health concern than a criminal justice issue. This process led to the formation of an inter-ministerial committee in 1970 to develop policy and programs to deal with issues created by individuals who were constantly in conflict with the law because of their misuse of alcohol.

Bill 101 led to the creation of non-medical detoxification centres in Ontario. These centres provided care and rehabilitation in judicial districts having more than 1,000 arrests per year for public intoxication as an alternative to incarceration. "Non-medical" meant staffed by specially trained paraprofessionals, rather than by medically trained personnel, with no administering of medication to assist with the pain of withdrawal. This is the pattern most provinces eventually followed across Canada, though British Columbia, Quebec, and Prince Edward Island still use primarily medical withdrawal management programs staffed by nurses and related health care professionals. These facilities provide not only addiction-related psychosocial support, but also pharmacological intervention (prescription medications) for distressing withdrawal symptoms. The remainder of the Canadian withdrawal management programs are located in close proximity to parent hospitals, so that any necessary backup medical support is immediately available if a crisis situation arises.

The choice of a non-medical detoxification process in most Canadian jurisdictions occurred essentially for two reasons. First, it became apparent that most people could be detoxified safely in a non-medical facility, and second, with the removal of public drunkenness from the criminal statutes, it became necessary to provide a relatively inexpensive alternative to the historical remedy of the "drunk tank." Detoxification centres were intended to provide a link in the continuum of care for chronic alcohol-using offenders by receiving clients from police and, when possible, referring clients to recovery homes that would provide longer-term shelter and rehabilitation. However, smaller communities with no large public drunkenness issues were forced to make other arrangements for detoxification services, usually on an ad hoc basis. Typically, persons in these situations are detoxified in local community hospitals, but often without the benefit of a carefully designed withdrawal management program. Initial detoxification programs were designed exclusively for men, and it took over a decade in Ontario, once withdrawal management programs were established, to begin to include women and to develop women-specific resources for this component of the continuum of care (Watt, Saunders, Chaudron, & Soden, 1988).

Withdrawal management centres are crisis-care units that operate 24 hours a day, seven days a week, 365 days a year. In most cases they have evolved to become more than simply places to "dry out." They are now a core component in the continuum of care, acting as a gateway to other services, as well as remaining a safe haven. The overall population of detoxification centres is considerably different from that envisioned and experienced in the early 1970s. Whereas the original residents were largely chronic abusers, residents now represent a greater range of social and economic strata and age groups, as well as both sexes.

This integral component of the treatment system, while rudimentary in its approach, has continued to grow and evolve. As a result of increasing demand but reduced ability to meet the needs of clients, in-home detox emerged as an experiment in some communities, particularly in rural and more isolated areas. This programming option is actually now more common in larger urban centres that also have specific withdrawal management facilities. Daytox is a non-medical withdrawal management alternative that treats clients in an outpatient setting during the course of the day, allowing clients to go home each evening only to return the next day to continue to receive assistance and social support until they are fully detoxified (Alwyn, John, Hodgson, & Phillips, 2004). As well as being an option where there is no residential withdrawal management program available, daytox can be used with individuals who do not experience severe withdrawal symptoms, and who have a relatively stable environment and supportive social network (Williams, 2001). Not surprisingly, the lower operating costs associated with outpatient care seemed to drive the emergence of such programs, and this is expected to continue as health care costs continue to be scrutinized (Bischof, Richmond & Case, 2003). However, non-residential arrangements such as daytox can allow parents to continue to care for their children when they are not in treatment, diminishing the risk that they will be taken into care. Similar arguments can be made for maintaining employment. However, family support and relative stability in life are essential in an individual being assessed for a home detoxification program (Zinn, 1997).

In 1996, the Timmins Withdrawal Management Project was created as a partnership among social service agencies, the Ontario Addiction Research Foundation, and corrections services to provide a mobile, in-home outreach detoxification program. During the first two years of operation, the program was able to attract hard-to-reach populations, including women, First Nations clientele, youth, and the elderly, all of whom had traditionally exhibited reluctance toward in-patient care. In fact, 40 percent of the entire treatment population consisted of these demographic groups, compared to just 17 percent in the Timmins in-patient detoxification centre (Stuart, 1998). Vancouver opened a daytox centre in 2002 that continues to operate. Originally intended as a pilot project, the facility has been able to maintain operations due to its promising outcomes and fiscal structure: the centre costs approximately 60 percent less to run than traditional residential detoxification centres (Kent, 2002). In 2008, following the success of Vancouver's operation, a similar program opened in Surrey, where Fraser Health officials estimated that one-third of all clients receiving detoxification services could be appropriately treated in an outpatient setting. Both of these programs offer education, counselling, treatment, and follow-up support, and nurse case managers provide initial assessments, treatment planning, and case management to clients as they move through the program. By incorporating alternative therapies, individual and group supports, and relapse-prevention strategies, the program encourages participation by clients who have not succeeded in traditional program models. Similarly, the flexible hours and individualized treatment allows clients to maintain employment or continue academic pursuits that may otherwise be abandoned during hospitalization (Surrey Now, 2008).

Another initiative arose in the three Prairie provinces—Manitoba, Saskatchewan, and Alberta—in response to concerns raised by increasing methamphetamine use (crystal meth). Each of these provinces created legislation and new facilities to allow parents to forcibly send and confine their teenage children to youth detoxification centres for a limited stay, a measure called "involuntary confinement." In Alberta, the legal process is driven by parents who bring evidence to the courts and, in turn, if the judge finds in favour of the parents, the teenager can be confined for detoxification for up to 15 days. In Manitoba and Saskatchewan, the courts have more limited powers. Judges can order a youth to be taken for assessment, with an addiction specialist and/or physician making the final decision on whether the youth will be confined. In Saskatchewan, two doctors must assess the youth, and both must agree that involuntary confinement is necessary. Otherwise, the teen is released. The maximum length of confinement is also 15 days. Similarly, in Manitoba, the teen's drug problem is assessed by two addictions specialists. Those experts then decide whether to issue a stabilization order to confine the youth for up to seven days. In Alberta and Manitoba, only parents can seek a court order for their child, while in Saskatchewan, police officers and youth workers can also order a youth into assessment.

A final and controversial withdrawal management option is rapid detox/ultrarapid detoxification. This treatment is for those dependent on opioids, and at this time in Canada, it is offered only by private clinics. The cost can thus range from $3,000 to $10,000. Normally, withdrawal from opioids results in severe flu-like symptoms, with pain reported to be as severe as that experienced by those with bone cancer. These symptoms peak two to five days after the last administration of the drug, and then gradually diminish over seven to ten days. In rapid detoxification, only a one-night residential stay is required. In this program, withdrawal is precipitated by opioid antagonists (either naltrexone or naloxone) after the client is sedated. The most severe withdrawal phase is thus compressed to just hours, and the entire process, into only two days. The discomfort is avoided by deeply sedating the patient in rapid detox, or anaesthetizing the patient in ultra-rapid detox, during the worst phase of the withdrawal period (Gevirtz, Frost, & Kaye, 2011). It has been found that for many who undergo ultra-rapid detoxification and experience a diminished use of opioids in the short-term, the initial gains fade with time and many users return to use patterns similar to before the procedure, particularly if no counselling component accompanies the post-treatment period (Krabbe et al., 2003; McGregor, Ali, White, Thomas, & Gowing, 2002; Rothenberg et al., 2002). As well, a few deaths resulting from the procedure have been reported (Dyer, 1998; Hamilton et al., 2002). Where no evidence of contraindication exists, the risk of death is assumed to be related to the use of general anaesthetic and not the administration of the antagonists. However, the fact that 1 in 500–1,000 patients die for unknown reasons following the detoxification is a troubling statistic (Coleman Institute, 2014).

5.2 ADDICTION-SPECIFIC RESOURCES
Community-Based (Outpatient) Treatment
Day Treatment
Harm Reduction
Concurrent Disorder Programs
Short-Term Residential Treatment
Recovery Homes
Alternative Living Environment and Therapeutic Communities
Addiction Supportive Housing (ASH)
Managed Alcohol Programs: Non-Abstinence Residential Programs—The "Wet Shelter"
Drug Treatment Courts

Intervention programs may be outpatient or residential, community-based or institutional. Outpatient programming allows a person to live at home and attend treatment sessions during the day or evening. Residential programs provide overnight accommodation to clients for varying periods, from a few weeks to a year. Community-based programs are generally not-for-profit incorporated or sponsored services, non-medical in nature, and operated by a voluntary board of directors. Contrarily, most institution-based programs are medical programs administered through and usually in hospitals. The community versus hospital distinction often revolves around the extent to which the program is affiliated with hospitals for fiscal and/or administrative purposes.

Community-Based (Outpatient) Treatment
This treatment is provided on a non-residential basis, usually in a regularly scheduled session of 1–2 hours per week, though sometimes two times per week. Treatment may entail individual and/or group sessions to explore all aspects of the person's substance abuse and related problems. Sessions offer information and strategies to assist each individual in her or his recovery process. This is the least intense and intrusive treatment intervention option, primarily offered by non-medical, community-based counselling agencies. Appropriate matches for this service include clients who

- are free of any significant medical problem;
- are self-motivated;
- have a support system in place, including family, friends, or work;
- live within easy access to the facility; and

- have not yet had their personal or work life extensively affected by their substance use.

Day Treatment

This more intensive, structured non-residential treatment is typically provided five days per week or four or five evenings per week for 3–4 hours per session. The concept of using day treatment as an alternative to in-patient programs emerged in the late 1960s, but it has never been prominent in Canada. Treatment involves group activities ranging from formal group treatment sessions, to education groups, to recreational activities. As clients are home weekends, evenings, and/or days, the home environment must be stable with support from family and friends. This treatment option allows the social aspect of addiction to be acknowledged and addressed early in the treatment process.

Day treatment is appropriate for individuals who are able to maintain social competence despite their dependency. Day treatment programs operate under a philosophy that attempts to develop a sense of community support and responsibility so that a person may attain balanced health and wellness. Day treatment is one means of providing a short-term, intensive, and structured period of treatment while keeping treatment costs down, especially in comparison to an in-patient stay in a more institutional setting.

An option that has traditionally received much less attention but has great merit as an alternative is evening-care programming. Intensive treatment programs offered in the evening may be desirable given the high proportion of people in addiction programs who are employed. Intensive evening programs may be more responsive to the time constraints of particular clients than programs operating during normal business hours. This option also appeals to those who do not wish their workplace to know about their personal problems or who need to continue to work throughout their treatment.

Harm Reduction

A comparatively newer, more specialized form of community-based counselling that has taken root throughout Canada is based on harm reduction. This initiative is a response to AIDS and HIV and is foremost about reducing the spread of potentially deadly communicable diseases, preventing drug overdose deaths, increasing substance users' contact with health care services along with more traditional drug treatment programs, and reducing the consumption of illicit drugs in the streets.

Harm reduction interventions have proven successful in decreasing the spread of HIV/AIDS and hepatitis while decreasing overdoses and overdose deaths in nations around the world. The most common forms of harm-reduction programs include needle exchanges, methadone maintenance, and methadone treatment programs. Heroin prescription and safe injection sites are viewed as being even more controversial and thus are fewer in number worldwide (Watkin et al., 2010). In fact, Canada has only one safe injection site and one heroin prescription site, both located in Vancouver, and despite overwhelming empirical support for their effectiveness, it took court rulings to ensure both could offer their life-saving services to vulnerable drug-dependent persons (Rowe & Gonzalez, 2010).

Concurrent Disorder Programs

Another specialized form of community-based counselling entails work done by agencies whose clients have both an addiction and a mental health issue. Services offered by institutional and community-based psychologists, psychiatrists, social workers, and nurses have long been a part of the extended continuum of care. Traditionally, these helping professionals dealt with either the mental health issue or the addiction issue alone, rarely together. However, beginning this century, many more specific programs have begun to emerge that address both issues simultaneously (Kimberly & Osmond, 2010).

Concurrent disorder programs move beyond working only with the addiction issue and provide counselling that also addresses issues such as depression, loneliness, suicidal ideation and attempts, paranoia, and violent behaviours. Whether these behaviours are primary or secondary to the use of psychoactive agents is no longer an issue. Rather, the mental health problems are categorized as coexisting with the drug misuse or abuse, and vice versa, and thus intervention focuses on both. Mental health agencies had traditionally provided a wide range of individual and group counselling techniques, including behaviour modification, assertiveness training, leisure counselling, relaxation techniques, communication skills, and, when needed, pharmacological interventions. However, they did not typically directly address any addiction issues their clients had, and thus long-term outcomes were not as favourable as they could have been. Agencies providing concurrent disorder programming work with clients who historically fell through the gaps of the addiction and mental health systems, as one system often did not wish to work with the client until the issues relating to the other system were resolved. This, of course, left clients with both issues typically receiving no care and thus deteriorating in their mental health and drug use.

Short-Term Residential Treatment

The first formal treatment environments to emerge in North America, after Alcoholics Anonymous, were three in-patient treatment programs: Pioneer House (1948), Hazelden (1949), and the Willmar State Hospital (1950). Prior to these, the only type of residential programming that treated those with alcohol issues were sanatoriums or rehabilitation farms, where alcohol-dependent individuals were sequestered from their environments for health reasons. These early programs were founded on the principles and philosophy proposed by AA, and took on the moniker of the Minnesota Model, following the same guidelines:

- Alcoholism is an involuntary, primary, chronic, progressive biopsycho-social, spiritual disease.
- Recovery is contingent upon abstinence from all non-medical drugs.
- Recovery is best achieved through the Twelve Steps of AA and immersion in a community of shared experience, strength and hope.
- Focus of the residential rehabilitation process should be on the direct treatment of the disease.
- Addiction needs to be treated in an environment of dignity and respect.
- Motivation or lack of motivation at point of intake is not a predictor of outcome success, and motivation is as much the responsibility of the treatment setting as the individual (Cook, 1988; McElrath, 1997).

Success entailed not only attending AA meetings as an integral part of the residential treatment process, but also continued attendance on completion of rehabilitation.

Currently these treatment services are provided for less than 42 days, though average program length in Canada is typically 21–28 days. These short-term intensive treatment programs are either affiliated with hospitals and take a medical orientation or operate as community-based programs that still follow the Minnesota Model principles. Programs are not restricted to particular groups, and they receive referrals from all segments of the health and social service network and also the workplace. Given the range of expertise within these facilities, they are capable of providing comprehensive client assessments and offer a wide variety of treatment modalities. Almost all programs now also provide aftercare support in the form of relapse-prevention or alumni groups, with many offering family information nights or weekends. Unfortunately, the residential component of hospital-based programs makes them much more expensive in comparison to day treatment or community-based outpatient options, though 12-step based programs and other non-medical programs are less expensive to operate.

In-patient residential treatment offers a wide variety of services, including medical evaluation, assessment of the extent of the drug dependency, detoxification in some facilities, individual and group counselling, drug education, spiritual guidance, family involvement, vocational guidance, and even employer involvement. The centres provide a safe, relatively stress-free environment in which the person can recover from the physical and emotional effects of prolonged drinking and/or substance abuse. Planning for rehabilitation on return to the natural environment is also typically part of the process. Education regarding the effects of drugs varies from centre to centre, but usually includes the short- and long-term physiological, social, spiritual, and psychological effects of drug use. There is also often attendance at a 12-step group that is either recommended or mandated, even in programs not premised on the philosophy of Alcoholics Anonymous.

Treatment staff's efforts to involve families and employers in the intervention process reflect the increasing awareness of the social-emotional environmental aspects that affect and are affected by clients' behaviour. This logical extension of increasing involvement of the client's social world in the intervention process has also encouraged a significant increase in the options for help available following the in-patient experience. For example, in some institutions clients are informed that a successful recovery process can involve two full years of active participation while the client is living in his or her natural environment. Even more progressive residential programs have developed specific information and counselling programs for family members of those in residence.

In Canada, as a result of treatment costs, standardized provincial assessment outcomes recommend that only those with severe or chronic addiction issues be referred to residential programs. This has forced many programs to develop two-tier admission policies: one for those who are receiving treatment through universal health care and one for those who are paying for the treatment through workplace or personal extended health care benefits. This, in turn, has led to the slow but steady growth of private fee-for-service short-term residential programs, many of which that operate without oversight, with costs running as high as $30,000.

Recovery Homes

For many struggling with ongoing issues in their recovery, the ability to avoid a relapse is often jeopardized by untenable housing or an unsupportive living environment. Recovery residences, also called social model recovery, or sober living houses, are designed to provide safe and supportive housing to help individuals initiate and sustain recovery, primarily through peer-to-peer interactions guided by a staff who themselves have recovery histories. They are gender-specific residential programs in which the goal is to provide a safe, supportive, therapeutic program of addiction education and life skills counselling. They provide an array of services to individuals with addiction problems within a structured environment, either prior to or after the person has attended a withdrawal management program and/or received more intensive treatment from a short-term residential program. In some jurisdictions, these homes are classified as supportive housing programs (Polcin, Mericle, Howell, Sheridan, & Christensen, 2014).

Programs are developed to assist the recovering person in personal growth and positive lifestyle change. Recovery homes have a comparatively long history, with many facilities first developed in the 1960s and early 1970s (Ogborne, Annis, & Sanchez-Craig, 1978). In the United States, the use of AA as the foundation for programming in this environment became known as the Oxford House approach. Recovery homes are centres from which individuals can re-establish themselves in the community. A typical stay can range from three to six months. Therapeutic efforts are focused on providing social support and linking this with the social reality of the living circumstances, working with the residents through the actual living problems as they present themselves. The intent is for the facility to provide a bridge between initial intensive treatment and returning to the community. Residents assume a major share of the daily chores and functions of the house, and are encouraged and assisted in finding employment in the local community, thereby actively contributing financially toward their own room and board. Recovery homes also offer group and individual counselling that focuses on physical, emotional, educational, and employment objectives. Alcoholics Anonymous and Narcotics Anonymous meetings also tend to be a core feature of recovery home programs. Staffing is frequently done by recovering persons who share their own life experiences with new residents and who act as role models and sounding boards (Polcin, 2009).

Typical sessions offered can include the following:

- education on the process of drug dependency
- exercise, nutrition, and health issues
- problem solving and decision-making skills
- information on retraining and job search skills
- appropriate use of leisure time
- goal setting
- communication and assertiveness
- stress management
- avoiding relapse

Recovery homes also place an emphasis on knowledge gained through one's recovery experience. Residents draw on that experience as a way to help others. As well, for those who retain family supports, weekly family education sessions may be a component to aid family, friends, and significant others in learning how to deal with their feelings and to help them provide support for clients during their ongoing recovery. Numerous recovery homes also provide non-residential services, indicating a willingness to diversify and attract clients for whom a completely residential service may not be totally appropriate. As well, many offer follow-up programs for clients who have returned to the community to live. Costs of staying at a recovery home are typically geared to an individual's income, with subsidies often provided through local social-assistance programs if an individual in unable to pay.

Alternative Living Environment and Therapeutic Communities

For many persons with a substance abuse problem, the environment they live in is counterproductive to their successful treatment and recovery. These persons have unstable home lives and/or no support from family and friends. Others who come into treatment have no real home, no role models for healthy living, or need to relearn or learn socialization skills. Alternative living environments and therapeutic communities provide a protective living environment for people whose substance abuse is not an isolated problem but a major disruption of their entire lives. These programs help in setting limits and defining behaviour while satisfying daily needs and desires in a quasi-home setting. Relationships that develop provide a basis on which the members can learn or relearn how to live with others. Real-life issues of daily existence take precedence at these facilities. Many alternative living settings are affiliated with a religious order, with the most prominent being the Salvation Army.

Although the term was first used in 1946, the therapeutic community (TC) movement evolved mainly during the 1960s as an alternative to institutionalized psychiatric care (Main, 1946; Manning, 1989). In the United Kingdom, TCs originally provided an optional form of treatment not only for addiction, but also for personality disorders and related mental health diagnoses. In the United States, they evolved as an alternative to involuntary detention under civil commitment laws (De Leon, 1988). The major proponent was Charles Dederich, who developed Synanon in an attempt to provide a safe haven for chronic opioid users within a positive living environment. Recovering drug-dependent persons viewed the therapeutic community treatment modality as a mutual aid endeavour to treat the whole person, whose criminal thoughts and lifestyle were at the root of drug use. They believed that the best way to counter antisocial thinking and exploitative social interaction was to immerse formerly drug-dependent persons, mainly heroin users, in a community-based, therapeutically oriented social environment. In this setting, every aspect of maladaptive behaviour and thinking would be exposed and subject to correction by other recovering persons, who would recognize the distorted ways of thinking and social interaction that are common in drug addiction. Therapeutic communities were seen as a viable treatment alternative for individuals whose substance use made them eligible for detention in the criminal justice system. Their originators saw programs evolve that had an intense structure, peer-enforced values, and active confrontation of any behaviour deemed disruptive or regressive. The intent at Synanon in particular was to change the personality so that the individual remained drug- and crime-free (Barnett, 2009; Mandell, Olden, Wenzel, Dahl, & Ebener, 2008).

Therapeutic communities operate from the perspective that substance use is a problem of the whole person. The goal of the TC is not just to eliminate the substance use behaviour, but to refocus the individual. Thus all activities are designed to be psycho-educational, emphasizing personal behavioural, attitudinal, and value change to support lifelong abstinence (De Leon, 1997). These facilities focus on the here and now, on truth and honesty, and on personal responsibility and community involvement. Participants contribute to all activities of daily living in the TC. As a result, they adopt various social roles and become active participants in the process of changing themselves and others (Barnett, 2009).

Peer membership provides the primary source of instruction and support. Participants have a shared responsibility to observe and authentically react to each other's actions. Each participant aims to model the change process. Not only do they provide feedback about what others can change, but they also model change behaviour in themselves. Group formats are used for education, training, and other therapeutic activities. Shared norms and values, rules, and regulations serve as explicit guidelines for self-help and teaching how to live right. Participants must reinforce these guidelines. Learning occurs not only through skills training but also by adhering to the procedures and systems of the TC (De Leon, 1995). The model has even been applied to a correctional setting in Missouri, where inmates with extensive histories of crime and drug use who wish to alter their behaviour can volunteer to be housed together under the same principles and guidelines as a community-based TC (Barnett, 2009). Over 65 nations on all five continents have programs that follow the core principles of the therapeutic community model (Bunt, Muehlbach & Moed, 2008).

Addiction Supportive Housing (ASH)

Addiction supportive housing programs are another component of the treatment continuum that recognizes the importance of safe and sustainable housing in the recovery process. Part of the Housing First initiative, these programs, while still limited, provide longer support in a therapeutic environment than shortterm residential programs or recovery homes. The goal is to encourage program participants to develop long-term skills that are necessary to maintain their own residence. Increasingly, the value of supportive housing initiatives is being recognized across service sectors, as addiction is frequently intertwined with issues of poverty, homelessness, and mental health (DiLeo, 2003; Rickards et al., 2010). In fact, substance abuse is a primary predictor of homelessness (Dickson-Gomez, Convey, Hilario, Corbett, & Weeks, 2007; Edens, Kasprow, Tsai, & Rosenheck, 2011). By providing housing supports, ideally in conjunction with, but not contingent on, addiction treatment, service providers can increase the probability that someone who is marginally housed or homeless will follow through with addiction treatment. This is particularly crucial after a person receives his or her initial assessment and is placed on a waiting list due to a lack of available resources (O'Connell, Kasprow, & Rosenheck, 2013; Winn et al., 2013). Clients who have participated in supportive housing programs demonstrate a reduction in contact with the criminal justice system and residential treatment while improving their income levels, access to food, and housing stability (Hickert & Taylor, 2011).

Housing First programs can also be considered a component of harm reduction (Collins et al., 2012; Larimer, 2012; Pauly, Reist, Belle-Isle, & Schactman, 2013), as permanent housing is viewed as a human right and not an earned privilege contingent on abstinence or treatment participation (van Wormer & van Wormer, 2009). What distinguishes some Housing First programs is that they do not make admission contingent on sobriety or treatment attendance but rather target chronically homeless people who are frequent users of publicly funded health and criminal-justice resources. A study in Seattle, Washington, reviewed the use and cost of services before and after program admission among 95 participants in a

Housing First program, 39 of whom were wait-listed and all of whom had severe alcohol problems. The results revealed the following:

- Monthly median costs among admitted participants decreased from $4,066 in the year before admission to $1,492 after six months in housing and $958 after twelve months in housing.
- Even after accounting for housing program costs, total mean monthly spending on housed participants compared with wait-listed participants was $2,449 lower after six months.
- Both costs and crisis-services use decreased the longer the person remained housed.
- The number of drinks per day among housed participants decreased from 15.7 prior to housing to 14.0 at six months, 12.5 at nine months, and 10.6 at twelve months.

Both costs and alcohol consumption further decreased the longer participants were in supportive housing. This indicates that the provision of supportive housing for chronically homeless individuals can substantially reduce the cost of and burden on health and criminal justice services (Larimer et al., 2009).

In the Ontario ASH initiative, two living options are available to clients who have typically completed an addiction treatment program yet still remain at risk of homelessness. One is the transitional house option, which is gender-specific communal living with up to four individuals per house. Clients are required to attend weekly house meetings, be involved in a community support program, such as a 12-step group or an aftercare program, and participate in the general upkeep and chores of the house. This very much resembles an alternative living environment, though under much smaller parameters and less direct supervision. The other option is independent living in a single unit. Clients are required to attend a weekly one-to-one counselling session with an ASH counsellor. The single units are, however, a harm-reduction-based approach and the requirements for remaining in the program are much more individualized and client centred, though all clients must be participating in the program and be actively working on some type of change goal. Both the transition home and single units are subsidized, geared-to-income rental units. The initial six-month evaluation of this initiative indicates that the program is reaching a group that had historically been hard to serve. Improvements were found in increased levels of health and functioning and in reductions in substance use, use of emergency departments, hospital admissions, and encounters with the criminal justice system (Johnston Consulting, 2014).

Managed Alcohol Programs: Non-Abstinence Residential Programs—The "Wet Shelter"

Harm reduction initiatives have historically been outpatient and community-based with the goal of reducing negative health, social, and economic outcomes. Until the early 1990s, the policy throughout Canada was to confiscate any drug, including alcohol, from an individual seeking a shelter bed for a night. This precluded many chronic alcohol users from using the shelter system, including during cold Canadian winters. Influenced by harm-reduction advocates, staff at Seaton House, a large shelter in Toronto, adopted a policy where any alcohol coming into the shelter would not be confiscated and poured down the drain, but rather collected, labelled, stored, and returned to the owner the next morning when he or she left the shelter for the day. After a coroner's inquest into the freezing deaths of three homeless men in Toronto, Seaton House expanded its approach to include supervised consumption of alcohol on site, an ongoing initiative in which residents are provided with a regulated amount of alcohol each hour. The idea was to keep residents from leaving the shelter and putting themselves at risk in order to find a drink, and also to reduce the consumption of harmful alcohol-based products such as hand sanitizer and mouthwash.

Two other communities in Ontario—Ottawa and Hamilton—followed Toronto's lead in establishing addiction-related residential programs where the consumption of alcohol is a core part of the daily routine (Table 5.2). At the Shepherds of Good Hope in Ottawa, clients are individually assessed to determine the appropriate amount and how frequently it should be administered to meet health needs. Clients have a choice of 12 percent white or red wine. No more than 5 oz. is given at one time, with the exception of the first drink of the morning, which can be up to 7 oz. Between 7:30 a.m. and 9:30 p.m., participants can receive a maximum of 14 drinks, which by standard levels seems excessive. However, some individuals in the program had consumption levels as great as 48 standard drinks a day (Inner City Health, 2010). Claremont House in Hamilton has moved to the point where residents are involved in brewing their own alcohol as part of their residential responsibilities, with the enhancement of the quality of life of residents being the ongoing mission of the organization.

The primary purpose of managed alcohol programs (MAP) is to offer continuing health and housing services for individuals who have a history of homelessness and alcohol abuse along with chronic health issues, and who are often deemed to be near the end of their lives. The aim of this new component of the continuum of care is to provide humane treatment and reduce harm to the clients by eliminating the need to binge drink and to drink non-beverage alcohol products. Nursing, medical, and rehabilitation care are provided, along with a regular but limited amount of alcohol. MAP programs provide residents with permanent rather than transient housing, similar to the Housing First philosophy, though some, like The Annex at Seaton House, remain shelters. Some MAPs offer private rooms, though the standard is shared accommodation, with all programs staffed 24 hours per day. Care plans are individualized and include a recreational component. The overall goal is to improve the quality of life of clients while allowing them to live in a respectful, supportive environment (Podymow, Turnbull, Coyle, Yetisir, & Wells, 2006). Along with improving quality of life and stabilizing housing, managed alcohol programs have also been shown to reduce the amount of alcohol consumed (Pauly et al., 2013) and be more cost-effective than acute and crisis use of the health care system (Larimer et al., 2009). The benefits and risks of managed alcohol programs are outlined in Table 5.3.

TABLE 5.2: MANAGED ALCOHOL PROGRAMS IN CANADA

City	Name of Program	Number of Beds	Date Established
Toronto	The Annex	140	1996
Ottawa	Shepherds of Good Hope (The Oaks)	30 in the Oaks 12–16 MAP reserved	2001
Hamilton	Claremont House	16 + 1 palliative care	2005
Thunder Bay	Shelter House (Kwae Kii Win)	15	2012
Vancouver	The Station	80	2012

TABLE 5.3: RISKS AND BENEFITS OF MANAGED ALCOHOL PROGRAMS

Risk	Single Heavy Drinking Episode	Non-Beverage Alcohol Consumption	Drinking in Unsafe Settings	Chronic High-Volume Alcohol Consumption
Potential Harms	violence, injury, poisoning, seizures, legal issues	exacerbate chronic diseases, poisoning	violence, injury, freezing, conflict with the law	cirrhosis, cancer, housing and social problems
MAP Benefits	smooth drinking pattern, fewer injuries and seizures, secure housing, improved relationships	reduced consumption of non-beverage alcohol	shelter from cold, protected supply of alcohol, personal safety, food	housing security, reduced consumption, improved nutrition
MAP Risks	higher blood alcohol concentration if drinking continues outside of program	increased ethanol consumption if drinking continues outside of program	less exercise and weight gain	fewer days of abstinence contribute to liver disease risk

Source: Stockwell, Pauly, Chow, Vallance, & Perkin (2013)

Drug Treatment Courts

One of the more recent developments in addiction treatment is the use of drug courts or drug treatment courts (DTCs), which aim to reduce substance use and provide rehabilitation to persons who resort to criminal activity to support their addictions (CADTP, n.d.). First established in Miami, Florida, in 1989, the inaugural Canadian drug treatment court opened in 1998 in Toronto. DTCs are premised on the theory that substance use and criminal behaviour can perpetuate a vicious cycle. To break this cycle, treatment and rehabilitation outside of the traditional prison system are often required. In this way, DTCs represent a partnership between the criminal justice and substance abuse treatment systems (Barnes, 2009).

Justice Barnes (2009) identified the following principles and objectives of DTCs:

- increase public safety
- help participants reduce or eliminate drug use
- help participants reduce or eliminate criminal behaviour
- help reunite participants with their families
- help participants become productive members of society
- have participants experience an overall improvement in personal well-being

Although unstandardized and with no universal model (United Nations Office on Drugs and Crime, 2005), there are established international guidelines that each drug treatment court strives to uphold. There is also recognition that they can and should be tailored to individual jurisdictional needs (CADTP, n.d.). The guidelines include:

- integrating addiction treatment services with justice system case processing
- using a non-adversarial approach to allow prosecution and defence counsels to promote public safety while protecting participants' Charter right
- identifying eligible participants early in their contact with the criminal justice system so that they can be placed in the drug treatment court program as promptly as possible
- providing access to a continuum of drug, alcohol, and other related treatment and rehabilitative services
- monitoring compliance by frequent drug testing
- developing a coordinated strategy governing drug treatment court responses to participants' compliance and non-compliance
- applying both sanctions and rewards, swiftly, certainly, and consistently, for both non-compliance and/or compliance

- ongoing judicial interaction with each drug treatment court participant
- monitoring and evaluating the achievement of program goals and gauging their overall effectiveness
- continuing interdisciplinary education promoting effective drug treatment court planning implementation, and operations
- forging partnerships among courts, treatment and rehabilitation programs, public agencies, and community-based organizations to generate local support and enhance program effectiveness
- ongoing case management providing the social support necessary to achieve social reintegration
- being appropriately flexible in adjusting program content, including incentives and sanctions, to better achieve program results with particular groups, such as women, indigenous people, and minority ethnic groups

Although drug treatment courts are recognized as specialized programs, an even more specific court process is the family drug treatment court (FDTC). In addition to the need for substance use treatment, FDTCs also recognize the role of trauma in both addiction and child welfare contexts (Drabble, Jones, & Brown, 2013). While research evaluating the effectiveness of these courts is even sparser than that for DTCs, preliminary data has been positive regarding decreased substance use, improved mental health, improved housing stability, and engagement in employment or education (Powell, Stevens, Lo Dolce, Sinclair, & Swenson-Smith, 2012). It is noteworthy, however, that the positive results do not necessarily include higher parent-child reunification rates (Young, Wong, Adkins, & Simpson, 2003), despite this being a preferred outcome. There may also be variation in the outcomes based on the structure of the FDTC itself (Worcel, Green, Furrer, Burrus, & Finigan, 2007), which is why further research is needed.

Lastly, it is important to note the potentially preventative role that DTCs play, especially among juvenile populations. Criminologists have historically maintained that conflict with the law among young offenders is a strong predictor of adult criminal behaviour, as 68 percent of adult crimes are committed by individuals formerly involved in the youth justice system (Kempf-Leonard, Tracy, & Howell, 2001). The overlap with substance abuse is also relevant, since people abusing substances are three to four times more likely to commit a crime (Bennett, Holloway, & Farrington, 2008). While research in this area is also sparse, one program evaluation did find that participation in juvenile DTCs reduced subsequent adult felonies, though not misdemeanours (Carter & Barker, 2011).

5.3 IN-PATIENT VERSUS COMMUNITY-BASED OUTPATIENT CARE

Many controversies exist within the addiction field. Among the most prominent is the in-patient/outpatient treatment argument. The traditional approach, especially with long-term substance abusers, had been in-patient residential programming, however, research over the past four decades has tended to indicate that this is not the most efficient method of intervention and it is definitely not the most cost-effective.

The first studies were conducted in the Maudsley Hospital in London, England (Edwards & Guthrie, 1966, 1967; Edwards et al., 1977). A one-year follow-up study of men dependent on alcohol reported that there was no significant difference in outcome between those who had received community-based outpatient counselling and those who had received several months of in-patient treatment. Helen Annis (1984), of the Ontario Addiction Research Foundation, conducted an extensive review of the in-patient versus community counselling question at that time. Her conclusions were quite decisive:

- In-hospital alcoholism programs of a few weeks to a few months duration show no greater success in producing abstinence than do periods of brief hospitalization of a few days.
- The great majority of alcohol-dependent persons seeking treatment for alcohol withdrawal can be safely detoxified without pharmacotherapy and in non-hospital-based units.
- Detoxification with pharmacotherapy on an ambulatory basis has been demonstrated to be a safe alternative at one-tenth the cost.
- Partial hospitalization (day treatment) programs have been found to have equal or superior results to in-patient hospitalization in producing abstinence among clients at one-half to one-third the cost.
- Controlled trials have demonstrated that community-based outpatient programs can produce comparable results to in-patient programs. One estimate placed the cost saving at $3,700 per patient (1984 dollars) compared with the typical course of medical in-patient treatment.

A growing body of evidence suggests that if clients could be matched on clinically significant dimensions to a range of treatment alternatives, much higher overall improvement rates in the alcoholism treatment field would be observed.

Another major critique of residential programming was that moving to a special treatment environment, where the client's residence is temporarily changed, brings with it a set of limitations on the impact of the intervention. It is argued that the residential shift is an artificial one, and the impact of the treatment is heavily affected by this limitation. It is further contended that the transfer of a client's treatment into the natural world needs to occur for the impact to be most successful. However, in-patient programs do provide environments where there are fewer urges or opportunities to use drugs, and limit the negative social issues associated with drug use. Nance (1992) agreed that there were shortcomings to in-patient care including cost, lack of matching client to level, intensity, and duration of treatment, and overly simplistic treatment regimens. However, he stated that in-patient care offered several significant advantages as a treatment format by providing the following:

- protection from further drug use
- the opportunity for clients to focus solely on their substance abuse problem
- a focus on ego strengthening and learning how to control compulsive behaviours
- maximum treatment retention

The short-term protection of a residential setting also enables those clients with the greatest needs and most substantive environmental pressures to do as well as clients with more initial strengths, often by eliminating the extra environmental risks faced in the community (Witbrodt et al., 2007). Residential treatment has been demonstrated to assist in moving clients along in their preparedness to change and also in instilling a sense of hope and resiliency (Shumway, Bradshaw, Harris, & Baker, 2013). As well, Finney, Hahn, and Moos (1996) found in-patient treatment to be more cost-effective than outpatient treatment one-third of the time.

With the emergence of daytox options in Canada, controversy has also arisen in withdrawal management. As previously discussed, although the primary consideration of outpatient detoxification programs is their cost-effectiveness when compared to in-patient settings, some suggest that the client's personal characteristics may be more important than setting in predicting treatment success (McLellan, Luborsky, Woody, O'Brien & Druley, 1983; Hayashida, 1998; Hayashida et al., 1989). This contention is supported by research that finds no difference in recidivism rates among those receiving alcohol detoxification in hospitals, recovery homes, or outpatient centres (Smart, Gray, Finley, & Carpen, 1977). One fairly robust clinical audit of an at-home detoxification program in England found that 96.6 percent of suitable candidates completed their programs successfully, but results were very much contingent on the client having a suitable caretaker in the home and not having a severe mental health issue (Callow, Donaldson, & de Ruiter, 2008). Another contention is that for home-based detoxification to succeed, primary care physicians must support these endeavours (Roche, Watt, & Fischer, 2001). In their interviews with general practitioners in Australia, general physicians did not feel that the necessary policies, infrastructure, or remuneration strategies were in place to support effective and widespread at-home detoxification. Similar studies in Wales, however, found that physicians were supportive of such treatment, and some even volunteered their time to provide in-home detoxification services to appropriate clients (Middlemiss, 2002; Stockwell, Bolt, & Hooper, 1986; Stockwell, Bolt, Milner, Pugh, & Young, 1990).

Residential rehabilitation is a vital component of the addiction treatment continuum of care, not as an alternative to community treatment, but as one potential element of a successful recovery journey. However, unless there are pressing reasons for residential care, community-based counselling results are typically equivalent, at a much lower cost and with far less disruption to a client's life. Shorter and less-intensive approaches are not only most cost-effective but are also more effective in absolute terms (Miller & Hester, 1986b; Witbrodt et al., 2007). An exception is concurrent disorder treatment programs, where longer residential care is associated with longer periods of abstinence and lower risk of homelessness (Brunette, Drake, Woods, & Harnett, 2001). Of course, it makes little sense to talk about length or intensity of treatment without considering what kind of treatment is being offered. Some modalities lack evidence for effectiveness at any length or level of intensity.

It is tempting to assume that more treatment is better treatment, and that longer or more intensive interventions will yield superior outcomes. However, there needs to be a continuum of care in place to allow for the widest possible range of services. A balance is required between community and institutional treatment. A client's needs must always be the first item on the agenda, and clients should be matched to treatment according to their specific needs.

5.4 ADJUNCT RESOURCES
Budgeting and Financial Counselling
Employment Assistance/Vocational Training
Legal Assistance
Marital and Family Counselling
Medical Services
Mutual Aid/Self-Help Groups
Recreational/Leisure Programs
Social Assistance

Treatment of a substance abuse client often entails working with issues beyond those that deal exclusively with psychoactive drugs. Substance abusers tend to encounter other problems of daily living that require resolution before they can fully overcome their addiction.

Budgeting and Financial Counselling
Substance abusers often accumulate significant debt by diverting much of their money toward their drug of choice, or simply through financial mismanagement or neglect. As part of the entire recovery process, attention may

need to be concentrated at some point on budget counselling and assistance in debt management or consolidation. This type of assistance is generally free through registered credit counselling services, which are most often affiliated with family services agencies or financial institutions such as credit unions. Regardless of the service provider, it is important that the credit counsellor has completed the Accredited Financial Counsellor of Canada (AFCC) certification program.

Employment Assistance/Vocational Training

During the course of treatment, some clients will come to the realization that they need to enter a new field of employment or look for a more stable employment option. Of these clients, a proportion will also require additional assistance because of physical or psychological limitations that played a part in their becoming drug dependent or are a result of chronic abuse. Other clients would benefit from aptitude testing, additional education, or specific skills training or retraining. Thus, the vocational segment of the initial assessment can again be accessed in helping to establish an employment plan as part of the extended continuum of care.

Legal Assistance

Unfortunately, many persons become involved in the addiction treatment system as a direct result of coming into conflict with the law. For others, the dramatic changes they personally undergo as a result of treatment lead them to significant life changes that necessitate legal action. Thus, a high rate of separation, divorce, and child custody claims can occur among substance abusers before, during, and after, their recovery process, especially if family counselling was not part of the formal treatment process. Other frequent legal problems include driving while intoxicated, assault, and civil litigation claims, as well as theft and break and enter charges for those who committed crimes to support a drug dependency. As many substance abusers often require legal advice but do not have sufficient funds to pay for a lawyer, counsellors should also be aware of good legal aid lawyers and community and legal clinics that will provide legal counsel without charging a fee.

Marital and Family Counselling

Additional therapy beyond substance abuse counselling is often required for families, especially if it was not part of the formal addiction treatment process. This may entail couples counselling, sexual counselling, sessions on parenting, grief counselling, and, for some, separation and/or divorce counselling. Support for spouses and children of substance abusers should be a core feature of any community's continuum of care. Typically, in North America, family treatment occurs outside the addiction treatment system, though in some nations, such as Norway, family members of the person with the alcohol or other drug problem are also entitled to take sick leave from work to accompany the person to treatment and receive counselling.

Medical Services

Too often persons suffering from an addiction have poor health, and thus part of the recovery process is dealing with the physical aspect of wellness. Medical attention may be required for emergency treatment of injuries or severe medical conditions, such as hepatitis or HIV, as part of a comprehensive assessment. However, clients often have more common problems, such as gastrointestinal complications, liver disorders, a cardiovascular problem, or even cancer due to their historic drug use, which have not been properly addressed. As well, medical support may be necessary to facilitate a complete recovery from substance abuse problems in deal with issues as fundamental as nutrition and fitness counselling. Addiction medicine is a specialized area of practice, one that not many physicians are well versed in and one for which not all hospitals have dedicated staff.

Mutual Aid/Self-Help Groups

Self-help groups hold a unique distinction: not only are they a method of peer-based helping, but also, for some, a cultural experience. The original substance-related self-help group and the association responsible for the growth of addiction services in North America is Alcoholics Anonymous (AA). From it has sprung Narcotics Anonymous, Nicotine Anonymous, Gamblers Anonymous, Overeaters Anonymous, Cocaine Anonymous, and many other similar 12-step recovery groups. As well, a series of addiction-specific non-12-step groups has arisen in response to the limitations of AA, thus further enhancing the support offered by this adjunct component of the continuum of care. Self-help groups can be used as an entry point into treatment, including non-addiction-specific groups, as well as a maintenance and relapse-prevention service. In communities where there are few or no drug-specific services, there is still likely to be an AA group. In larger communities, AA groups meet seven days a week. Membership is voluntary and fees are based primarily on a "pass-the-hat," pay what you can format. However, self-help groups have moved beyond AA and addiction-related themes and offer support in areas ranging from mental health to physical health to parenting support. Those involved in providing assistance should be familiar with the continuum of care offered by mutual aid/self-help groups.

Recreational/Leisure Programs

Quitting or moderating the use of a drug often constitutes a major change in a person's lifestyle, and thus he or she must develop constructive uses of leisure time to replace the heavy drug use. Studies have found that participating in sober recreational activities was correlated with ongoing sobriety six months after treatment (Zemore & Kaskutas, 2008) and with improved quality of life (Muller & Clausen, 2014). Low-cost recreational options include the YMCA/YWCA, where subsidies are often available, local recreation centres, and board of education programs offered through high school facilities. Leisure counselling may help a person choose an appropriate activity or to engage in activities initially only with other recovering persons. As well, some communities have developed leisure activities and clubs specifically for those in recovery.

Social Assistance

Social assistance refers to the provision of monetary or in-kind supports to low-income individuals to achieve a minimum income standard established by law or convention. While this is most often associated with financial support, employment support, child care, food subsidies, and transportation assistance are also subsumed under this category. The relationship between social assistance and addictions is complex. First, social assistance is certainly not a resource everyone with an addiction issue requires. In fact, it is a major myth that addiction only occurs to those with economic issues or challenges. However, addiction certainly can lead to the loss of economic supports, and there is a correlation between poverty and addiction. Social assistance is therefore an adjunct resource to support some people undergoing addiction treatment and to aid in their re-establishing themselves financially on completion. A quasi-experimental study in 1998 demonstrated that when people receiving substance abuse treatment had access to social assistance caseworkers to assist with "medical screenings, housing assistance, parenting classes and employment services," they showed "significantly less substance use, fewer physical and mental health problems and better social function at 6-months" compared to the control group (McLellan et al., 1998, p. 1489). Social assistance recipients typically also receive drug benefit coverage, which has important implications for treating addictions. A number of pharmacological therapies for smoking cessation, opioid dependency, and alcohol abuse are also covered for social assistance recipients under drug formularies.

5.5 RELAPSE PREVENTION

Follow-up, aftercare, or, as it has become more prominently known, relapse prevention are different names describing similar programming activities. Relapse poses a fundamental barrier to the treatment of addiction. Depending on the definition one uses for recovery, statistics indicate that up to 90 percent of clients have the potential to lapse or to relapse (Brandon, Vidrine, & Litvin, 2007; Carroll, 1996; Marlatt, 1985). Relapse itself is a process rather than a discrete event and is now considered, not as a failure, but rather as a setback. Thus, aftercare needs to be a continuation of work initiated during the initial treatment regimen, with a focus on resettling and reintegrating individuals back into society. The goal is to provide continuing encouragement, support, and additional services as needed following a client's completion of a treatment plan. Preventing relapse or minimizing its extent is a necessity for successful, long-term change (Csiernik & Troller, 2002; Hendershot et al., 2011).

Relapse prevention entails supporting the client after treatment and monitoring progress, so if an issue does arise, an appropriate referral can be quickly made. Relapse-prevention programs also offer clients contacts and a support system after treatment so that an early intervention can be made in the event of a lapse or relapse. The actual length of the follow-up period will vary in how often contact is made and for how long it is kept, with the most significant restriction being staff resources. A minimally acceptable aftercare program would be a monthly contact for one year, with the provision that the client can contact the relapse-prevention worker whenever needed. A two-year follow-up is preferable, though some programs have moved to a five-year plan, encouraging those with longer recovery histories to facilitate relapse-prevention groups for more recent clients, as well as to join alumni groups for their own growth and development (Noone, Dua & Markham, 1999).

Various studies have demonstrated the utility of relapse prevention (Bennett et al., 2005; McKay et al., 2011; Witkiewitz & Bowen, 2010). However, it can be difficult empirically to disentangle the effects of aftercare itself from what motivated the client to participate in it. Despite the potential for aftercare to sustain treatment gains, not all treatment providers routinely include it as part of their continuum of care, and clients must often seek out this care separately at the end of their treatment program.

DISCUSSION QUESTIONS

1. (a) Identify, from your own community, one example of each of the addiction-specific treatment resources discussed in the chapter.
   (b) What client attributes would lead you to refer a client to each of those resources?
2. Identify one example of each of the adjunct resources (section 5.4) from your community.
3. From your perspective, which are superior in-patient or outpatient/community-based programs? Specify the needs that each kind of program addresses.
4. What agencies offer relapse-prevention counselling in your community? Which modalities are used in the different programs?
5. What gaps exist in your community's continuum of care that need to be addressed with additional resources?

Chapter 6
PREVENTION

6.1 INTRODUCTION
Universal Prevention
Selective Prevention
Indicated Prevention

School-based drug education remains the great hope for preventing psychoactive substance abuse, for the longer drug use can be delayed, the less likely it is to become a lifelong issue (Christensen & Kohlmeier, 2014; Jit, Aveyard, Barton, & Meads, 2010; Norström & Pape, 2012; Odjers et al., 2008). Prevention initiatives offer a tangible approach to diverting the development of substance use before it becomes a habit and develops into an addiction. The International Narcotics Control Board (2014) states that, while "the phenomenon of drug abuse requires societies to dedicate resources to evidence-based prevention, education and interventions ... [and] although such activities can be resource-intensive, studies have shown that for every $1 spent, good prevention programmes can save governments up to $10 in subsequent costs" (p. 1). The route to substance abuse and addiction is a complex interaction between individual biological and psychological factors, developmental maturation, family variables, and each individual's social context (Hays, Hays, & Mulhall, 2003; Vimpani, 2005). There are three levels of prevention:

- Primary: Occurs before a person begins to use substances. The goal is to prevent or delay the onset of first use.
- Secondary: Occurs once a person has begun to experiment with drug use. The goal is to prevent more frequent, regular use.
- Tertiary: Occurs after substance use has become problematic. The goal is to reduce the harm associated with use or, if possible, achieve complete abstinence.

The goal of psychoactive drug-abuse prevention can be very narrow, as in complete abstinence. It can also be more broad, and defined as a reduction in the prevalence of the misuse and abuse of drugs, or the reduction in the incidence, duration, or intensity of undesirable developmental outcomes, through a sustained change in drug-using behaviour (Dumka, Roosa, Michaels, & Suh, 1995; Shepard & Carlson, 2003; Siegal et al., 2001). The use of psychoactive substances is a widespread phenomenon with a peak risk between the ages of 10 and 20. The preadolescent years from 10 to 12 are a particularly vulnerable period for the development of early substance abuse (Segal & Stewart, 1996; Skara & Sussman, 2003). In Canada, 60 percent of those between the ages of 15 to 24 are drug users (Canadian Centre on Substance Abuse, 2008). Research indicates that even delaying alcohol use onset to age 13 can significantly reduce the risk of severe alcohol problems in later adolescence, and that subsequent delays in onset of use provide additional protection from later problems, such as committing a crime or contracting a sexually transmitted disease (Odjers et al., 2008; Werch et al., 2001). Those working to minimize this harm need to consider which level of intervention they wish to take. Is the focus of the psychoactive drug prevention program on

- those who chose to abstain from drug use;
- those who chose to postpone drug use;
- those already using drugs;
- those experiencing difficulties with their current drug use;
- those experiencing difficulties with the use of drugs by relatives or friends; or
- the larger family system (Griffin & Svendsen, 1992; United Nations Office on Drug and Crime, 2004)?

Prevention efforts should start early and continue through adolescence and into adulthood. Prevention initiatives must also be repeated: they do not work in isolation. There are two principal prevention strategies—risk avoidance and risk reduction—that are used to influence three distinct subpopulations: non-users, low-risk users and at-risk users (British Columbia Ministry of Children and Family Services, 1996). The risk continuum (Figure 6.1) illustrates the different types of strategies used to influence people's behaviour, depending on their level of risk for alcohol or other drug problems. The risk continuum is a useful tool to help understand the levels of risk and also to demonstrate the relationship between prevention and treatment.

There are three prevention focuses that can be adopted within the risk continuum: (1) universal, (2) selective, and (3) indicated or targeted.

FIGURE 6.1: THE RISK CONTINUUM

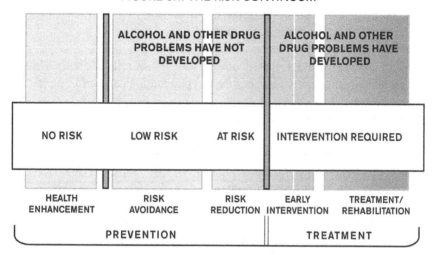

Source: British Columbia Ministry of Children and Family Services (1996)

Universal Prevention

These are activities that target the entire population, such as all Grade 9 students or all parents of high school students, with the aim of promoting the health of the population or preventing or delaying the onset of substance use (health enhancement). Activities are targeted to a general population that has not been identified or pre-selected on the basis of individual risk. There is generally no indication that any particular member of these groups is using psychoactive drugs, or at risk of using, but engaging in this type of prevention has definite benefits compared to the costs (Dumka et al., 1995; Shenassa, 2002). Universal prevention consists of activities and intervention that are applicable to everyone in the group, so this approach avoids labelling (Bauman et al., 2000; Durlak, 1998; Foxcroft, Ireland, Lowe, & Breen, 2002).

However, while the majority of adolescents are able to negotiate the transition to adulthood without major crisis, some are innately unable to handle the stresses and strains of the teenage years. Others lack adequate family support through this developmental stage, and some simply become involved with a problematic peer group, which can continue into adulthood. These individuals will need different approaches than a basic universal prevention program (Tobler, 2000).

Selective Prevention

A more intensive approach targets specific subgroups deemed to be at greater risk (risk avoidance and risk reduction), including those with

- academic problems;
- family issues and dysfunction;

- issues of poverty;
- problematic social environments; and
- a family history of substance abuse.

Program recipients are targeted not because of specific individual needs assessment or diagnoses, but because of epidemiologically and empirically established risk.

Compared to universal programs, selective programs have

- smaller numbers of participants per group;
- recipients who are known and who are specifically recruited to participate in the intervention;
- longer and more intensive structure;
- more intrusive intervention, with a goal of changing existing behaviours in a positive direction;
- a higher degree of skill among program leaders and staff;
- a greater cost per participant; and
- a greater likelihood of demonstrating change.

As selective programs do not individually assess participants, it is critical to be clear on the variables and characteristics being considered for group selection, and some general screening should occur (Kumpfer, Alexander, McDonald, & Olds, 1998).

Indicated Prevention

Indicated prevention is for those who are already using or involved with psychoactive drugs, but who are typically not yet dependent, though are at a high risk to be so in the future. This type of programming is individualized and can include a formal counselling or treatment component for the student and also for the family as warranted. Individual rather than group work is recommended with this population, as bringing them together can normalize their behaviour and increase substance use. Indicated prevention also targets injection drug users (IDUs) and teaches them harm-reduction techniques with or without a goal of abstinence. These are the most costly types of programs (Catalano et al., 1993; Cuijpers, 2003; Greenberg, Domitrovich, & Bumbarger, 2000; Kumpfer et al., 1998; Roberts et al., 2001).

Ultimately, the utility and feasibility of community intervention and prevention programs depend greatly on matching students to an appropriate program, as indiscriminate application of a program to an entire community benefits only a few and can actually harm others. The most comprehensive approach is a multiple gating intervention strategy (MGIS) that combines and integrates universal, selective, and indicated prevention programs to maximize their collective impact, though this requires a coordinated effort among multiple partners, including the school system, police, and community-based health and social services (Dishion & Mc-Mahon, 1998).

6.2 PROGRAM COMPONENT OPTIONS

Components of a psychoactive drug prevention program can be divided into three core areas: (1) knowledge, (2) attitudes and values, and (3) skills.

Knowledge
- the concept of abstinence and alternative behaviours to drug use
- definitions of drugs and psychoactive drugs, drug misuse, and abuse and drug dependency
- how different contexts and situations influence personal values, attitudes, beliefs, and behaviour in relation to drug use
- how different drugs can affect a person's ability to perform tasks
- the impact of media messages on the health behaviour of individuals and societies
- the importance of self-esteem, positive self-concept, and identity
- the rights and responsibilities of interpersonal relationships

Attitudes and Values
- a value stance regarding drug use and the confidence to act on those values
- the significance of social and cultural influences on beliefs
- empathy and acceptance of a diverse range of people
- individual responsibility for health and universal health protection
- personal beliefs about drugs and their effects on decisions

Skills
- the ability to communicate constructively with parents, teachers, and peers
- giving and receiving care in a variety of health-related situations
- setting short- and long-term health goals
- demonstrating conflict, aggression, stress, and time-management skills
- identifying and assessing personal risk and practising universal protection
- developing assertiveness and dealing with influences from others; working effectively with others; and coping with change, loss, and grief (Minnesota Department of Education, 1992; Tobler, 1993; Tobler & Stratton, 1997; United Nations Office on Drug and Crime, 2004)

Prevention programming for youth may be classroom-based, school-wide, or applied in multiple settings, including the community. Prevention programs can be presented by appropriately selected and matched peers, teachers, program staff, outside speakers, police, parents, or professional counsellors. A thorough prevention program framework

- addresses protective factors, risk factors, and resiliency;
- seeks comprehensiveness;
- ensures sufficient program duration and intensity;
- uses accurate information;
- sets clear and realistic goals;
- monitors and evaluates the project;
- addresses sustainability from the beginning;
- accounts for the clients' stage of psychosocial development;
- recognizes youth perceptions of substance use;
- involves youth in program design and implementation;
- develops credible messages delivered by credible messengers;
- combines knowledge and skill development;
- uses an interactive group process; and
- provides sufficient attention to teacher/leader qualities and training (Roberts et al., 2001).

Again, the issue of program intent must be clearly specified, as the program will

- increase the knowledge about drugs in adolescents;
- increase the knowledge about drugs in adults;
- increase the knowledge about drugs in families;
- reduce the use of drugs;
- delay the onset of first drug use;
- reduce abuse of drugs; or
- minimize the harm caused by the use of drugs (Cuijpers, 2003).

Actual prevention strategies options are quite broad and, of course, are not equally applicable to each of the three prevention focuses:

1. *Information strategies*: Teaching facts about the legal, physiological, and psychological consequences of psychoactive drug use and abuse using didactic presentations, discussions, and multimedia presentations.
2. *Normative education*: Adolescents and adults alike typically overestimate the level of drug use among their peers and the general population, which leads to inaccurate normative expectations and a set of expectations of drug use. Normative education makes students aware that most people do not use drugs and do not think drug use is "cool,"

countering the myth that everyone is doing it through use of national and local surveys.

3. *Perceived harm education*: Entails teaching participants about the risks and short- and long-term consequences of alcohol and other drug use. The message is best received when it comes from a credible source and is reinforced in multiple settings.

4. *Social influence education*: Teaches individuals to recognize external influences, such as social and peer pressure (role models, peer attitudes) to use drugs, and to develop cognitive skills to resist these influences.

5. *Advertising pressures education*: Teaches individuals to recognize the purposes and effects of advertising and other media, and the cognitive skills to resist these influences.

6. *Protective factors*: Teaches, supports, and encourages the development of positive aspects of life, such as helping, caring, goal setting, and challenging students to live up to their potential, and facilitating affiliations with positive peers.

7. *Resistance (refusal) skills*: Teaches students and adults how to recognize and resist pressure from others to use drugs, including learning to resist peers effectively and assertively while still maintaining friendships by using behavioural examples, homework, and even older peers. Common techniques include:

   • teaching students to recognize high-risk situations
   • increasing awareness of media influences
   • developing direct refusal skills

8. *Competence enhancement skills training*: In this approach, drug use is conceptualized as a socially learned and functional behaviour that is the result of the interplay between social and personal factors. Those with poor personal and social skills are more susceptible to influences that promote drug use, and are also more motivated to use drugs as an alternative to more adaptive but typically more difficult to master skills. This approach teaches generic social and personal skills.

9. *Persuasion strategies*: Influencing attitudes or behaviours regarding drugs through persuasive messages.

10. *Counselling strategies*: Peer, self-help, or professional counselling programs for those experiencing both drug and non-drug-related personal and family problems (targeted prevention).

11. *Tutoring/teaching strategies*: Peer or cross-age tutoring or teaching to assist in enhancing academic achievement.

12. *Peer group strategies*: Attempts to strengthen or exploit natural peer group dynamics to inhibit drug use. This is primarily targeted at students.

13. *Family strategies*: Efforts aimed at strengthening parenting skills and family relationships to address student drug issues.

14. *Recreational activities*: Programs to occupy leisure time and provide alternative activity other than drug use.

15. *Harm minimization/harm reduction*: The goals of this approach do not focus on abstinence but rather on imparting information to reduce the harm stemming from substance use and to promote safer drug-using skills, though abstinence remains an option as the ultimate risk-reduction goal. This approach does not condone drug use but acknowledges that it exists and responds to it by providing accurate information about drugs, combined with the opportunity to learn appropriate skills to allow young people to become more discerning in their drug use, leading to the minimization of drug-reduced harm. This includes the following:

   - decision-making and problem-solving techniques for handling situations in which a choice needs to be made
   - stress management to allow participants to learn how to recognize positive and negative stress and how to develop skills to manage stress
   - anger and anxiety management skills
   - communication skills and social competence to help students learn to listen, express themselves effectively, and avoid being misunderstood; the importance of core verbal skills should not be underestimated here
   - personal and social skills to teach effective social interaction skills, including how to make friends and reduce anxiety when interacting with those they do not know or know well
   - assertiveness skills (peer resistance) in learning how to express needs and likes/dislikes, stand up for oneself, and resist pressure to do things you do not want to do

16. *Affective education*: Focuses on enriching the personal and social development of prevention program participants by developing positive self-esteem, good interpersonal skills, and decision-making ability so that individuals will be less likely to use or abuse psychoactive substances. The intent is to increase self-understanding and acceptance through values clarification and decision making to improve interpersonal relationships by fostering effective communication. It can include both affective skill-building strategies, which are systematic efforts to improve affective skills related to drug use (such as communication skills, decision-making skills, and self-assertion), and affective experiential strategies, which are attempts to provide positive or growth-inducing affective experiences.

17. *Resilience development*: A selective prevention approach that entails achieving positive outcomes despite the risk situations in which people must live. It involves the development of social competence; increasing bonding;

communicating high expectations for academic, social, and work performance; maximizing opportunities for students' meaningful participation in the school environment or employees in a work environment; and creating partnerships with families and community resources. Resilience is conceptually distinguished from risk reduction, as it focuses on developing people's interests and strengths to promote their healthy development. Resilience education is the development of decision-making and affective skills within each person and connectedness among people in the context of a healthy and democratic learning environment. Resilience education can lead to higher levels of internal locus of control, concern for others, conflict-resolution skills, and a fuller sense of school as community. At the curriculum level, young people show more participation, higher self-efficacy, better decision-making skills, and less involvement with outside negative activities. The educator becomes a facilitator of learning rather than only an imparter of knowledge as the use of this approach is more problem-solving-and process-orientated (Botvin, 1990, 2000; Botvin & Griffin, 2004; Brooks, 2006; Brounstein & Zweig, 1999; Brown, 2001; Griffin & Svendsen, 1992; Hawthorne, 2001; Poulin & Nicholson, 2005; Schaps, DiBartolo, Moskowitz, Palley, & Churgin, 1981; Shope, Elliot, Raghunathan, & Waller, 2001).

Finally, there are questions that must also be at the forefront of programming decision making. How culturally and gender sensitive should the program be? Is there a need to include or enhance the program for those of minority status or those who face additional challenges? Cultural sensitivity in this field entails adapting prevention curricula to accommodate the intended audience, including surface structure, which involves matching curricula to superficial demographics, such as language. However, the more difficult component is adapting curricula for deep structure, which needs to take into account cultural, social, historical, environmental, and psychological factors (Blake, Amaro, Schwartz & Flinchbaugh, 2001; Catalano et al., 1993; Davis et al., 2004; Foxcroft, Ireland, Lister-Sharp, Lowe, & Breen, 2002; Foxcroft, Ireland, Lowe, & Breen, 2006; Guthrie & Flinchbaugh, 2001; Hawkins, Cummins, & Marlatt, 2004; Hecht & Raup-Krieger, 2006; Kulis et al., 2005; Resnicow, Soler, Braithwaite, Ahluwalia, & Butler, 2000; Schinke et al., 1988; Schinke, Di Noia, & Glassman, 2004; Schinke & Schwinn, 2005; Unger et al., 2004).

6.3 EFFECTIVE PROGRAMMING

Results! Why, I have gotten a lot of results.
I know several thousand things that won't work.
—Thomas Edison

Prevention interventions need to be intensive and extensive to achieve positive outcomes. Targeted programs do better than universal programs at obtaining

316   Substance Use and Abuse

specific objectives, with parental involvement making a significant difference in overall outcomes regardless of which approach is taken (Hayward, Cook, & Thorne, 1994). Effective programs for youth are typically led by teachers and supported by specialists from the treatment community, with police retaining a core educational function relating to illicit substances (Allott, Paxton, & Leonard, 1999). An effective global plan would have a balance between universal, selective, and targeted programs.

In general, effective comprehensive youth development programs should foster and promote the following:

- bonding
- resilience
- social competence
- emotional competence
- cognitive competence
- behavioural competence
- moral competence
- self-determination
- spirituality
- self-efficacy
- clear and positive identity
- belief in the future
- recognition for positive behaviour
- pro-social norms
- opportunity for pro-social involvement (Catalano, Berglund, Ryan, Lonczak, & Hawkins, 2004; Nation et al., 2003)

Prevention programs should aim to both reduce risk factors and enhance protective factors by employing a variety of prevention strategies:

- helping students recognize internal pressures, such as wanting to belong to the group, along with external pressures, such as peer attitudes and advertising, that influence them to use alcohol, tobacco, and other drugs
- facilitating development of personal, social, and refusal skills to resist these pressures
- teaching that using alcohol, tobacco, and other drugs is not the norm among teenagers, correcting the misconception that everyone is "doing it," and promoting positive norms through bonding with school and constructive role models (normative education)
- providing developmentally appropriate material and activities, including information about the short-term and long-term consequences of alcohol, tobacco, and other drugs

- using interactive teaching techniques, such as role play, discussion, brainstorming, and co-operative learning
- actively involving the family and the community so that prevention strategies are reinforced across settings
- including facilitator training and support to ensure that curricula are delivered as intended
- containing information that is easy for facilitators to implement and both culturally and gender-relevant for participants
- being developmentally appropriate
- engaging parents in reinforcing ideas discussed in class, including refusal skills as part of family homework assignments
- promoting positive relationships between parents and children to enhance family norms, including communication skills to allow parents to communicate with their children as they move into adolescence
- teaching parenting skills, including positive discipline and adequate supervision
- including community resources to support and reinforce concepts being taught
- including school and workplace policies on alcohol, tobacco, and drug use
- providing important health information that people need to make decisions about use and non-use
- encouraging and supporting drug-free activities and situations, emphasizing not only the skills required for participation but also the personal, social, and spiritual dynamics associated with choice
- developing guidelines for safe, healthy, and appropriate behaviour for family members
- encouraging broader skills beyond substance use refusal, including promoting positive, healthy lifestyles; development of positive personal, social, and spiritual support systems; and promoting healthy lifestyles that include good nutrition, stress management, and lifelong exercise and activity (Brounstein & Zweig, 1999; Griffin & Svendsen, 1992)

An Australian study conducted by Midford and colleagues (2002) indicates that effective school-based drug education should be based on the following:

- evidence-based
- involvement of parents and the wider community
- drug education as an entire school initiative
- taught in a sequentially, developmentally appropriate school health curriculum

- based on students' expressed needs and responsive to their developmental, gender, cultural, language, socio-economic, and lifestyle differences
- initiated before drug use begins
- harm-minimization focus
- interactive teaching techniques
- use of trained peer facilitators to lead discussions
- the classroom teacher as central in the education process and supported by regular training and up-to-date teaching resources from community experts
- practical, immediate, relevant information on the harms associated with drug use, influences that promote drug use, and normative student drug use
- drug resistance, along with more general social skills training, including the values, attitudes, and behaviours of the broader community
- consideration of the interrelationship among the individual, social context, and drug in determining drug use
- emphasis on drug use that is most likely and most harmful

Effective school-based programs are also supported by policies that prohibit smoking, drinking, and other drug use by students on school property and extend to teachers or members of the community using the school for a function. The messages should be positive (school premises are drug-free) rather than negative ("Just Say No") with consequences for violation of the policy clearly presented. Fully comprehensive and integrated programs involve the entire community; make use of multiple strategies; design ongoing activities that target audiences from the very young through older citizens; allow adequate time for prevention efforts; and seek to integrate prevention strategies into family, school, religious, and other community environments (Paglia & Room, 1999; Wagner, Tubman, & Gil, 2004). What has yet to be established is how social media can best be incorporated into these initiatives.

6.4 INEFFECTIVE PROGRAMMING

For young people, smoking, drinking, and other drug use are key to distinguishing their identities and their subculture from those of adults. Thus, even good prevention programming has much to overcome to prevent drug use. One of the difficulties with school-based drug education is that it is an attempt by the adult world to have an impact on youth. Most universal drug-prevention initiatives have not been able to demonstrate ongoing effectiveness; they simply have not shown long-term impacts, though it has been argued that some of this may be a result of how success has been conceptualized and how the evaluations have been analyzed. Most universal drug education initiatives have had, at best, minimal impacts on behaviour, with typical initiatives achieving only short-term delays in the onset of substance use by non-users and short-term reductions in use by current users. Programs tend not to work because there is inappropriate initial selection of the program, inadequate stakeholder involvement (including the school system), insufficient attention to program fidelity, and improperly conducted evaluation (Case & Haines, 2003; Cuijpers, 2002; Derzon, Sale, Springer, & Brounstein, 2005; Dusenbury, Brannigan, Falco, & Hansen, 2003; Faggiano et al., 2006; Foxcroft et al., 2006; Foxcroft, Lister-Sharp, & Lowe, 1997; Gorman, 1997, 2002; Hawthorne, 2001; MacKinnon & Lockwood, 2003; White & Pitts, 1998).

The seminal piece on what not to do regarding illicit drug prevention programming was written in 1975 by de Haes and Schuurman. They randomly assigned 1,035 Dutch youth ages 14–16 into four groups. Two groups involved one-shot approaches, led by outside experts. The first stressed the dangers and moral dimensions of illicit drug use and was called the "warning/mild horror" approach. The second was a factual psycho-educational approach that provided accurate information to participants. The third group consisted of 10 1-hour small group sessions led by teachers in which general issues of adolescence were discussed rather than only drug use and prevention. The fourth group of youth were a control group who received no additional education. Regardless of which approach was used, those already using drugs were not deterred and continued to use. However, three months after the initiatives were completed, follow-up questionnaires found significant differences between those who had not been using at the time they participated in the program. Control group use had increased 3.6 percent and was considered a baseline increase resulting from natural curiosity and experimentation. The "warning" group's drug-using rate three months after the intervention had increased at double the rate of the control group to 7.3 percent, while the "fact" group also had more new drug users than the control group, at 4.6 percent. Only in the discussion group was the number of new users less than that of the control group, one-third that of the warning group (2.6 percent).

Similarly, evaluations of early intervention programs focused on information dissemination, alternatives approaches, and affective education, typically in a non-integrated manner, have consistently failed to show any long-term effects, with some studies indicating, as was found by de Haes and Schuurman, that factual initiatives alone actually increased drug use (Foxcroft et al., 2002, 2006). Nearly half of all implemented drug education prevention programming focuses only on providing knowledge while alternative methods promoting risk and protective factors are used much less. Studies examining the effectiveness of drug education have led to the conclusion that neither information alone nor affective programs nor social skills–alone programs—including the original DARE, Life Skills Training, the Seattle Social Development Project, ATLAS, SUCCESS, or Learning for

Life—have had significant impacts (Allott et al., 1999; Brown, 2001; Clark et al., 2010; Gorman, 2003; Lynam et al., 1999; Perry et al., 2003; Sobeck, Abbey, & Agius, 2006; West & O'Neal, 2004).

As well, there is no evidence that approaches promoting no use of any drug are more successful than alternative options, as most of the research has focused only on abstinence and not openly broached other strategies to reduce use. A focus on no-use drug education has resulted in decreased educator credibility, with students losing trust in adults because no-use programs have punitive zero-tolerance policies, but adults do not abide by the same guidelines. In a no-use context, young people cannot seriously engage with educators in the necessary and complex process involved in their own cognitive and emotional development regarding such a socially pervasive issue as drug use. Furthermore, fewer than one in five prevention programs has been actually implemented as designed. The main deficits are a lack of teacher training and materials, the use of some but not all lessons, and limited teaching strategies (Hallfors & Godette, 2002). While schools attempt to engage students by encouraging curiosity and risk taking as part of their personal development, when it comes to drug prevention, the typical message has been no, abstinence-only, and zero tolerance (Brown, 2001; Gorman, 1997; Marsiglia, Holleran, & Jackson, 2000).

Psychoactive drug-prevention programs shown not to produce significant changes include the following:

- single-shot assemblies and testimonials by former drug dependent persons that reinforce a negative norm that everyone uses drugs
- programs presented independently and in a non-integrated manner
- projects with inadequate facilitator training, preparation, and instruction manuals
- sessions where there is inconsistency between presenters' messages
- initiatives that take a fragmentary approach and are not coordinated with other existing community prevention efforts
- undertakings in which abstinence is the primary criteria of success
- presentations that focus on fear arousal, using scare tactics and moralistic appeals that assume fear or negative consequences will prevent use, disseminating only information that using drugs is dangerous
- programs with curricula that rely solely on accurate information about drugs, their effects, and their dangers
- projects that focus only on affective education, working to promote self-esteem and emotional well-being without providing training in resistance skills and normative education
- undertakings with only a social influence component
- sessions that spend too much time focusing on those who are using drugs

- presentations based exclusively on strategies to enhance an adolescent's character or personality
- initiatives that do not respond to youth of varying ages, from different settings, and of different ethnic backgrounds
- programs that do not specifically identify and offer additional services to at-risk children and their families
- enterprises that start too late, as kindergarten is the appropriate starting point for school-based prevention programs
- projects with an inadequate or insufficient evaluative component
- programs with insufficient implementation, program fidelity, and curriculum (Bosworth, 1998; Botvin, 1990; Donaldson, Graham, Piccinin, & Hansen, 1995; Gorman, 2003; Griffin & Svendsen, 1992; Midford et al., 2002; Mohai, 1991; Resnicow & Botvin, 1993; Tobler, 2000)

In general, school-based programming has been too narrow. The process that local schools use in developing their own substance abuse curriculum includes high levels of involvement by a variety of personnel, but low levels of training, little use of resources outside of the school's immediate sources, and poor training of teachers who will be implementing the curriculum (Bosworth, 1998). As well, most of the literature supporting resistance training is American-based, and there is a different culture of violence and gangs in the United States than exists in other nations. Thus, the importance of resistance skills training may be overstated as is the importance of peers in determining drug use (Allott, Paxton & Leonard, 1999; Oster, 1983).

Resources used in conducting drug-prevention programs should not do the following:

- glamorize drug use and drug users as cool or sophisticated
- exaggerate and misrepresent the dangers of drug use as these contradict participants' knowledge or belief based on their own experiences
- use graphic images that portray drug use as dangerous or exciting
- present frightening case studies that are too far removed from the reality of participants' lives
- present emotionally loaded videos and personal anecdotes
- romanticize drugs using slang or street names without using the pharmacological names as this highlights a drug's positive side
- inform students on how to obtain, make, or use potentially harmful substances
- use images of drug use that can be appealing

- use one-off or standalone activities rather than activities that contribute to an ongoing comprehensive, developmentally appropriate program
- use only passive participation, such as lectures and teacher-centred discussions and dialogues (United Nations Office on Drugs and Crime, 2004)

There is no one best prevention strategy, and programs must be matched to the target. Thus, the first step in any programming plan should be a needs assessment to determine what is missing. To minimize the risk of a drug-prevention program being ineffective, the goal should be clearly articulated from the commencement of the initiative.

6.5 FAMILY PROGRAMMING

Parents can inhibit their children's substance use directly. They can reinforce their children's involvement in positive alternatives, yet many parents feel ill equipped to do so as there is no formal training in this skill, just as there is no formal training to become a parent (Dusenbury, 2000). Parents are powerful socializing agents in the lives of their children, and they are in a unique position to engage children in ongoing rather than singular dialogues about risky situations and decision making (Dufur, Parcel, & McKune, 2013; Miller-Day, 2002). Family-based prevention promotes healthy functioning in children primarily by addressing the risk and protective factors that characterize parents and families. Family interventions are generally the most effective strategy for changing the behaviour of high-risk young adolescents (Becker, Hogue, & Liddle, 2002; Davis et al., 2004; Dusenbury, 2000; Hays et al., 2003; Kumpfer & Alvarado, 2003; Kung & Farrell, 2000; Montoya, Atkinson, & McFaden, 2003; Redmond, Spoth, Shin, & Lepper, 1999; Vakalahi, 2001). Selective prevention initiatives that have also shown promise include working to decrease the use of substances by pregnant women and after the birth of a child. The work continues through the child's early education, including the development of parenting skills. The goal of family skills programs is not only to decrease substance abuse, but to positively affect parent-child family relations by increasing family cohesion, decreasing family conflict, and decreasing family health and social problems overall. Such programs should provide parents with the skills and opportunities to strengthen positive family relationships and family supervision and monitoring, and assist the family in communicating values and expectations. Though there is great range in the actual content of family skills, there are four primary approaches:

1. information only
2. parental skills
3. parent support

4. family interaction (Allott et al., 1999; United Nations Office on Drugs and Crime, 2009, 2013).

Box 6.1 provides a best practices program outline designed by the United Nations Office on Drugs and Crime to address this area.

A significant issue is the level of parental participation, as universal prevention initiatives usually attract very few parents. As well, the greater the parental use of alcohol, tobacco, and other drugs, the lower the rates of participation in any type of programming. Attempts at school-based initiatives tend to attract only the most motivated parents and to have high drop-out rates (Allott et al., 1999; Toomey et al., 1996). Parents who engage in universal drug-prevention programs prefer those that promote communication with their child, do not require much time to complete, and can be completed at home, typically through joint homework assignments. In these instances, materials should be enjoyable, easy for families to use, complement school-based activities, provide information to parents, and strengthen family communication (Bickel, 1995; Biglan & Metzler, 1998). However, as children grow into adolescence, this approach becomes less attractive, and older adolescents are more hesitant and resistant to engage in this type of program, which also requires teacher co-operation and coordination with other classroom activities (Spoth & Redmond, 2000).

An alternative that is not as comprehensive but has been used with positive outcomes is direct mailing of information, materials, and activities to parents for use in guiding discussions with their teenagers. A review of this method indicates that it did not alter parental behaviours, nor did the technique alone have a dramatic effect on adolescent drug use. However, it did enhance overall family functioning of those who chose to participate and opened up communication between parents and children (Bauman et al., 2000).

Recognized family factors that inhibit drug use include the following:

- close, mutually reinforcing parent-child relationships
- positive discipline methods
- monitoring, behavioural management, and supervision of children's activities outside the home (parental monitoring is the strongest preventative factor of any parenting variable)
- family involvement and advocacy in the community (Bahr, Hoffman, & Yang, 2005; Bry, Catalano, Kumpfer, Lochman, & Szapocznik, 1998; Case & Haines, 2003; Dishion & McMahon, 1998; Griffin, Botvin, Scheier, Diaz, & Miller, 2000)

However, as much as most families work to prevent their children from engaging in drug use, a minority of families actually contribute to their children's substance use and abuse through a variety of dynamics. These range from genetic predisposition to environmental factors, including being tolerant to use, modelling use, inconsistent discipline, poor supervision, unrealistic expectations, ineffective parenting, family isolation, family instability, conflict, family disorganization, marital discord, criminality, influencing peer selection (including condoning peers who use drugs), stress, faulty and harsh parenting, and, of course, physical, psychological, and sexual abuse (Bahr et al., 2005; Case & Haines, 2003; Dusenbury, 2000; Gardner, Green, & Marcus, 1994; Kumpfer & Alvarado, 2003; Kumpfer & Kaftarian, 2000; Lochman & van den Steenhoven, 2002). In these instances, a universal prevention approach would not be appropriate. Rather a selective or targeted approach would be necessary that

- enhanced family functioning, including teaching stress management strategies and conflict resolution options;
- addressed risky parenting behaviours, including discipline and increased monitoring of activities;
- included both mothers and fathers in the programming, along with the children; and,
- targeted decreasing parental use of psychoactive drugs (Bahr et al., 2005).

Research has indicated that in these circumstances, parental skills workshops, parent training, and family skills training have all decreased child substance use (Lochman & van den Steenhoven, 2002). These sessions have included resilience training, behavioural parent training, in-home family support, and family therapy. However, there are significant barriers to obtaining family involvement, including the following:

- unclear definitions and expectations
- lack of information
- inherent family-school system tensions
- the family and/or school system's lack of acknowledgement of the significance of alcohol and other drugs in both the family and the school system
- additional work for teachers and other school officials
- lack of coordination with other school events/educational efforts (Bickel, 1995; Biglan & Metzler, 1998; Perrino, Coatsworth, Briones, Pantin, & Szapocznic, 2001).

As well, most schools are not in a position to add a distinct family program to their curriculum. Thus, these initiatives, while they may begin within the school and should be coordinated with schools, usually occur in the community within a social agency. Despite the difficulties in establishing and implementing selective prevention programs that target high-risk families, these have been shown to have an impact on adolescent substance use. To be most successful, programs should begin work with high-risk families before and immediately following the birth of a child (Dusenbury, 2000).

The focus of successful selective programs has been on skill development and not only education. This allows for practice and feedback, assigning homework, and then helping family members refine skills that work while modifying those that are not improving (Etz, Robertson, & Ashery, 1998). The most effective strategies include parents and children in individual and group training sessions. In these interventions, work is done individually with the parents and the children, and then the entire family is brought together to practice skills and strategies (Hogue, Liddle, Becker, & Johnson-Leckrone, 2002). However, selective prevention programs are still not always sufficient, and the ability to incorporate targeted prevention programming with specific therapeutic interventions can be a valuable addition (Dusenbury, 2000).

Families least likely to engage in prevention programming are those that are disorganized with poor communication; have significant family conflict; have unreliable and inconsistent supports; and divergent expectations—exactly the group most in need. High-risk families may not resist participating. However, the qualities that make their children susceptible to substance abuse are the exact ones that limit their participation in prevention programs (Garnier & Stein, 2002). Thus, families may need support to achieve a minimal level of health and positive functioning to allow them to even participate in prevention programs. Pre-intervention programs may be necessary in these cases, as the family may be facing more pressing stressors than the risk that a child may be or is using drugs. This may necessitate crisis intervention or family therapy as a precursor to and component of the prevention program (Perrino et al., 2001).

Recommendations for engaging high-risk families in prevention programming are as follows:

- have a leader who is positive; who can remain hopeful and optimistic under trying circumstances; who is not into power and control; who is confident without being aloof; who focuses on family strengths, not deficits; and who has a high level of energy, creativity, and enthusiasm for the group
- clearly convey the purpose of the program to parents—why it is important to their children and to them
- build relationships of mutual trust, respect, and equality; be sincere in the relationships built; and have a positive community profile—small things such as calling parents after a session, thanking them for attending, and asking if they had any questions were seen as critical to long-term parental commitment, as

was dropping by the home when a session was missed to inquire if everything was okay

- create parent ownership and group bonding
- provide easy access to meetings, incentives, and reminders, including child care for those with younger children
- provide in-home sessions to those who missed some to keep them on pace with others in the group
- be flexible yet persistent (St. Pierre & Kaltreider, 1997)

Issues of race and culture are just as important when developing programs for families as they are when creating them for individual students or school systems. However, the greatest preventative factor appears to be affectionate parents who are attentive to their children, spend time with them, are aware of their activities, and set boundaries with a degree of flexibility (Bahr & Hoffman, 2010; Turner, 2000; Turner, Wieling, & Allen, 2004).

An interesting finding is that one of the most substantive ways for parents to decrease substance use among their children is to have dinner with them. As frequency of family dinners increases, reported drinking, smoking, and other drug use decreases. Compared to teens who participate in frequent family dinners (five to seven times per week), those who have infrequent family dinners (fewer than three times per week) are twice as likely to have used tobacco or marijuana, and more than one and a half times likelier to have used alcohol. Of course, this is a correlational finding and not causation, for the actual factor decreasing risk of use is family engagement. Being together is what decreases risk; speaking and listening to one another and giving children undivided parental attention. Cellphones and tablets need to be set aside and not only for dinner, but for regular, shared family activity. Children and youth need boundaries and established rules that are fair and consistently applied. They also need parents to set appropriate examples. The work in this area has led to the fourth Monday of September in each American state being proclaimed CASA Family Day—A Day to Eat Dinner with Your Children (National Center on Addiction and Substance Abuse, 2009, 2012).

One final debate involving families and prevention relates to harm minimization and alcohol and to setting appropriate boundaries and examples. An ongoing question in the field of prevention is whether parents should enforce an abstinence approach or provide alcohol and supervise their children's underage use of the drug. While there is variance by culture, adult supervised drinking overall tends to lead to higher levels of harmful alcohol use than in families where alcohol is not supplied by parents or where children are allowed to drink with their parents at home. While this runs contrary to some cultural beliefs, research findings provide little support for parental supervision of alcohol use as a protective factor for adolescent drinking. Providing opportunities for drinking in supervised contexts does not inhibit alcohol use or harmful use among adolescents. Even after adolescents begin to drink, adult supervision of alcohol use appears to exacerbate continued drinking and the harms associated with drinking. Parental supervision of children's drinking at a young age can establish a developmental process by which progression to unsupervised drinking occurs more rapidly than in families where alcohol use in not openly supported. Alcohol use in a supervised setting and subsequent alcohol use outside a supervised setting both influence the progression to misuse in adulthood compared to families where parents adopt a no-use expectation at home with their adolescent children (Gilligan, Kypri, & Lubman, 2012; Komro, Maldonado-Molina, Tobler, Bonds, & Muller, 2007; Kypri, Dean, & Stojanovski, 2007; Lundborg, 2007; McMorris, Catalano, Kim, Toumbourou, & Hemphill, 2011; van der Vorst, Engels, & Burk, 2010). Similar findings have also been noted with tobacco use (Gilligan, Kypri, & Lubman, 2012; Mahabee-Gittens, Xiao, Gordon, & Khoury, 2013).

BOX 6.1: PRINCIPLES OF A GOOD FAMILY SKILLS TRAINING PROGRAM

CONTENT AND SKILLS FOR PARENTS

Parents should learn and practice how to

- display affection and empathy appropriately to each other, their children, and other people;
- use positive attention and praise, consistent with desirable behaviour that has been communicated clearly to the child, including telling children that they are behaving well at appropriate times;
- appropriately express their feelings and emotions, talk about their own and their children's feelings, and help their children to recognize and express their emotions;
- identify and model behaviour that corresponds to the values and norms they want to transfer to their children
- learn new coping, resiliency, and anger-management skills to avoid further stress, and use fair-conflict strategies to eliminate verbal and physical fighting;
- use responsive play skills, allowing children to lead play activities and learn to manage their children while they lead in play; and
- have expectations that are appropriate to the age and developmental level of their children.

TEACHING PARENTS TO PROVIDE STRUCTURE
Parents should learn and practice how to
- use age-appropriate discipline methods, including teaching children about the consequences of their behaviour;
- establish clear rules and values for appropriate behaviour and help children understand the rules and values of the family and community;
- recognize possible problems and problem situations in the family and in the community (excessive or inappropriate Internet/social media use, neighbourhood environment) and how to protect their children;
- recognize what their good qualities are as parents and build on these qualities;
- reach agreement with each other on core issues of child rearing, parenting style, and family life and put them into practice, or, in the case of a single parent, consciously decide on core issues by themselves;
- monitor children's whereabouts, activities, friends, and school and academic performance;
- support children in reaching the goals that both parents and children think are important and praise them for doing so;
- manage conflicts in the family, solve arguments, and demonstrate forgiveness;
- protect children from involvement in parental arguments and help them to understand the reasons for them; and
- provide structure for family life in general, including having meals together at certain times of the day, and establishing times for doing homework and going to bed.

TEACHING PARENTS TO BECOME INVOLVED IN THEIR CHILDREN'S SCHOOL AND STUDIES AND IN THE COMMUNITY
Parents should learn and practice how to
- monitor and assist their children in the school and with their homework; and
- co-operate and communicate with the school and recreation and health centres in the community on matters involving their children.

Source: United Nations Office on Drugs and Crime (2009)

6.6 WHAT WORKS
The impacts of drug education on drug use have historically been minor and short-lived. This is not only due to poor initiatives but also to inherent

contradictions between the objectives of prevention and those of education. The first seeks to empower children and youth to think for themselves; the latter seeks to influence them to implement ready-made decisions. There are also inherent contradictions within prevention programs themselves. Some aim to limit young people's autonomy in their choice of friends and substances by extending autonomy in decision making. Programs encourage conformity to non-drug-use values by discouraging conformity to drug-using peers. They encourage the development of teamwork and social solidarity without acknowledging that youth may choose to accompany their peers as often as not, based on the situation. What appears to work best in keeping those who do not use drugs from starting to use are small, universal, interactive school-based programs that involve parents. Components that should be included are the following:

- Knowledge: Information about short-term and long-term health consequences
- Attitudes about drug use: feedback from school surveys of peer drug use, analysis of media and social influences that promote pro-drug attitudes, perception adjustment regarding actual peer use
- Drug refusal–based interpersonal skills: drug refusal skills, assertiveness skills, communication skills, safety skills (ways to intervene in a drinking/drugging and driving situation)
- Intrapersonal skills: coping skills, stress reduction techniques, goal setting, decision-making/problem solving
- Active involvement: student-generated role plays, participation among peers, supportive comments from peers, peer modelling of appropriate behaviour, rehearsal of drug-refusal skills, sufficient practice time, developmentally appropriate activities (Bahr et al., 2005; Baker, 2006; Case & Haines, 2003; Ma & Thompson, 1999; Marsiglia et al., 2000; Piper, Moberg, & King, 2000; Sale, Sambrano, Springer, & Turner, 2003; Tobler, 2000; Tobler & Stratton, 1997)

Successful universal prevention programs

- strengthen social competency;
- strengthen emotional competency;
- strengthen behavioural competency;
- strengthen cognitive competency;
- strengthen moral competency;
- enhance self-efficacy;
- increase healthy bonding with adults, peers, and younger children;
- expand opportunities and recognition;

- are consistent in program delivery;
- are at least nine months in duration with booster sessions;
- deliver the same message in multiple settings (school, home, community); and
- have a social influence component that increases awareness of the social influences promoting drug use, alters norms regarding the prevalence and acceptability of drug use, and provides formal drug resistance skills (Catalano et al., 2004; United Nations Office on Drugs and Crime, 2004).

However, in the majority of cases, drug problems disappear spontaneously when young people grow up. The proportion of adults with drug problems that continue past the age of 24 is small compared to the number of initial users. Thus, it may be more beneficial to examine programs for those with continuing problems and to develop more intense prevention programs for those with a high risk of ongoing problems (Cuijpers, 2003). Universal programs that are theoretically sound with empirical support have distinct limits: they are unlikely to reach those youth at the highest risk of using drugs and engaging in other anti-social behaviour, including those no longer in school, leading to a prevention conundrum. Those students at highest risk are often disconnected from the schools that offer the supports they require due to intellectual, academic, or family issues and are most likely to be absent or suspended from school (Cunningham & Henggeler, 2001). Thus, those most in need are least likely to benefit from universal prevention programs.

In the criminal justice literature, the offending population consists of two subgroups: a large group of individuals who experiment with illegal activities for a short period during adolescence who naturally or spontaneously stop; and a smaller group of offenders who begin earlier, continue for a longer period, and offend at higher rates, and are responsible for the majority of youth crime. A similar pattern exists among substance users, and thus targeting more prevention services toward higher risk youth has programming utility (Gottfredson & Wilson, 2003).

There is no single program that can prevent multiple high-risk behaviours. A package of coordinated, collaborative strategies and programs is required. Multifaceted interventions that target multiple risk and protective factors focusing on the influence not only of peers but also of parents, siblings, and other adults are the most likely to succeed with a higher risk population (Greenberg et al., 2000).

Program delivery is also important to consider. A tolerant atmosphere free of moralizing or scare tactics should be created in which an open dialogue between program leaders and students can occur. The program should be built around an active learning model that includes small-group discussions and role play rather than passive lectures and films. Presenters are best when participants can trust them and when they can present information in an accurate and unbiased manner. Teachers can also be assisted by peer leaders, though the peer's social group and who he or she is presenting to also need to be considered. Finally, anything taught in the school has greater impact when it is reinforced in the community by not only parents, but also the media and health policies (Centre for Addiction and Mental Health, 1999).

The goals of alcohol and drug prevention programs for youth have to be realistic to be effective. The main thrust, especially with those at higher risk, should be preventing or reducing harms associated with alcohol and other drug use as opposed to preventing use completely, with resiliency-focused programming having great potential. An attainable positive goal is to delay a young person's first use, to limit overall use, and to shape his or her drug use in a safe way. Programming should be comprehensive and include school-based initiatives in combination with family programming and broader community campaigns, while also including special programs for those at greater risk or who are already using in a problematic manner. Whenever possible, young people should be directly involved in the program planning and implementation to identify the issues, develop solutions, and deliver messages to their peers. Zero tolerance and hardline approaches do not work and can be counterproductive, punishing students who are still in the experimental stage and discouraging students already using from seeking help to minimize harm or to seek counselling support (Centre for Addiction and Mental Health, 1999).

6.7 WHAT TO DO

Before beginning a new program, answer the following questions:
- What is the purpose of the program?
- What is it that you are asking and wish to evaluate?
- Who is the population you wish to change?
- How will success be defined?
    through abstinence
    decreased/controlled use
    harm reduction
    psychosocial factors, such as coping
    change in knowledge or attitudes
    refusal skills
    resilience
    family functioning

The optimum evaluation has a pre-test and a post-test component. It includes both qualitative and quantitative data collection using a range of instruments, including, but not limited to the following:

- questionnaire survey
- interviews
- direct observation
- analysis of institutional records (secondary data analysis)
- focus groups
- measure of actual drug use (and which drugs)
- measures of intended drug use (and which drugs)
- measure of attitude toward drug use (and which drugs)
- drug knowledge (which drugs)
- affect (attitudes toward oneself, family, and school)
- academic performance and attendance
- family cohesiveness.

It is highly recommended that a triangulation approach be taken when evaluating any program with multiple measures from multiple viewpoints (Liddle & Hogue, 2000; MacKinnon & Lockwood, 2003; Schaps et al., 1981).

In determining what type of program to develop, the following five issues must be considered:

1. Outcome focus:
   (a) abstinence
   (b) harm minimization
   (c) harm reduction
2. Program focus:
   (a) universal
   (b) selective
   (c) indicated
   (d) multiple gating
3. Population focus:
   (a) students
   (b) families
   (c) adults
4. Program strategy:
   (a) adopt existing program
   (b) adapt existing program
   (c) develop own program
5. How will issues of gender and cultural sensitivity be addressed?

To aid with this process, the Canadian Centre on Substance Abuse (2010a) developed an evidence-informed tool that can be used when planning, implementing, or evaluating substance abuse prevention initiatives (Figure 6.2).

FIGURE 6.2: PLANNING, SELF-ASSESSMENT, AND ACTION SHEET

	Fully in place	Partly in place	Under development	Not done
A. Assess the situation				
1. Determine youth substance use patterns and associated harms				
2. Learn factors linked to local youth substance use problems				
3. Assess current activities, resources and capacity to act				
B. Organize the team and build capacity				
4. Engage youth partners in the initiative				
5. Develop organizational structure and processes				
6. Build and maintain team capacity				
7. Clarify team members' perceptions and expectations				
C. Plan a logical and sustainable initiative				
8. Ensure the plan addresses priority concerns, factors and current capacity				
9. Develop a logic model showing how initiative will bring desired change				
10. Plan for sustainability of the initiative				
D. Coordinate and implement evidence-based activities				
11. Promote quality of existing and planned initiatives				
12. Strengthen coordination among local initiatives				
13. Give attention to community policies and processes				
14. Monitor the initiative				
E. Evaluate and revise initiative accordingly				
15. Conduct a process evaluation of the initiative				
16. Conduct an outcome evaluation of the initiative				
17. Account for costs associated with the initiative				
18. Revise initiative based on the evaluations				

Source: Canadian Centre on Substance Abuse (2010a)

DISCUSSION QUESTIONS

1. (a) Which of the prevention initiatives discussed in the chapter have you been previously exposed to?
   (b) Which did you find effective? Why?
   (c) Which did you find ineffective? Why?
2. What barriers would you anticipate in developing a prevention program for:
   (a) grade-school children?
   (b) high school students?
   (c) families?
3. Based on the readings, your experiences, and the barriers any prevention initiative faces, design an outline for an effective prevention program and the steps you would take to implement it.

Chapter 7

BECOMING A COMPETENT ADDICTION COUNSELLOR: LEGAL, ETHICAL, AND PRACTICE CONSIDERATIONS

7.1 PSYCHOACTIVE DRUGS AND THE LAW
  History
  Penalties
  Alcohol
  Tobacco
  Cannabis

History

Since the early 1970s drug offences have accounted for more than one-third of the growth in the incarcerated population in Canada, with the rate for drug arrests increasing 1,000 percent between 1980 and the end of the century. Over the past two decades, Canada has had the highest number of drug arrests per capita of any nation other than the United States (Grant, 2009; Motiuk & Vuong, 2002; Riley, 1998). Contemporary Canadian drug legislation traces its origins to the Opium Act of 1908, which created the first drug prohibition of the 20th century while also formally regulating alcohol and tobacco sales. Other opioids and cocaine were added in 1911, with cannabis being made an illicit substance without any parliamentary debate in 1923. Six years later, the Opium and Narcotic Act was introduced and became Canada's primary drug legislation of the 20th century. Since then Canada has become a signatory to all three major international drug laws, which prohibit and regulate psychoactive substances: the Single Convention on Narcotic Drugs (1961), the Convention on Psychotropic Substances (1971), and the Convention against Illicit Traffic in Narcotic Drugs and Psychotropic Substances (1988) (the Vienna

Convention). These treaties significantly determine which drugs will be allowed to be legally used and which are to be banned, not only in Canada but around the globe. For example the Single Convention, which limits the production and trade in prohibited substances to the quantity needed to meet the medical and scientific need of each nation, has incorrectly labelled cannabis as a narcotic and thus purposefully shaped international drug policy regarding this drug for over half a century (Solomon, Richmond, & Usprich, 1989).

In 1961, in response to the Single Convention on Narcotic Drugs, the Canadian government introduced the Narcotic Control Act, which made the simple possession of cannabis an indictable offence along with drugs such as heroin and cocaine, while increasing the maximum jail sentence for trafficking to 14 years from 7 for all narcotic substances. Between 1969 and 1973, the Commission of Inquiry into the Non-Medical Use of Drugs (the Le Dain Commission) examined the use of psychoactive drugs in Canada and recommended changes to the legislation that took on more of a public health orientation rather than an exclusive criminal justice focus. Despite some sympathy for the Committee's paradigm-shifting recommendations, Canada's drug laws remained unaltered.

In 1987, in response to the Reagan administration's reaffirmation of the War on Drugs in the United States, which actually officially began during President Nixon's time in office, Canada's federal government introduced a new drug strategy in an attempt to address not only the supply, but also the demand component of the drug equation. Not only were new enforcement initiatives introduced, but funding was also provided for new treatment and prevention programs. As well, a decision against random drug tests for civil servants was made, and instead, employee assistance programs were introduced for all employees and their family members, establishing a new timbre for the era (Standing Committee on National Health and Welfare, 1987).

However, nearly a decade later, a much more conservative legislation was passed to close the 20th century. In a ploy used over time in numerous local and national jurisdictions, the Chrétien Liberals, in attempting to demonstrate to the Canadian electorate that they were "tough on crime," opted to revert to a less progressive philosophical stance and return to viewing drug use primarily as a criminal rather than a health or social issue. This led to the development of the Controlled Drugs and Substances Act (CDSA), which moved Canadian drug policy back towards a prohibitionist orientation, with the CDSA only minimally addressing the long-term financial and human costs of treating drug users primarily as criminals. The importation, exportation, production, distribution, and possession of drugs and substances in Canada, including obtaining multiple prescriptions from one or more physicians (double doctoring), all became governed by the provisions of the CDSA, which replaced the Narcotic Control Act and parts III and IV of the Food and Drugs Act on June 20, 1996 (Riley, 1998). In 2012, additional amendments were made to the law by the Harper government, the most contentious of which was the addition of mandatory minimum sentencing for an accused convicted of serious drug-related offences including trafficking, possession for the purpose of trafficking, importing and exporting, and production of drugs listed in Schedule I and Schedule II of the CDSA. The legislation also moved GHB and Rohypnol, as well as all of the amphetamine drugs, from Schedule III to Schedule I so that the new harsher penalties could be applied. However, with the election of a new Liberal government in 2015, changes in drug laws are anticipated.

Penalties

The Controlled Drugs and Substances Act allows for three different charges to be laid pertaining to drugs: (1) summary conviction, (2) indictable, and (3) hybrid or Crown election offences. Summary conviction offences encompass the most minor offences in the Criminal Code, with the penalty typically being a fine of up to $5,000 or six months in jail or both. If an individual is convicted of a summary offence as an adult, the person may be eligible for a pardon three years from the time the sentence is completed, typically at the conclusion of probation. Indictable offences are harsher, with lengthier incarceration periods and greater financial penalties. If you are prosecuted by indictment, you are entitled to trial by jury for most offences. If convicted of an indictable offence, the individual may still apply for and receive a pardon but must wait a minimum of five years once the sentence is completed. Drug-related offences may be prosecuted either by summary conviction or indictment, at the discretion of the Crown prosecutor. These are referred to as hybrid offences (Table 7.1) (Jourard, 2014). As well, the CDSA also includes provisions for the forfeiture of property and proceeds of drug offences on conviction. In the 2012 amendments, minimum sentencing penalties were introduced for trafficking in, production of, or importing or exporting marijuana, hashish, cocaine, or heroin. As well, the maximum penalty for cultivation of marijuana was increased from 7 to 14 years. However, in R. v. Lloyd, the British Columbia Provincial Court found the mandatory minimum sentence provision for drug possession for the purpose of trafficking to be a violation of the Charter of Rights and Freedoms, and the same may occur to other new amendments as they face Charter challenges.

TABLE 7.1: DRUG OFFENCE CHARGE AND PENALTY

Offence Description	Controlled Drugs and Substances Act Section	Summary, Hybrid, or Indictable
Possession of marijuana (up to 30 g) or hashish (up to 1 g)	4(1)	S
Possession of marijuana or hashish	4(1)	H
Possession of cocaine or heroin	4(1)	H
Possession of amphetamines, LSD, mescaline, or psilocybin	4(1)	H
Trafficking in marijuana or hashish or possession for the purpose of trafficking (up to 3 kg)	5	I
Trafficking in marijuana or hashish or possession for the purpose of trafficking (over 3 kg)	5	I
Trafficking in cocaine or heroin or possession for the purpose of trafficking	5	I
Trafficking in amphetamines, LSD, mescaline, or psilocybin or possession for the purpose of trafficking	5	H
Trafficking in barbituates or anabolic steroids or possession for the purpose of trafficking	5	H
Importing, exporting marijuana or hashish, or up to 1 kg of heroin or cocaine	6	I
Importing, exporting heroin or cocaine (more than 1 kg)	6	I
Importing, exporting amphetamines, LSD, mescaline, or psilocybin	6	H
Cultivation of marijuana	7	I
Production of hashish	7	I
Production of cocaine or heroin	7	I
Production of amphetamines, LSD, mescaline, or psilocybin	7	H
Production of barbituates or anabolic steroids	7	H

Minimum Penalty*	Discharge Available	Maximum Penalty: Summary Conviction	Maximum Penalty: Indictable Conviction
	yes	6 mos./$1,000 fine	
	yes	6 mos./$1,000—1st offence; 1 yr./$2,000—subsequent offence	5 yrs. less a day
	yes	6 mos./$1,000—1st offence; 1 yr./$2,000—subsequent offence	7 yrs.
	yes	6 mos./$1,000—1st offence; 1 yr./$2,000—subsequent offence	3 yrs.
	yes		5 yrs. less a day
1 yr. if you commit the offence (a) for a criminal organization, (b) use, or threaten violence in its commission (c) carry, use or threaten to use a weapon in its commission, or (d) within the previous 10 years, you were convicted of a designated substance offence*; 2 yrs. if you commit the offence (a) in or near a school or any other public place usually frequented by minors, (b) at a prison, or (c) with the assistance or involvement of a minor			life imprisonment
same minimums as noted above			life imprisonment
	yes	18 mos./$5,000 fine	10 yrs.
	yes	1 yr./$5,000 fine	3 yrs.
1 yr. if you commit the offence (a) for trafficking, (b) you abuse a position of trust or authority while committing the offence, or (c) you have access to an area that is restricted to authorized persons and use that access to commit the offence			life imprisonment
2 yrs.			life imprisonment
	yes	18 mos./$5,000 fine	10 yrs.
(i) 6 mos. if there are between 6 and 200 plants and the production is for trafficking; (ii) 9 mos. for between 6 and 200 plants, the production is for trafficking, and any of the following apply: *(a) you use real property that belongs to a third party to commit the offence, (b) the production could endanger the security, health, or safety of minors at or close to the offence location, (c) the production constitutes a potential public safety hazard in a residential area, or (d) you set or place a trap, device, or other thing that is likely to cause death or bodily harm to another person in or close to the offence location, or permit such a trap, device, or other thing to remain or be placed in that location or area,* (iii) 1 yr. for between 201 and 500 plants; (iv) 18 months for between 201 and 500 plants and any of the factors (a through d, in italics, above) apply; (v) 2 yrs. for more than 500 plants, or (vi) 3 yrs. for more than 500 plants if any of the factors (a through d, in italics, above) apply	no longer available (since November 6, 2012)**		14 yrs.**
1 yr. if the production is for trafficking; 18 months if the production is for trafficking and any of the four factors (a through d, in italics) noted above under cultivation of marijuana apply			life imprisonment
2 yrs.; 3 yrs. if any of the four factors (a through d, in italics) noted above under cultivation of marijuana apply			life imprisonment
	yes	18 mos./$5,000 fine	10 yrs.
	yes	1 yr./$5,000 fine	3 yrs.

Under the Controlled Drugs and Substances Act, unlawful possession of either heroin or cocaine is a criminal offence punishable on indictment by imprisonment for up to seven years or on summary conviction for a first offence to a fine of up to $1,000 or imprisonment for up to six months, or both. A subsequent offence is punishable on summary conviction by a fine of up to $2,000 or imprisonment for up to one year, or both. Trafficking, possession for the purpose of trafficking, possession for the purpose of exporting, production, import, and export are indictable offences punishable by up to life imprisonment. In contrast, amphetamines and their derivatives are punishable on indictment by imprisonment for up to three years and on summary conviction to a fine of up to $1,000 or imprisonment for up to six months, or both. Trafficking, possession for the purpose of trafficking, possession for the purpose of exporting, production, import, and export offences are punishable by imprisonment for up to 18 months or on indictment by imprisonment for up to 10 years, while for khat it is a maximum of only three years (Government of Canada, 2015). However, regulations within the legislation do allow for the prescription of some otherwise illicit drugs for treatment or therapeutic purposes, including both methadone and heroin (Riley, 1998). This clause allowed the North American Opiate Medication Initiative (NAOMI), which evaluated the feasibility and effectiveness of heroin-assisted treatment (HAT) in the Canadian context, to proceed.

Benzodiazepines and barbiturates are governed by Schedule IV of the CDSA, and convictions pertaining to trafficking and possession are similar to khat. Psychotherapeutic agents, including all of the tricyclics, MAOIs, and SSRI antidepressants, are subject to the provisions of the Food and Drugs Act and Food and Drug Regulations applicable to drugs listed in Schedule F to the Regulations. The Regulations generally require that the sale or distribution of Schedule F drugs be made pursuant to a prescription. Violation of the act or regulations is an offence punishable on indictment by a fine of up to $5,000 or imprisonment for up to three years, or both, and on summary conviction for a first offence by a fine of up to $500 or imprisonment for up to three months, or both. A subsequent offence is punishable by a fine of up to $1,000 or imprisonment for up to six months, or both (Government of Canada, 2015).

With a few minor exceptions in northern Canadian communities and Alberta, possession and sale of inhalants is not regulated. However, the abuse of a solvent may be taken into consideration when dealing with young offenders and children found in need of protection under provincial legislation. As well, gammahydroxybutyrate (GHB) is governed by the provisions of the Controlled Drugs and Substances Act, with its possession punishable by imprisonment for up to three years on indictment or on summary conviction to a fine of up to $1,000 or six months imprisonment, or both for a first offence, and a fine of up to $2,000 or up to one year imprisonment, or both for a subsequent offence. Offences of trafficking, possession for the purpose of trafficking, possession for the purpose of exporting, production, import, and export of GHB are punishable on indictment by imprisonment for up to 10 years and on summary conviction by imprisonment for up to 18 months (Health and Welfare Canada, 2009).

Alcohol

The sale and use of alcohol is subject to federal, provincial, and territorial legislation, including the sale to minors and use in public places. In the Northwest Territories, alcohol use is restricted by the municipality and not by the territorial government, with individual communities having the right to ban alcohol completely if the local government wishes. Distinct offences related to underage drinking include possessing, consuming, purchasing, attempting to purchase, or otherwise obtaining liquor outside of the home. In some jurisdictions, parents or guardians may legally supply liquor at home to an underage person, but in others, supplying liquor or selling liquor to a minor is an offence regardless of the relationship between provider and consumer. Currently, in all provinces and territories, the legal drinking age is 19 with the exception of Alberta, Manitoba, and Quebec, where the legal drinking age remains 18.

While the laws respecting alcohol are determined by the province or territory and not by the federal government, alcohol is still governed by the Criminal Code of Canada. Thus, across the country it is an offence to drive with a blood alcohol level (BAL) of .08 percent or greater and to drive while impaired, even if one's BAL is less than .08 percent. Nine of the 13 provinces and territories impose administrative licence suspensions on drinking drivers at .05, with Saskatchewan currently having the lowest limit at .04. All except Nunavut have a zero BAL for drivers under the age of 21. As well, most provinces and territories have introduced 90-day administrative licence suspensions effective almost immediately after a driver registers a BAL over the statutory limit or fails to provide a breath sample. Section 253(1) of the Criminal Code establishes the offence of operating a motor vehicle while impaired by alcohol but also by other psychoactive agents:

> 253. (1) Every one commits an offence who operates a motor vehicle or vessel or operates or assists in the operation of an aircraft or of railway equipment or has the care or control of a motor vehicle, vessel, aircraft or railway equipment, whether it is in motion or not,
>
> (a) while the person's ability to operate the vehicle, vessel, aircraft or railway equipment is impaired by alcohol or a drug; or
>
> (b) having consumed alcohol in such a quantity that the concentration in the person's blood exceeds eighty milligrams of alcohol in one hundred millilitres of blood.

Section 254 of the Criminal Code gives police officers the authority, under certain circumstances, including random automobile stops, to test individuals through the use of breathalyzers and sobriety tests. In Ontario, when a police officer conducts a breathalyzer test and an individual's results are over the legal limit, the police officer has the power to request that the person surrender their driver's licence under section 48(3) of the Ontario Highway Traffic Act. Further, section 255 of the Criminal Code establishes different punishments for those convicted under section 253. Anyone who causes bodily injury to another while impaired and is found guilty can be imprisoned for up to 10 years. If you kill another person while operating a motor vehicle and are impaired, you can be incarcerated for life.

Tobacco

The Federal Tobacco Act allows retailers to sell tobacco products only to individuals who have reached the age of 18. However, five provinces—Nova Scotia, New Brunswick, Newfoundland, Ontario, and British Columbia—increased the age limit to 19 based on arguments arising from the availability-control theory that indicate the later a person is legally able to use a socially sanctioned drug, the less likely they are to begin. As well, since second-hand smoke has the potential to harm non-smokers, including children, many municipalities and provinces have enacted bylaws that restrict or ban smoking in public places, including restaurants and bars. At the federal level, the Non-Smokers' Health Act bans smoking in all federally regulated workplaces and bans smoking on trains, planes, buses, and ships (Health Canada, 2009).

Cannabis

Cannabis is regulated under the Controlled Drugs and Substances Act. Interestingly, and perhaps due to the continuing ambiguity surrounding the status of this psychoactive substance, the legislation established distinct penalties for the possession, distribution, and production of cannabis apart from other illicit substances. For example, the offence of simple possession of 30 g or less of cannabis or 1 g or less of hashish is a summary conviction offence that typically does not result in a criminal record. However, possession of more than those amounts without the intent to traffic is a dual offence under CDSA. It may be either a summary conviction or an indictable offence and, on conviction, will result in a criminal record (Health Canada, 2009).

Marijuana is not an officially approved drug or medicine in Canada. However, despite the Harper government's prohibitionist stance and view that cannabis is an illicit substance, the Federal Court of Appeal has ruled that it may be prescribed by a physician to individual clients. While the federal government repealed the Marihuana for Medical Purposes Regulations (MMPR) in 2014, it was stayed by the federal court, allowing individuals with an Authorization to Possess to possess up to 150 g. As well, individuals with a medical need who have the support of a licenced health care practitioner may register and receive cannabis to aid in the treatment of their recognized medical condition (Health Canada, 2014b). However, the Canadian Medical Association does not officially support the use of medical marijuana, and no physician is obligated to complete the forms necessary for an individual to access the drug (Canadian Medical Association, 2015). Changes in cannabis legislation are anticipated with the election of a new federal government in 2015.

7.2 ETHICAL CONSIDERATIONS
Teleological versus Deontological Ethical Decision Making
Ethical Decision-Making Approaches
Canadian Addiction Counsellors Certification Federation
   Canon of Ethical Principles

Ethics is a branch of moral philosophy concerned with human conduct and moral decision making, with being a good person and doing the right thing. An ethic is a statement of the most fundamental principle of professional counselling conduct. It is an attempt to answer the question of what is right and wrong in a consistent and systemic manner. The study of ethics is a discipline examining our values, beliefs, morals, and the justification of these. Ethics frame the rules of conduct by which we live our lives and conduct our counselling practice. When thinking about ethics, the question typically arises: How should we think? What are the values and attitudes that should shape the concepts through which we define ourselves, the world in which we live, and thus our work as professional counsellors?

To join a profession entails subscribing to some common ethical values, yet values do not always lead to desired behaviours, and counselling professionals can have their values depart greatly and gravely from societal values or even the values of other professions. We see this in conflicts regarding right-to-life decisions, reproductive freedom, minority rights around fundamental issues of what is a family and who should be considered eligible for marriage, and, of course, in addiction around issues such as harm reduction, mandated detoxification treatment for youth, and the imprisonment of individuals because of behaviours caused by their drug use. Ethics are also often closely linked to societal values and are reflected in statutes, policies, and the criminal justice system.

The following are examples of unethical counselling behaviour:

- violation of confidentiality
- exceeding one's level of professional competence
- negligent practice
- claiming expertise one does not possess

- imposing one's values on a client
- creating dependency in a client
- conflict of interest
- questionable financial arrangements/financial exploitation

and lastly, one that appears totally obvious, yet is one that still too frequently violated:

- sexual harassment of or activity with a client

In essence, any activity by a counsellor that leads to exploitation, insensitivity, incompetence, irresponsibility, or abandonment of a client is unethical behaviour. Most counselling professions have prescribed ethical codes, as does the addiction field, and a formal college to protect the public from unethical and unprofessional behaviour. However, in the case of addiction, there is no mandatory association to which one must belong to qualify as an addiction counsellor. Nor is there a uniform ethical code that all counsellors working in the addiction field are obligated to follow or an association that members of the public can turn to if they have concerns regarding the practice of an addiction counsellor, though a voluntary association and ethical code are in place.

There is also a more subtle ethical issue in the addiction field that relates to how voluntary the consent is to treatment. The subtle coercion that often precedes seeking treatment may be an invisible barrier to forming a therapeutic alliance with a client. There are three distinct forms of constraint that may affect the counselling relationship: (1) judicial, (2) institutional, and (3) relational. The coercive aspect of treatment can consist of any one or a combination of all three of these forms of constraint. Judicial constraint refers to any mandate from the criminal justice system to seek treatment or a specific form of treatment, either as a condition of sentencing or to avoid sentencing. This can take different forms, such as therapeutic remands, conditions of a probation order, conditions of a conditional sentence of imprisonment, or coercive treatment mandates ordered through drug treatment courts. Institutional constraint is coercion exerted within any institutional setting, such as a workplace to preserve employment, or a school to maintain enrolment. The third form of coercion, relational, applies to any form of constraint in which the drug user is encouraged or pressured to seek treatment by people in his or her immediate environment, such as family members, friends, or workplace colleagues. Even if this form of constraint is not as obvious as those exerted by a court or correctional facilities, it must be considered by practitioners who are evaluating the motivation of the person seeking treatment. The recognition of these three forms of coercion is vital for practitioners to incorporate into their assessment of the client's environmental context (Quirion, 2014).

Teleological versus Deontological Ethical Decision Making

While competent practitioners easily avoid ethical problems, ethical dilemmas are more likely to create a lose-lose situation in which any action will have some negative consequences. There are two basic approaches to ethical decision making when one is faced with an ethical dilemma: (1) teleological, and (2) deontological.

Teleological ethical decision making is goal directed and is consequentialistic in its approach. The focus is on the anticipated outcome of a given situation or action. This approach is most concerned with overall consequences rather than the outcome for a specific individual, thus making it utilitarian in its orientation. Teleological ethics draws its name from the Greek *telos*, which refers to an archery target. A teleological approach is one that orients each action or activity toward a goal or a target that is deemed to be good. A teleological ethic orients actions to ends and chooses those means that lead to a desired outcome identified with "the good." Thus, actions taken under this ethical decision-making framework are good by virtue of the consequences they produce. We should act in a certain manner because it will produce the most positive results. Teleological ethical approaches, being consequential in nature, focus on the expected outcomes, leading to cost-benefit and cost-effectiveness-based courses of action. This model has been regularly followed by health care and social services professionals as it fosters general benevolence.

In contrast, deontological ethical decision making is concerned with balancing rights and duties, and tends to reject purely outcome-orientated considerations. While not ignoring outcomes entirely, this philosophical approach states that certain kinds of actions are either inherently right and good, or wrong and bad. It proclaims that we do the right thing because it is in fact the right thing to do. The right thing to do is typically based on an external authority, such as the Ten Commandments, or the code of practice of a professional body, such as social work, psychology, or addiction counselling. Deontological is derived from the Greek work for duty, and thus this approach is orientated less to goods or harms produced by actions and more toward the basic principles of right and wrong. In and by themselves, the consequences of an action do not determine whether the action is ethically right or wrong. Rather, this perspective maintains that whether an action is ethical depends on whether it is in accordance with, and is performed out of respect for, certain absolute and universal principles.

The classic though simplistic example illustrating the difference between these two approaches is found in the scenario in which one has the opportunity to return in a time machine to murder Adolf Hitler's mother, so that Hitler is never born. From a teleological perspective, this could be argued as ethical behaviour, as it would prevent the murder, death, and suffering of millions. However, from a deontological viewpoint, the argument would be that murder is wrong regardless of the situation and cannot be justified even under these circumstances.

Few of us are purely teleological or deontological ethical decision makers, but rather follow both paths at different times and in different situations. What is critical is to appreciate which philosophical approach we are using and why, and to be able to document the process of our decision making. Ethical guidelines are just that, guidelines, and at times counsellors are faced with lose-lose situations in which ethical implications are unavoidable.

SITUATION ONE: THE LIMITS OF CONFIDENTIALITY

Debbie Woods calls your agency and asks to speak to an addiction counsellor. You arrange to meet with Debbie the next day and find out that she does not personally have an addiction issue, but is looking for your assistance in obtaining a divorce from her husband of 12 years. During the course of your assessment, Ms. Woods confides that she wants a divorce because of her husband's excessive drinking. She states that he drinks heavily four to five times a week even if he has a scheduled flight. Ms. Woods tells you that her husband is a commercial pilot and recently returned from a 21-day vacation during which time he entered an in-patient treatment facility under an assumed name. He did not complete the program, but left after two weeks. As the counsellor, you are aware of aviation regulations that forbid a pilot from drinking for several hours prior to a flight.

You further explore the issues of Debbie's husband causing harm if he drinks and flies. Ms. Wood becomes quite agitated and says that this session is confidential. "I don't want you reporting anything to anybody. We're here to discuss my problem. If he loses his job, he won't be able to support himself let alone provide assistance for me and our children."

What action can you take?
What will you do?

SITUATION TWO: TESTING THE LIMITS OF CONFIDENTIALITY

Violet Woodlands calls your agency and asks to speak to an addiction counsellor. You arrange to meet with Violet the next day and find out that she does not personally have an addiction issue but is looking for your assistance in obtaining a divorce from her husband of 12 years. During the course of your assessment, Ms. Woodlands confides that she wants a divorce because of her husband's excessive drinking and behaviour toward their children. She states that he drinks heavily four to five times a week, even if he has a scheduled flight. Ms. Woodlands tells you that her husband is a commercial pilot and recently returned from a 21-day vacation during which he entered an in-patient treatment facility under an assumed name. He did not complete the program, but left after two weeks. He returned home, and during a drinking episode, hit the oldest child, age nine, so hard that the child's shoulder was partially separated. As a professional counsellor, you are aware of aviation regulations that forbid a pilot from drinking for several hours prior to a flight and about the need to protect children.

You further explore the issues of Violet's husband causing harm when he drinks excessively. Ms. Woodlands becomes quite agitated and says this session is confidential, and that it says so in everything she has read about counselling. "I don't want you reporting anything to anybody. We're here to discuss my problem. If he loses his job or goes to jail, he won't be able to support himself, let alone provide assistance for me and our children."

What action can you take?

What should you do?

Were there any differences in the course of action you took with Debbie as compared to Violet?

Ethical Decision-Making Approaches

Ethical dilemmas arise when there is a conflict in the following:

- problem definition
- goal setting
- priority setting
- decisions on means
- decisions on strategy
- decisions on outcomes

Proposed by the following:

- client
- counsellor
- family system
- criminal justice department
- employer/school

For each relates to different assumptions about the following:

- human nature
- values

- criminal justice/workplace/school issues
- the personal-work/school interface

Along with determining if you are a teleological or deontological decision maker, a variety of ethical decision-making formats have been proposed to assist practitioners in making good ethical decisions. Kitchener's model (1984) is a bottom-up process based on the assumption that some clinical decisions cannot be made by simple reasoning alone. Its intent is to provide counselling professionals with a systematic ethical decision-making process. The model proposes that ethical decision making always begins by thoroughly examining the particular facts of a situation, and that the more experience a counsellor has with potential ethical dilemmas, the more likely he or she will be able to act appropriately using ordinary moral and common sense. It is a hierarchically tiered model, so that if a decision cannot be made at a lower level, one can move up and engage in ethical reasoning at a higher level of abstraction (Figure 7.1).

The intuitive level is derived through a counsellor's post-secondary education in combination with one's immediate personal response to a situation. It is what "feel's right" based on an individual's values, ethical behaviour, life experiences, education, and supervisory experiences. This is the most biased and responsive level of reasoning and occurs at the lowest level of abstraction or at a pre-reflective state. Relying solely on intuition does not allow individuals to critically evaluate their decisions.

The critical-evaluative level consists of a series of options to provide a clearer rationale when making ethical decisions, with the goal of protecting the interests of all persons involved in the decision-making process. Generally these are organized using a deontological process established by a governing professional body and presented in a formal set of rules or guidelines. Counsellors are urged to follow these guidelines and sanctions are typically applied if they are not adhered to. The ethical principles arising from the ethical rules component of the critical-evaluative level are established beliefs about specific modes of conduct, and are somewhat more general than ethical rules found in codes of ethics. Autonomy is the basis for the preferred rights of clients found in ethical codes, including such concepts as self-determination, confidentiality, and informed consent. Autonomy does not imply unlimited freedom, as people do not have the right to infringe on the rights of others or to cause them harm. Non-maleficence is the process of doing no harm, while beneficence entails promoting the wellness of others. Justice is the principle of treating people equally by treating them according to their needs, while fidelity involves loyalty on the part of the counsellor to the client's best interests. Of course none of these principles are absolute or perfect. While always relevant in every situation, a principle must be overturned when a stronger ethical one is in conflict with it.

Finally, if one is still uncertain of how to act, the addiction counsellor can move to the top of Kitchener's model, to ethical theory. This tier is applied when intuitive thought, ethical codes, and ethical principles fail to resolve an ethical dilemma—when the lose-lose situation leads to a stalemate. There are two principles in this final and top tier. Universalizability is the broad-based use of a principle that can be applied fairly similarly in all cases, implying that an act is ethical only if it can be generalized to all similar cases. In contrast, the balancing principle, derived from teleological thought, states that the potential for good in all aspects must be balanced against the potential for harm. Thus, the final stage also allows the addiction counsellor to include consideration for what action would bring about the most good for the most people in the decision-making process.

FIGURE 7.1: KITCHENER'S MODEL OF ETHICAL JUSTIFICATION

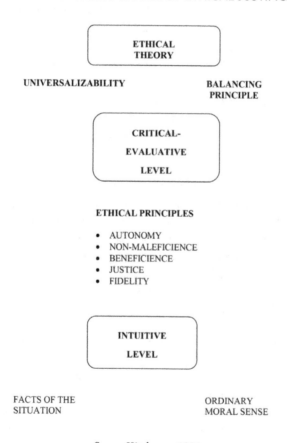

Source: Kitchener, 1984

Loewenberg and Dolgoff (2008) have proposed a much simpler process—one that allows practitioners to compare the source of the conflict and determine which course to take based on its level. The higher level takes precedence over the lower when faced with a lose-lose situation.

The following are listed from most to least important when resolving an ethical dilemma:

Ethical Principle 1: Principle of the protection of life
Ethical Principle 2: Principle of equality and inequality
Ethical Principle 3: Principle of autonomy and freedom
Ethical Principle 4: Principle of least harm
Ethical Principle 5: Principle of quality of life
Ethical Principle 6: Principle of privacy and confidentiality
Ethical Principle 7: Principle of truthfulness and full disclosure

SITUATION THREE: SELF-DETERMINATION

Mary Popovich was born on August 10, 1949. During her childhood, she moved several times before her family settled in St. Catharines, Ontario. Her father died when she was six and her mother remarried. Mary completed Grade 8 and then obtained an office job. She was 22 when she was first admitted to St. Michael's Hospital in Toronto. Her case history described her as "pale, underweight, preoccupied, and vague." Her diagnosis was possible schizophrenia. Electroconvulsive therapy was ordered, which was the acceptable standard of the time.

Mary lived in a boarding house for one year, but ended up in the North Bay Psychiatric Hospital. Her prognosis did not appear favourable. During the 1960s, Mary was in and out of hospital. She gave birth to a healthy baby boy, whom she put up for adoption. Mary's symptoms were controllable with psychotherapeutic drugs, but without supervision, she stopped taking her medication and began drinking. She began slowly, but over time has developed a serious substance dependency.

In the 1980s, Mary became an active outpatient. She did well for several years, but in the 1990s, she stopped attending clinic appointments to get her medication and began self-medicating with alcohol and street drugs. She was finally evicted from her accommodation in 2005 and began to live on the street. She became a permanent fixture around the corner from the women's withdrawal management program, and once or even twice a year, she would admit herself to be detoxified before returning to the street. These self-admissions have tended to occur during the winter months and have increased in recent years. Her homelessness also caused her to be admitted to the hospital with breathing problems. She was also suffering from liver problems, kidney problems, and cardiovascular problems and was malnourished. She was transferred to the Queen Street Mental Health facility in Toronto, and then to the Hamilton

Psychiatric Hospital. Once there, she refused to accept any ongoing treatment. She was subsequently released.

On her return to the community, she occasionally dropped in to the Centre for Hope for companionship, the occasional meal, and even for a place to sleep when it got too cold outside. One day, Mary suddenly refused to go inside. Already street-weary, she became even more short-tempered and difficult to interact with. Some days she would talk with anyone, but at other times, she would refuse to communicate. The Centre's alleyway soon became her permanent home.

In the mornings, staff from the withdrawal management centre would hose down the area where she had slept because of the smell. They grew increasingly concerned as she appeared to be ill with a chronic cough, but Mary continued to refuse assistance. It is now early November and winter conditions are encroaching. Mary has not given any indication that she will be moving indoors.

What is your course of action?

SITUATION FOUR: DUAL RELATIONSHIPS

John Kowalski, who began his recovery as a result of your intervention, is a volunteer with your facility. He has an excellent reputation as a caring volunteer and is considering taking early retirement to formally study addiction counselling. He is held in high regard by board members, staff, fellow volunteers, and clients.

Cheryl Hillwards voluntarily sought counselling. She has worked for Union Chemical for five years, since completing college. She has a variety of problems, including inappropriate use of prescription drugs and interpersonal issues, all of which appear to stem from a lack of self-confidence and self-esteem. After an initial assessment, Cheryl is assigned to John Kowalski's voluntary peer-led group for ongoing support as part of a larger professional treatment program. John notices that Cheryl has difficulty establishing friendly relationships with any of the men in the group. During the course of her ongoing group sessions, he publicly compliments her on her appearance to bolster her self-esteem and provides supportive hugs at the end of sessions. After one particular session, Cheryl admits that she is attracted to him. John immediately transfers Cheryl to another group.

After six months, John calls Cheryl to see how she is. He then asks her if she would like to go out with him on a date.

Are there ethical dilemmas arising out of this situation?

What additional issues would arise if John were a paid staff member rather than a volunteer?

Canadian Addiction Counsellors Certification Federation Canon of Ethical Principles

Despite the lack of professional college, many practising in the addiction field in Canada have voluntarily joined the Canadian Addiction Counsellors Certification Federation (CACCF) and ascribe to the Federation's Canon of Ethical Principles (2010). CACCF promotes, certifies, and monitors the competency of addiction specific counsellors in Canada, using current and effective practices that are internationally recognized. This association serves as a voluntary professional body that certifies professionals working in the addiction field and offers a Canon of Ethical Practice consisting of 12 principles:

1. Believe in the dignity and worth of all human beings, and pledge my service to the well-being and betterment of all members of society
2. Recognize the right of humane treatment of anyone suffering from alcoholism or drug abuse, whether directly or indirectly
3. Promote and assist in the recovery and return to society of every person served, assisting them to help themselves, and referring them promptly to other programs or individuals when in their best interests
4. Maintain a proper professional relationship with all persons served, assisting them to help themselves, and referring them promptly to other programs or individuals, when in their best interests
5. Adhere strictly to established precepts of confidentiality in all knowledge, records, and materials concerning persons served, and in accordance with any current government regulations
6. Ensure that all interpersonal transactions between myself and persons served are non-exploitive and essential to their good recovery
7. Give due respect to the rights, views, and positions of any other alcoholism and/or drug counsellors and related professionals
8. Respect institutional policies and procedures, and cooperate with any agency management with which I may be associated, as long as this remains consistent with recognized standards, procedures, and ethics
9. Contribute my ideas and findings regarding alcoholism and other drug addictions and their treatment and recovery, to any body of knowledge, through appropriate channels
10. Refrain from any activities, including the abuse of alcohol, drugs, or other mood-altering chemicals where my personal conduct might diminish my personal capabilities, denigrate my professional status, or constitute a violation of law
11. Avoid claiming or implying any personal capabilities or professional qualifications beyond those I have actually attained, recognizing that competency gained in one field of activity must not be used improperly to imply competency in another

12. Regularly evaluate my own strengths, limitations, biases, or levels of effectiveness, always striving for self-improvement and seeking professional development by means of further education and training

7.3 PRACTICE CONSIDERATIONS: ADDICTION COUNSELLOR COMPETENCIES

Frontline addiction counsellors have difficult and stressful positions. However, not only are there no mandatory ethical guidelines to support them in their practice, as discussed above, there are also no national educational or practice standards required for those working in this field. Canada's substance abuse workforce is currently unregulated, meaning that persons working in the field of substance abuse are not required to conform to any standardized qualifications or professional standards. However, in this century, both in Canada and internationally, there has been an increasing interest in workforce development issues stemming from a growing need to ensure services are being delivered in accordance with the highest possible standards and practices, while creating supportive and satisfying work experiences for those who are employed in this demanding arena (Canadian Centre on Substance Abuse, 2007, 2014b; Pernell-Arnold & Finley, 2012).

In March 2005, the Canadian Centre on Substance Abuse (CCSA), a national agency that was created as part of the 1987 Drug Strategy, took the lead in coordinating a workshop and national survey to identify the needs of the addiction workforce (Ogborne & Graves, 2005). Arising from this was the formation of the National Advisory Group on Workforce Development (NAGWD) in 2006, whose responsibilities included development, implementation, and ongoing evaluation of a broad national strategy on workforce development across the continuum of services related to substance use. A primary focus of the committee was to identify core knowledge and practice competencies needed by the substance abuse workforce, with a goal of enhancing professionalism within the field by supporting the adoption of evidence-informed practice and supporting the hiring and retention of skilled practitioners (Canadian Centre on Substance Abuse, 2007).

The result has been the development and subsequent revision of a set of core knowledge and practice competencies that any professional working in the addiction field should become familiar with and adept at (Canadian Centre on Substance Abuse, 2010b, 2014b). Competencies are essential skills, knowledge, attitudes, and values, with competency-based education being an approach that advocates for and attempts to provide precise measurable knowledge, skills, and behaviours by the end of a course or educational program (Richards & Rodgers, 2001). Competencies are specific, measurable skills and/or knowledge needed to effectively perform a particular function or role (Marrelli, 2001;

Mirabile, 1997). They do not equate to increased job performance but rather are areas in which addiction counsellors should have and gain expertise during their professional careers (Boyatzis, 2008). No one counsellor can be expected to have expert proficiency knowledge in all competencies. Some competencies will not pertain to the responsibilities of every counsellor, but rather they are areas pertinent to the entire field of addiction.

Technical competencies are the specific, measureable knowledge and skills required when applying specific technical principles and information in a job function that are typically learned in an educational environment or on the job. They are considered to be the hard skills of the profession. Complementing these are behavioural competencies, which are the abilities, attitudes, and values required to perform effectively in a specific position. These soft skills involve performing in the role of an addiction counsellor and complement the technical competencies (Canadian Centre on Substance Abuse, 2010b, 2014b).

The Canadian Centre on Substance Abuse (2010b, 2014b) has developed 17 technical (Box 7.1) and 18 behavioural (Box 7.2) competencies that those working in the addiction field should become adept at. The aim of these competencies is not to be proscriptive but rather to enhance professionalism within the field by providing tools and resources to identify knowledge and skill sets for allied professionals, support employers in hiring and staff development, and assist educators and trainers in developing strategies for learning to provide Canadians with a more consistent quality of service delivery from the substance abuse workforce. To further this goal, a joint initiative has been undertaken by the Canadian Centre on Substance Abuse (CCSA) with the Canadian Addiction Counsellors Certification Federation (CACCF) to address the need for the regulation of addiction counsellors, and to create a certification process not only for the benefit of those working in the field but also for the protection of the public.

BOX 7.1: TECHNICAL COMPETENCIES

As the CCSA reminds us, "Understanding substance use and understanding concurrent disorders are the two foundational technical competencies upon which the others rest. If one does not grasp the key points for these two competencies, one will be less effective in implementing the other technical competencies."

1. *Understanding substance use*: Background or contextual knowledge of substance use, as defined in the Competencies, required to properly inform more specific aspects of a professional's work with clients and their families.

2. *Understanding concurrent disorders*: Knowledge and skills required to properly inform more specific aspects of a professional's work with clients with co-occurring substance use and mental illness, or substance use and mental health issues.

3. *Case management*: Facilitating a substance use client's movement within and between service providers. It includes maintaining accurate documentation, sharing client information appropriately and collaborating with other services providers.

4. *Client referral*: Collaborating with substance use clients, services, and supports to identify and access the best available resources to meet clients' needs.

5. *Community development*: Working together to identify community needs and resources, and to plan and support or guide collective action.

6. *Counselling*: Applying a comprehensive range of evidence-informed counselling styles, techniques, and methodologies aimed at improving the overall well-being of substance use and concurrent disorders clients.

7. *Crisis intervention*: Recognizing and responding effectively when a substance use or concurrent disorders client or associated group or community is in an unstable, risky, dangerous, or potentially dangerous situation.

8. *Family and social support*: Working with clients and individuals and groups most affected by the client's substance use and most able to either support or undermine the client's treatment goals.

9. *Group facilitation*: Using evidence-informed approaches to work effectively with substance use and concurrent disorders clients in group settings.

10. *Medications* (formerly pharmacology): The knowledge and skills required to understand and use medications in the treatment of clients with substance use or concurrent disorders and to understand and respond to the impact that medications could have on the client.

11. *Outreach*: Designing and delivering substance use and concurrent disorders services in the community to a broad range of clients, including those who might otherwise not seek or have access to those services.

12. *Prevention and health promotion*: Engaging with substance use and concurrent disorders clients, their families, and their communities to encourage the adoption of knowledge, behaviours, values, and attitudes that promote personal and community well-being.

13. *Program development, implementation, and evaluation*: Developing and implementing new substance use programs, modifying existing programs to respond to identified needs, and evaluating the outcomes of new or revised programs.

14. *Record keeping and documentation*: Creating and maintaining accurate, up-to-date, comprehensive client records able to withstand legal scrutiny.

15. *Screening and assessment*: Selecting, administering, and interpreting the results of evidence-informed tools and methods to measure a client's substance use and related concerns, and inform the care and treatment plan.

16. *Trauma-specific care*: Interacting with substance use clients to identify and consider the impact that overwhelmingly negative events have on functioning and the ability to cope, and then developing and delivering interventions that emphasize safety, choice, and personal control.

17. *Treatment planning*: Collaboratively developing a treatment plan based on screening and assessment findings, ensuring that activities and resources reflect the client's needs, strengths, and goals. The process also includes monitoring, evaluating, planning for discharge, and updating the treatment plan so that it reflects the client's evolving needs and goals.

Source: Adapted from Canadian Centre on Substance Abuse (2014b)

BOX 7.2: BEHAVIOURAL COMPETENCIES

1. *Adaptability/flexibility*: Willingly adjust one's approach to meet the demands and needs of constantly changing conditions, situations, and people and to work effectively in difficult or ambiguous situations.

2. *Analytical thinking and decision making*: Gather, synthesize and evaluate information to determine possible alternatives and outcomes and make well-informed, timely decisions, including critical thinking and reasoning.

3. *Client-centred change*: Enhance, facilitate, support, empower, and otherwise increase client motivation for positive change. Positive change is achieved by involving the client actively in the change process and encouraging the client to take responsibility for the outcomes he or she achieves. Clients may be individuals, groups, communities, or organizations.

4. *Client service orientation*: Provide service excellence to clients (which can include individuals, groups, communities, and organizations). Includes making a commitment to serve clients and focusing one's efforts on discovering and meeting client needs within personal, professional, and organizational capacities and boundaries.

5. *Collaboration and network building*: Identify and create informal and formal interdisciplinary networks and allied community groups to support the provision of client services and achievement of the organization's objectives. Clients include individuals, groups, organizations, and communities.

6. *Continuous learning*: Identify and pursue learning opportunities to enhance one's professional performance and development and the effective delivery of high-quality programs and services.

7. *Creativity and innovation*: Use evidence-based practices in innovative and creative ways to initiate both effective new ways of working and advances in the understanding of the field of practice. Innovation and creativity are

achieved in translating research into practice to optimize improvements in service delivery and professional practice.

8. *Developing others*: Facilitate and motivate sustained learning and create learning opportunities and resources, as well as promote and respect others' needs for ownership of learning outcomes. Includes creation of a continuous learning environment that fosters positive growth in both work and public contexts among peers, clients, client families, communities, and other groups (recipients).

9. *Diversity and cultural responsiveness*: Provide respectful, equitable and effective services to diverse populations, as defined by culture, age, gender, language, ethnicity, socio-economic status, legal status, health, ability, sexual orientation, type and mode of substance use, etc. Affirm and value the worth of all individuals, families, groups, and communities, and protect the dignity of all.

10. *Effective communication*: Articulate both verbally and in writing across a range of technologies in a manner that builds trust, respect, and credibility and that ensures the message is received and understood by the audience. Includes active listening skills (attending, being silent, summarizing, paraphrasing, questioning, and empathizing) and congruent non-verbal communication.

11. *Ethical conduct and professionalism*: Provide professional services according to the principles and values of integrity, competence, responsibility, respect, and trust to safeguard both self and others. Includes the development of professionalism and ethical behaviour in self and others (individuals, groups, organizations, communities).

12. *Interpersonal rapport/savvy*: Establish and maintain relationships based on mutual respect and trust, appropriate sensitivity and transparency, empathy, and compassion with clients, colleagues, professional associates, and the greater community. Encompasses skills of tact, diplomacy, and sensitivity in all encounters with others.

13. *Leadership*: Help others achieve excellent results and create enthusiasm for a shared vision and mission, even in the face of critical debate and adversity.

14. *Planning and organizing*: Identify and prioritize tasks, develop and implement plans, evaluate outcomes and adjust activities in order to achieve objectives.

15. *Self-care*: Deliberately and continuously apply professional and personal self care principles to oneself and, at times, others to sustain optimal productivity while maintaining physical, mental, spiritual, and emotional health.

16. *Self-management*: Appropriately manage one's own emotions and strong feelings; maintain a calm and tactful composure under a broad range of challenging circumstances; and think clearly and stay focused under pressure. Encompasses self-regulation and mindfulness.

17. *Self-motivation and drive*: Remain motivated and focused on a goal until the best possible results are achieved, with both passion for making a difference in the substance abuse field and persistence despite confronting obstacles, resistance, and setbacks.
18. *Teamwork and cooperation*: Work co-operatively and productively with others within and across organizational units to achieve common goals; demonstrate respect, co-operation, collaboration, and consensus-building.

Source: Adapted from Canadian Centre on Substance Abuse (2014b)

7.4 CONCLUDING THOUGHTS

Appendices A and B offer an overview of historical events pertaining to psychoactive drugs that are not only interesting but have also shaped current practice and policy in the addiction field and the world itself. Appendix A offers events relating to Canada while Appendix B provides some worldwide facts highlighting how drugs touch every facet of our lives.

In closing, Debbie Woods has provided you with only hearsay evidence and thus your only course of action is to work with her and support her working toward engaging her husband in the counselling process, as well as deal with his and their addiction issue. While you may have felt that you needed to act to protect innocent people, you neither have the authority nor sufficient information to proceed. However, in the case of Violet Woodlands, you are ethically, legally, and hopefully morally compelled to contact your local child welfare agency, or—even better—support Violet in making that contact herself, for when a minor is at risk, there is no alternative but to intervene regardless of what your client asks of you. The issue becomes less clear if the child is 17 rather than 9.

Mary's case asks you to reflect on client self-determination. Historically, the addiction field was very directive, and clients were told what was best for them. That has now changed, with a greater focus on clients' rights, harm-reduction approaches, and options other than abstinence. However, when does the need to protect your clients supersede their right to act in a manner they wish to? Do you have a moral obligation to intervene when someone is doing harm to himself or herself? What can you do if a person refuses your aid? Perhaps more importantly, how do you deal with your feelings and sense of professional responsibility when you are not allowed to provide the assistance you deem necessary?

Finally, there is the question of John's boundaries. The power differential that exists in professional counselling relationships quickly answers the question of whether one can have a relationship with a former client—the answer is no. (With a current client, the answer is definitely no!) However, John is not a professional counsellor. He does not belong to a professional association, nor is he bound by a college's rules and regulations. There is no government censure regarding his behaviour—a similar situation to what currently exists for addiction counsellors, and thus why having a professional body is essential to the future of the field.

Situations like those described above will always bring a challenge to working in the addition field. However, this a difficult yet vastly rewarding, noble, and gratifying calling that you are entering into as long as you take care of yourself first so that you can take care of others.

> At first people refuse to believe that a strange new thing can be done, then they
> begin to hope it can be done, then they see it can be done—then it is done and all
> the world wonders why it was not done centuries ago.
> —Frances Hodgson Burnett, *The Secret Garden*

DISCUSSION QUESTIONS

1. (a) What are your views on Canada's current drug laws?
   (b) If you had the opportunity to make a presentation to Parliament, what recommendations would you offer to change the current drug laws?
   (c) Knowing that your opinion must be based on facts, what information from the previous readings would you draw on to support the changes you are recommending?
2. (a) What are the greatest ethical challenges an addiction counsellor faces?
   (b) What ethical concerns do you have as you prepare to enter the field?
   (c) Are you more a teleological or a deontological ethical decision maker?
   (d) What actions did you take with Debbie, Violet, Mary, and John?
   (e) What self-care activities do you have in place for when you have to respond to a lose-lose ethical dilemma?
3. (a) Which of the competencies are your strengths?
   (b) Which of the competencies do you require more knowledge about?
   (c) Which of the competencies do you require more practice experience to master?
4. (a) What fears do you have about not being an ethical, competent counsellor?
   (b) What would you suggest if a client presented himself or herself with these concerns?

Appendix A

A HISTORY OF PSYCHOACTIVE DRUGS IN CANADA

4000 BCE	North American First Nations groups are using tobacco as a ritualistic substance.
1606 ACE	Samuel de Champlain's apothecary in Nova Scotia grows cannabis. Hemp is cultivated in Quebec to make rope for ships to sail back to Europe.
1665	Tea is introduced.
1668	The first brewery in Canada is established in by Jean Talon in New France.
1786	Molson's sells 34,069 L of beer in Montreal, whose population is approximately 9,000.
1828	The first acknowledged Canadian temperance meeting in Beaver River, Nova Scotia, is held on April 25.
1832	There are 100 temperance groups in Upper Canada, consisting of 10,000 members.
1835	The Total Abstinence Society is formed in St. Catharines, Ontario, and disallows not only liquor, but also wine, beer, and cider.
1846	Robert Smiley, of the *Hamilton Spectator*, writes in an editorial that the temperance movement is having little impact on the nation as alcohol consumption is at an all-time high. He estimates that the per capita consumption is at least 30 bottles of whisky and 14 bottles of beer a year for every man, woman, and child in Upper and Lower Canada, though it is probably much higher.
1847	Irish immigrant John Kinder Labatt and partner Sam Eccles purchase the London Brewery in London, Ontario.
1864	The Dunkin Act, or the Canada Temperance Act (1864), is passed, allowing any county or municipality to prohibit the sale of alcohol if supported by a majority vote.

1867	The patron of alcoholics and drug addicts, Alfred Pampalon, a Canadian, is born in Levis, Quebec. He is venerated by Pope John Paul II in 1991.
1868	The Indian Act outlaws alcohol on reserves.
1874	The first meeting of the Women's Christian Temperance Movement is held in Owen Sound, Ontario.
	Fellow band members kill 42 Blackfoot as a result of extended drinking bouts.
1875	Section 74 of the Northwest Territories Act prohibits the importation, sale, or possession of liquor under a general prohibition, except when imported under permit of the lieutenant-governor. Hamilton, Ontario, needing a facility for inebriates, builds a structure away from the economic centre of the city, on the edge of the Niagara Escarpment as a place to treat "drunks" after petitions from the Congregational Union of Canada to create a place of detention for inebriates. By 1914, it will be home to 1,300 patients, including those assessed as criminally insane. The facility will continue to treat alcohol-dependent persons on site and at a satellite location until December 2002, when the hospital administration decides it is no longer a cost-effective program and closes it with less than one month's notice to the community. In 2003, the original site of the facility becomes the home for a non-abstinence residential program, one of the first wet shelters in the country. It is then transferred to the downtown core of the city, as the site is redeveloped into a comprehensive mental health facility.
1876	The first Canadian anti-alcohol lobby group is formed, the Dominion Alliance for Total Suppression of Liquor Traffic.
1878	The Scott Act is passed, which enables any city to vote itself dry. The number reaches 62 in 1888, but then falls to 32 by 1892.
1881	Winnipeg's population is nearly 8,000. The city has 64 saloons, five breweries, and 24 wine and liquor stores.
1884	Of the 596 cases prosecuted by the North West Mounted Police (forerunners of the RCMP), 257 (43.1 percent) are for liquor offences.
1886	The *Lethbridge News* reports that two Mounties who had run out of money while drinking hold up a visitor from Saskatoon and then returned to the saloon to continue drinking.
1898	A national plebiscite on alcohol prohibition is held as a result of a petition from Manitoba. The vote is 278,380 for and 264,693 against, with only Quebec having a majority against. However, Prime Minister Laurier, whose governing Liberal Party holds power due to their sway in Quebec, deems that since only 23 percent of the electorate voted, he would not enact prohibition across Canada.

1901	Prince Edward Island becomes the first province to enact prohibition.
1906	The Adulteration Act, the forerunner to the Canadian Food and Drugs Act, is passed.
1908	An anti-opium law is passed, aimed primarily at Oriental railway labourers. The act is amended in 1911 to include cocaine and morphine.
	The Tobacco Restraint Act is passed, making it illegal to sell cigarettes to those under 16 years of age.
1911	The Temperance Movement and "Scientific Management," also known as Taylorism, lead to the creation of personnel departments and specialists emphasizing individual competitive performance as measured by impersonal scientific techniques. This, in conjunction with the growth of Workers' Compensation laws, combines to eliminate the open use of alcohol in most Canadian workplaces.
1915	On July 1, Saskatchewan closes 406 bars, 38 wholesale liquor dealers, and 12 clubs, replacing them with 23 provincial dispensaries. As a result the quality of the alcohol increases dramatically.
1916	Prohibition throughout Canada is enacted, allowing each province the right to prohibit the sale of alcoholic beverages.
	The Ontario Temperance Act is passed, allowing only beverages under 2.5 percent alcohol to be sold. Alberta and Manitoba follow suit, followed by Saskatchewan in 1917. However, each province continues to have functioning breweries operating under federal charter to supply alcohol for medical reasons and for sale through drug stores.
1917	With the passing of prohibition, drunkenness convictions in Manitoba drop from 7,493 in 1913 to 1,085; in Saskatchewan, from 2,970 to 434; and in Alberta, from 7,283 to 391.
	Prior to prohibition, Vancouver had approximately one saloon for every 300 Vancouverites, with no regulation of hours or sales. After prohibition, they are allowed to remain open but only to sell alcohol below 2.5 percent by volume. It is believed that intoxication cannot occur at this level, regardless of how much is consumed.
1920	The Manitoba Women's Christian Temperance Union investigates young people's excessive drinking of Coca-Cola in the province.
1921	Both Quebec and British Columbia adopt a government-controlled liquor distribution system.
1922	Pioneering feminist Emily Murphy publishes *The Black Candle*; in it she claims that marijuana turns its users into homicidal maniacs. Her book has a significant influence on political leaders.

1923	Without any debate in the Canadian Parliament, marijuana becomes classified as a narcotic under Canadian law. Possession becomes a criminal offence.
1925	Canada signs the International Opium Convention under the auspices of the League of Nations, introducing provisions that are later incorporated into the Single Convention on Narcotic Drugs of 1961, including the furnishing of statistics on the production and stocks of opium and coca leaf, the system of import certificates, and export authorizations for licit international trade in controlled drugs, including Indian hemp (cannabis).
1927	The Ontario Temperance Act is repealed and the Liquor Control Board of Ontario is established (LCBO). A quart of whisky sells for $3. Fifteen of Ontario's 64 breweries survive prohibition but are quickly excluded from the LCBO and form their own provincial distribution co-operative, which still exists today. The retail outlets for this co-operative are now simply known as "The Beer Store."
1929	Prince Edward Island is the only province to retain prohibition.
1931	Canada becomes a signatory of the Geneva Convention, which sets limits on the manufacture, regulation, and distribution of narcotic drugs to the amounts needed for medical and scientific purposes by introducing a mandatory system of estimates that continues to the present day.
1932	A federal ban of alcohol advertising is lifted in Canada.
1937	The first seizure of marijuana cigarettes in Canada occurs.
1941	The first AA group is established in Canada by a Toronto United Church minister, the Rev. George Little. Weekly dinner meetings would be launched two years later.
1948	After nearly half a century, Prince Edward Island ends prohibition.
1949	The Ontario Alcoholism Research Foundation (ARF) opens and is led by David Archibald, who has attended the School of Alcohol Studies at Yale University. His mandate is to determine the scope of alcoholism in Ontario. Focusing initially on outpatient treatment, ARF's first facility, Brookside Hospital, will open in 1951. In 1961, the name of the organization will be changed to the Alcoholism and Drug Addiction Research Foundation. ARF will become part of the Ontario Centre for Addiction and Mental Health in 1998.
1952	Psychiatrist Humphrey Osmond begins working with mescaline and LSD in an attempt to find a cure for schizophrenia at Weyburn Mental Hospital in Saskatchewan. He suggests that mescaline allows a normal person to see through the eyes of a person with schizophrenia, and suggests that it be used to train

doctors and nurses to better understand their patients. His research attracts the attention of Aldous Huxley, who volunteers to be a subject. In May 1953, Osmond will introduce Huxley to mescaline for the first time, an experience described in Huxley's book, *Doors of Perception*.

1953   Heightened interest in curbing the spread of communism in Asia leads American political and military leaders to forge ties with warlords in the Golden Triangle, which includes Laos, Thailand, and Burma. To strengthen these ties, the United States supplies the warlords with ammunition, arms, and air transportation for the production and sale of opium. As a result, increased amounts of heroin begin to flow into the United States and Canada.

1954   The Royal Canadian Mounted Police estimate that there are 3,000 heroin-dependent adults in Canada.

1956   A peyote ceremony takes place at the Red Pheasant reserve in Saskatchewan, organized by the Native American Church. Increasing concern regarding transnationalism among First Nations groups, a direct threat to federal government control, leads to increased RCMP monitoring of use of this legal drug.

1959   The federal government grants Native people the right to drink alcohol in their homes.

1960   The pass system is abolished in Canada, allowing First Nations individuals to travel outside their reserves without the permission of the Indian Agent or formal written documentation.

1961   Canada signs the Single Convention on Narcotic Drugs, which is established to streamline the mechanisms of drug control and to extend the existing control system to the cultivation of plants grown as the raw material of narcotic drugs. Its aim is to ensure the provision of adequate supplies of narcotic drugs for medical and scientific purposes, to prohibit all non-medical consumption of such drugs, and to prevent the diversion of such drugs into the illicit market.

1963   Federal Health Minister Judy LaMarsh states in the House of Commons that smoking contributes to lung cancer and other health problems.

1966   Forty-three percent of Canadian adults are smoking cigarettes. Between 1918 and 1966, Saskatchewan's population increased approximately 58 percent, while the number of alcohol-related charges and convictions increased approximately 1,500 percent. Between 1918 and 1966, Alberta's population increased approximately 200 percent while the number of alcohol-related charges and convictions increased approximately 2,000 percent.

1967   The Canadian Temperance Federation folds.

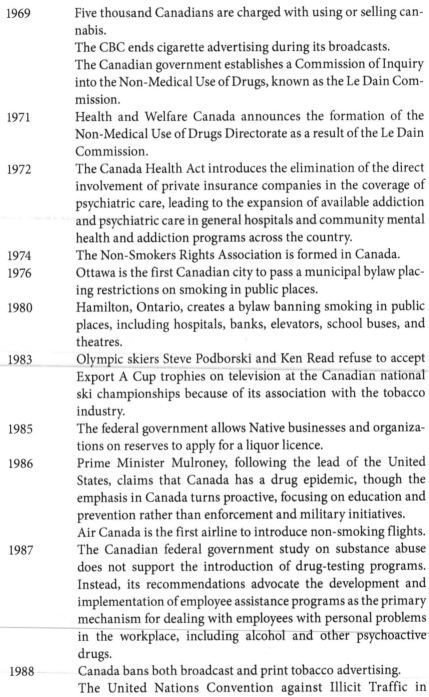

1969	Five thousand Canadians are charged with using or selling cannabis.
	The CBC ends cigarette advertising during its broadcasts.
	The Canadian government establishes a Commission of Inquiry into the Non-Medical Use of Drugs, known as the Le Dain Commission.
1971	Health and Welfare Canada announces the formation of the Non-Medical Use of Drugs Directorate as a result of the Le Dain Commission.
1972	The Canada Health Act introduces the elimination of the direct involvement of private insurance companies in the coverage of psychiatric care, leading to the expansion of available addiction and psychiatric care in general hospitals and community mental health and addiction programs across the country.
1974	The Non-Smokers Rights Association is formed in Canada.
1976	Ottawa is the first Canadian city to pass a municipal bylaw placing restrictions on smoking in public places.
1980	Hamilton, Ontario, creates a bylaw banning smoking in public places, including hospitals, banks, elevators, school buses, and theatres.
1983	Olympic skiers Steve Podborski and Ken Read refuse to accept Export A Cup trophies on television at the Canadian national ski championships because of its association with the tobacco industry.
1985	The federal government allows Native businesses and organizations on reserves to apply for a liquor licence.
1986	Prime Minister Mulroney, following the lead of the United States, claims that Canada has a drug epidemic, though the emphasis in Canada turns proactive, focusing on education and prevention rather than enforcement and military initiatives.
	Air Canada is the first airline to introduce non-smoking flights.
1987	The Canadian federal government study on substance abuse does not support the introduction of drug-testing programs. Instead, its recommendations advocate the development and implementation of employee assistance programs as the primary mechanism for dealing with employees with personal problems in the workplace, including alcohol and other psychoactive drugs.
1988	Canada bans both broadcast and print tobacco advertising.
	The United Nations Convention against Illicit Traffic in Narcotic Drugs and Psychotropic Substances is introduced to respond to transnational organized crime, drug trafficking, and the difficulties of pursuing persons involved in drug-

related crime and money laundering at the international level. The aims of the 1988 Convention are to harmonize the definition and scope of drug offences at the global level; to improve and strengthen international co-operation and coordination among the relevant authorities, and to provide them with the legal means to interdict international drug trafficking more effectively. Canada is one of the first nations to sign the Convention, which includes 119 narcotic drugs and 116 psychotropic drugs.

1989   Bill C-61 (Canada) is proclaimed on January 1. It provides additional powers to enforcement and prosecuting agencies, and fosters new investigative tools and techniques. Borrowing from American legislation, it allows for the confiscation of any assets earned through profits from drug trafficking.

The first needle-exchange program opens in Montreal.

1990   The Quebec Superior Court rules this unconstitutional, leading the federal government to appeal the provincial decision.

1991   Nearly 22,000 drug-related cases are handled by Canadian hospitals. This amounts to just under one case per 1,000 Canadians.

Sixty persons die of heroin overdoses in Toronto, with 510 deaths from illicit drug use across Canada.

Over 39,000 Canadians die directly or indirectly from smoking tobacco.

1992   There are 27 conventional breweries in Canada and 29 microbreweries.

Over 86,000 Canadians are hospitalized as a result of alcohol abuse.

Beer making and selling in Canada accounts for 1.6 percent of the national gross domestic product. Fifty-three percent of the cost is tax, with only two industrialized nations—Ireland and Norway—having higher levies.

Lung cancer, as a direct result of cigarette smoking, becomes the leading cause of cancer deaths among Canadian women.

Canadian police forces seize 115,081 kg of cannabis, 5,285 kg of cocaine, and 85 kg of heroin, while 2,170 prescription forgeries are detected.

1993   The smoking age in Canada is raised to 18.

Canada imports 68,038,855 kg of coffee. Approximately 60 percent of Canadians consume coffee, averaging three cups per day.

1994   Canada prohibits the use of vending machines to distribute cigarettes.

Imperial Tobacco produces 31 billion cigarettes in its two Canadian facilities located in Guelph, Ontario, and Montreal, Quebec.

Legislation requires cigarette packages to carry new warning messages, including:

- Cigarettes are addictive
- Tobacco smoke can harm your children
- Smoking can kill you
- Tobacco smoke causes fatal lung disease in non-smokers

1995   Changing attitudes concerning cannabis lead to the Canadian federal governments licensing of four individuals to grow cannabis for medical research purposes.

1996   The Ontario Human Rights Commission rules against Imperial Oil's drug-testing policy, indicating that testing employees is discrimination on the basis of disability.

Bill C-8, the Controlled Drugs and Substances Act, is passed. Little reform is contained in the bill, though cannabis possession is no longer an indictable offence. Persons charged with possession will no longer be fingerprinted, but conviction of a first offence will still entail a criminal record, a sentence of up to six months of incarceration, and/or a fine of up to $1,000.

The Ontario Medical Association states: "Parental tobacco use in the home, resulting in the inhalation of known carcinogens and asthmagens by children, is a form of physical abuse."

Over 100,000 Ontarians are charged with alcohol related provincial offences, including 88,100 persons charged with having a BAL of over .08.

1997   Ontario moves toward a maximum of 21 days for government funding of in-patient treatment beds.

It is estimated that Canada's 5,275 AA groups have a membership of just under 100,000.

The Canadian alcohol industry registers sales of $11.4 billion, employing 14,000 people and generating $3.34 billion in government revenue. The average Canadian spent $496 a year on alcohol.

Forty thousand Canadians will die prematurely as a result of cigarette smoking. That is the equivalent to one plane crash per day with all on board perishing, or roughly 20 percent of all deaths in Canada. Provincial and federal governments collect just under $4 billion from tobacco sales.

Khat is made an illegal substance to possess in Canada, immediately increasing the selling price by 100 percent.

The Concurrent Disorders Task Force of the Public Policy Committee of the Canadian Mental Health Association (Ontario Division) is established and clearly states that the term "concurrent disorders" refers to a combination of mental health and substance use problems.

1998   The first drug court opens in Toronto, Ontario. In the next decade, Vancouver, Edmonton, Calgary, Regina, Winnipeg, Ottawa, and the Region of Durham, Ontario will follow suit.

1999   Canadian Health Minister Allan Rock sanctions the testing of marijuana for medical purposes.

Fifty-six percent more Canadian women than men are prescribed benzodiazepines.

In St. Albert, Alberta, the Catholic school board introduces trained police dogs to hunt for drugs in students' lockers.

2000   The initial Canadian safe injection site clinic is proposed for Vancouver, based on a model established in Frankfurt, Germany, in 1994. Vancouver's mayor immediately objects to the idea, claiming that it would make Vancouver a magnet for drug addicts from across the country.

Supreme Court of Canada rules Canadians have a constitutional right to use cannabis as a medicine.

There are 15,709,000 prescriptions of benzodiazepines filled by Canadian retail pharmacies, an increase of 12.8 percent since 1996.

2001   The first legal marijuana grow-op under contract to Health Canada opens. Located in an abandoned mine in Flin Flon, Manitoba, and operated by Prairie Plant Systems, the 1,114-square-metre growth chamber supplies chronically ill Canadians with medical marijuana.

2002   Random drug and alcohol tests of Canadian workers and pre-screening of potential new staff are ruled an abuse of human rights by the Canadian Human Rights Commission. The commission states that an employee with a drug or alcohol dependency is disabled and should be assisted, not fired.

There are 12.2 billion cigarettes produced in Canada. The tobacco crop is worth $286 million and employs 14,000 people per year.

2003   Insite, Canada's first safe injection site facility, opens in Vancouver, British Columbia, though it does not receive permanent funding.

Rothmans Inc reports a profit of $93 million despite the decreasing number of smokers in Canada and pays a special dividend to its shareholders.

2004	Canada has the greatest estimate of cannabis use of any industrialized country: 16.8 percent of adults, four times the worldwide average of 3.8 percent.
2005	Abbotsford, British Columbia, passes a bylaw banning all harm-reduction facilities, such as needle exchanges and safe injection sites, in all zones of the city.
	The Supreme Court of Canada rules that the British Columbia government can sue cigarette companies for the cost of treating smoking-related illnesses dating back 50 years and into the future.
2006	The Supreme Court, in a four to three decision, rules that alcoholism and drug addiction are disabilities, and social assistance and other benefits cannot be denied because of these factors alone.
	The provincial governments of Alberta, Saskatchewan, and Manitoba all introduce legislation within two months of each other to allow parents to have their drug-using children forcibly confined and detoxified.
	Nine hundred Canadians are killed in traffic crashes involving drugged drivers.
	Heather Crowe, a lifetime non-smoker who became the public face in Canada of how second-hand smoke in the workplace can harm and kill non-smokers, dies of lung cancer.
2007	Per capita consumption of alcohol among Canadians is 8.1 L, an increase of 12.5 percent from the all-time recorded low of 7.2 L in 1997.
2008	The Liquor Control Board of Ontario has sales of $2.8 billion, and despite the economic crisis, it reports increased sales during the Christmas season.
	The city of Ottawa retrieves 507,692 needles, with approximately 273,000 returned by drug users in exchange for clean needles and another 230,000 returned via medical drop boxes.
	A community plebiscite on the Innu Nation reserve of Natuashish in northern Labrador goes into effect, prohibiting beer and liquor in the community. This band was formerly located on Davis Inlet and moved in 2002. Between 2008 and 2010, the prohibition, enforced by local RCMP constables, will contribute to a 50 percent decrease in suicides and violent crime.
	The number of recorded drug and alcohol deaths in Alberta more than doubles between 1998 and 2008. While Alberta's population grows 13 percent, the annual number of non-suicide deaths attributable to intoxicants increases from 210 to 437.
2009	A northwestern Ontario First Nation registers its first conviction under a bylaw banning inhalants. The bylaw prohibits the sale, manufacture, possession, and consumption of inhalants

in Wabaseemoong First Nation and is enacted "to protect the community and the community members against the injurious effects of intoxicating substance abuse." In its first test through the courts, Michelle Mandamin, 31, pleads guilty to bringing two 3.78 L cans of lacquer into the community.

The number of liquor-related offences in Nunavut's capital city rises 460 percent, with Iqaluit RCMP reporting 2,649 liquor offences in 2009, compared to 576 in 2008.

In a plebiscite, residents of Tuktoyaktuk, Northwest Territories, vote in favour of an alcohol possession limit of one 1.4 L bottle of hard liquor and 24 beers.

The Canada Border Services Agency (CBSA) stops approximately $240 million worth of illicit drugs from reaching the Toronto-area market, with more than half found in commercial shipments. Khat, most commonly detected, was involved in 1,400 incidents. There were also 245 cocaine seizures (totalling 798 kg); 123 marijuana finds (826 kg); 56 heroin caches (101 kg); 36 confiscations of hash (1,460 kg); and 22 incidents involving opium (273 kg). CBSA also reports 3,100 seizures of other drugs, including diazepam, amphetamines, and steroids.

2010   The Harper government attempts to legally close Insite, the country's only safe injection site located in Vancouver, just prior to the Olympic Games. The decision is overturned by the British Columbia Court of Appeals.

A national study concludes that family doctors too readily prescribe unnecessary drugs.

The Ontario Court of Appeals rules that denying long-term social assistance to alcohol- and drug-dependent persons is a violation of the province's Human Rights Code, because it discriminates on the basis of disability. Instead of receiving $585 per month through Ontario Works, individuals are now eligible for $1,042 through the Ontario Disability Support Program (ODSP).

There are approximately 3,200 retail outlets for alcoholic beverages in Canada, more than 30,000 on-premise accounts, and 35 Duty Free stores at border cities and airports. Liquor boards expect to reach $8 billion in retail sales, with profits of more than $2.5 billion.

Tobacco company R.J. Reynolds agrees to pay the Canadian government $324 million to settle a long-running case involving its role in cigarette smuggling.

2011   Canadians are the third highest per capita users of antidepressants among the 23-member Organisation for Economic Cooperation and Development (OECD).

The federal justice department concludes that harsher sentences, a key policy initiative of the Harper government, do not deter crime.

Nearly 89 percent of inmates within the correctional system of the Northwest Territories (NWT) are dealing with an addiction. Close to 62 percent of NWT residents between the ages of 15 and 24 are identified as having "heavy drinking habits," a label applied to those who indulge in five or more drinks in one sitting, at least once per month. NWT residents 15 years and older also report using cannabis at a rate of 20 percent, double the national average of 11 percent.

2012 Beer and liquor stores and agencies sell $20.9 billion worth of alcoholic beverages during the fiscal year, up 3 percent from the previous year.

British Columbia's underground cannabis industry is estimated to be worth between $3 and $10 billion a year.

Voters in Kimmirut, a southern Baffin Island community with a population of 410, decide to end a prohibition on alcohol. They establish an alcohol education committee to decide who possesses, purchases, or brings alcohol to the community.

The Quebec government announces the launch of a $60 billion lawsuit against 11 tobacco manufacturers. The lawsuit alleges that tobacco companies hid the health risks of smoking for several years and should be held liable.

2013 Between 2005 and 2013, the RCMP and Canadian military spend $11.4 million on search-and-destroy missions targeting cannabis in Canada, which leads to the eradication of 40,600 plants.

The Canadian Forces are working in conjunction with the US in counter-narcotic efforts in Central and South America. Canadian troops are training those from Chile, Brazil, and Colombia. The Canadian Special Operations Regiment, based in Petawawa, Ontario, is training the Jamaican Counter Terrorism Operations Group.

In response to losing at the Supreme Court of Canada, the Harper government introduces the Respect for Communities Act to ensure that communities can object to any proposed opening of a safe injection site.

Canada surpasses the United States in per capita consumption of opioids. It is followed by Norway, with 40 percent lower usage of opioids than Canada. Countries with approximately half the consumption rate of Canada are Switzerland, Austria, Germany, Australia, the United Kingdom, Belgium, New Zealand, Spain, and

Iceland. Those with about one-third of Canada's rate include France, Sweden, the Netherlands, and Finland. Countries with an even smaller fraction of our usage rate are Portugal, Israel, Italy, Greece, and Japan. The Japanese, for example, consume 29 times less opioids than Canadians per capita, while Cubans consume 376 times less.

The leading jurisdictions for per capita impaired driving offences are the Yukon, Northwest Territories, Nunavut, and Saskatchewan.

2014 British Columbia Supreme Court Chief Justice Christopher Hinkson grants an injunction allowing methadone-resistant individuals in Vancouver who participated in a clinical trial to continue to receive laboratory-manufactured pharmaceutical-grade heroin. The Canadian federal government, having lost several Supreme Court challenges relating to safer drug-use practices, did not appeal the injunction but will continue to vigorously defend the regulations in court.

The first drug treatment court in Atlantic Canada opens in King's County, Nova Scotia.

Tweed Marijuana, Canada's first publicly traded medical marijuana, ships its first orders to clients.

2015 Ontario bans smoking at children's playgrounds, publicly owned sports fields, and restaurant and bar patios, and prohibits the sale of tobacco on university and college campuses.

The number of babies born with Neonatal Abstinence Syndrome has jumped 15-fold in Ontario over the last two decades, reflecting the increased prescribing of opiates.

David Wilks, MP for the riding of Kootenay-Columbia, identifies himself as a person living in long-term addiction recovery in the House of Commons. He makes the following statement:

Mr. Speaker,

On January 27th and 28th of this year, individuals from across Canada came together in Ottawa to create a united vision for what addiction recovery means in Canada.

Hosted by CCSA, one of their declared visions was that recovery is real, available, attainable and sustainable.

Mr. Speaker, I bring this to your attention because just over 26 years ago, I took my last drink. My life had spiraled out of control. But, by the grace of God, I stand before you and all Canadians to give hope to all those who still suffer with addiction, that they can find a path which will provide them with a daily reprieve from their addiction.

Today I can tell you that I would not trade my best day drunk for my worst day sober.

Today I reach my hand out to help anyone in need, rather than pushing them away.

But most importantly I accept life as it is, not how I think it should be.

May we all come together and support those in recovery.

Justin Trudeau, elected Prime Minister of Canada, promises to legalize cannabis.

Appendix B
A GLOBAL HISTORY OF PSYCHOACTIVE DRUGS

50,000 BCE   Soil samples indicate that Neanderthals, in what is now Northern Iraq, used ephedra, an alkaloid that produces amphetamine-like effects.

10,000 BCE   Anthropologists believe that brewing alcoholic beverages began at this time in human civilization, prompting nomadic clans to settle and begin growing grain crops.

8000 BCE   Around this time the first batch of beer is brewed in the Mideast.

Cannabis is already being cultivated as a crop.

6000 BCE   Opium is being used medicinally.

There is evidence of breweries in Egypt.

5000 BCE   A Sumerian poem describing a boy's first use of alcohol is discovered.

Hemp is being cultivated in China.

4000 BCE   Cannabis is being used recreationally by cultures living along the Eurasian steppes.

3000 BCE   Tea has begun to be consumed socially in China.

The Egyptian *Book of the Dead* mentions the manufacturing of *Hek*, a beer-like beverage made from barley, bread, and water.

2737 BCE   Shen Neng, a Chinese emperor, lists marijuana as a cure for gout, rheumatism, female disorders, constipation, and absentmindedness in a book of medicines.

2500 BCE   Coca leaves found in burial chambers in Peru date back to this era.

The use of poppy seeds is confirmed in Europe in the area of present-day Switzerland.

2225 BCE   *The Code of Hammurabi*, written in Assyria, includes 282 paragraphs on rules for maintaining a beer shop.

2000 BCE	Egyptian soldiers are banned from drinking, followed by prohibition of drinking on the job for other workers.
	Indigenous peoples of the Andes are smoking Anadenanthera, a source of the potent hallucinogenic dimethyltryptamine (DMT), as indicated by radiocarbon dating.
1500 BCE	Egyptian engravings depict images of drunken members of the ruling class in the arms of their slaves.
	The Aztec civilization uses *psilcyben mexicana* mushrooms as part of religious ceremonies and for recreation.
	The Incas use coca leaves as an aid to working at high altitudes.
800 BCE	Distilled spirits are introduced to Western Europe as a remedy for most common ailments.
700 BCE	Assyrian tablets describe how to collect opium; similar methods remain in use today.
500 BCE	Homer discusses the effects of *nepenthe* in the *Odyssey*, effects similar to those associated with opium.
	Heroditus refers to drunkenness as a body and soul sickness.
400 BCE	Aristotle, in comparing licentiousness to drunkenness, notes that the former is a functional disorder while the latter results from an organic disorder. He views licentiousness as permanent but drunkenness as curable.
350 BCE	Alexander the Great dies at age 33 from alcohol-related causes during a wine-drinking contest.
300 BCE	First known use of coca as a stimulant by the Aymara of Bolivia occurs.
200 BCE	A capsule of the opium poppy is engraved on Jewish coinage.
98 BCE	Intoxicating liquors are made and sold in China under strict government regulation.
70 CE	Pedacius Dioscorides, a Greek physician living in Rome, writes that cannabis is an effective remedy for earaches.
250	The patron saint of wine producers, Saint Vincent of Saragossa, the earliest known Spanish martyr, is born at Heusca.
580	Saint Arnold, patron saint of Brewers, is born in Austria. He warned his parishioners not to drink water, which could be lethal at this time in Europe, but to drink beer, which, because it was brewed, was safe to drink.
711	The Moors introduce opium to Spain to be used as medicine.
950	A specially brewed beer served at weddings in England became known as bride's ale, the forerunner of today's translation: bridal.
1000	The Bible contains 17 specific references to wine, including Christ's first miracle and the recounting in Genesis of Noah's apparent drunkenness shortly after emerging from the Ark.

The brewing of coffee is first documented in Arabia.

Muslim traders first introduce opium to China.

1100   This is the first documentation of the making of brandy from wine in Italy.

1200   Marco Polo returns from the Orient with stories of a drug used by assassins to prepare them for the task. The translation becomes *haschishin* or hashish.

A contract signed in the Netherlands after 3:00 p.m. is considered invalid as citizens' minds are assumed to be clouded by beer. Average adult consumption in the Netherlands is more than 400 L per year, as water in cities is polluted, coffee and tea are not yet available, and milk is considered unhealthy.

1215   The Magna Carta is signed in England on June 15. The document has a clause referring to the proper size of beer handles.

1256   In Bohemia a brewery is constructed at Budweis.

1279   The Mongol Emperor Kubla Khan issues an edict condemning all dealers in alcohol to banishment or slavery.

1300   Hashish is introduced to Egypt.

1327   Legislation is introduced in England to curb intemperance.

1332   The first written documentation of the use of khat in Ethiopia dates from this time.

1400   The term "drug" comes into English usage. Its origins are believed to be the Dutch term for dried goods.

1493   Christopher Columbus introduces tobacco to the court of Spain.

1500   Whisky is produced in Scotland. Five years later its production will be placed under the jurisdiction of the Royal College of Surgeons.

1510   Benedictine is made at the French monastery at Fecamp.

1519   Tobacco leaves are imported to Europe.

1542   The Portuguese introduce tobacco to Japan.

1545   The Spanish bring cannabis to the Americas.

1551   The use of coca is condemned by the Catholic Church in South America.

1554   The first recorded coffee house opens in Constantinople, Turkey.

1560   Jean Nicot introduces tobacco to the court of France, while Walter Raleigh delivers it to England. Portuguese traders import tobacco to Africa from Brazil.

1563   The Portuguese explorer Garcia da Orta describes opium addiction in India: "There is a very strong desire for it among those who use it."

1590   English sailors receive about .6 L of beer a day as part of their ration. Under Mughal Emperor Akbar of India, opium is grown as a cash crop for international trade. It becomes a primary source of revenue for the British after they conquer India.

1592	H. van Linschoten of Holland describes opium use in India: "He that is used to eating it, must eat it daily, otherwise he dies and consumes himself … he that has never eaten it, and will venture to at first to eat as much as those who daily use it, will surely kill him: for I certainly believe it is a kind of poison."
1600	Persons convicted of excessive drinking in various parts of Europe are forced to walk about town for one day with only a barrel for clothing as a means to shame them into more moderate use. The British East India Company is formed and becomes involved in the opium trade in India, competing with Dutch and Portuguese interests. The German Order of Temperance is founded, with members pledging to never become intoxicated, which is defined as no more than 14 glasses of wine per day.
1603	Cultivation of tobacco becomes a crime in Japan. The law is repealed 22 years later and tobacco is turned into a cash crop.
1604	King James I of England writes *Counterblase to Tobacco*, condemning its use, and raises the tax on importing tobacco by 4,000 percent.
1605	Tobacco is introduced to India.
1606	Public intoxication becomes a criminal offence in England.
1608	Tobacco smoking is banned in Japan to counter an increasing number of fires.
1609	Henry Hudson meets a group of Delaware First Nations on an island and introduces them to gin. The island is named Manahachtanienk, which roughly translates into "place where we got drunk" and is currently known as Manhattan, which has since also become the name of an alcoholic beverage.
1610	Dutch traders introduce tea to Europe.
1611	The first commercial hemp crop is planted in Jamestown, Virginia.
1615	Coffee is introduced to Europe in Venice, Italy. The Persian Shah Abbas prohibits smoking as he fears it will affect the birth rate. Violators are forced to smoke pipes of camel dung.
1619	King James I prohibits cultivation of tobacco in England and declares the tobacco trade a royal monopoly.
1620	The Virginia colony ships 18,144 kg of tobacco to England.
1621	An English clergyman, Robert Burton, recommends the use of marijuana in the treatment of a variety of common maladies.
1623	Tobacco prohibition in Turkey is enacted due to the increasing number of fires caused by careless smoking.
1629	The ship *Arabella* arrives at the Massachusetts Bay colony, including in its cargo 42 tons of beer and beer-making equipment. Hemp is grown as a crop throughout New England.

1633	The death penalty is introduced for smoking in Turkey.
1634	Michael, the first Romanov czar of Russia, issues a decree prohibiting smoking. First-time offenders are to be whipped, second-time offenders, executed, while those using snuff are to have their noses amputated. Seven years later, the czar simply exiles tobacco users.
1635	In France, tobacco becomes a prescription drug.
1637	The first brewery in North America is established in Massachusetts.
1644	Tobacco smoking is banned in China. This practice is slowly replaced with opium smoking.
1658	Persons convicted of drunkenness are placed in the stocks in Maryland.
1660	Tobacco growing is banned in Scotland.
1675	Charles II of England calls for the suppression of coffee houses in London.
1679	Champagne is discovered by the Benedictine monk, Dom Perignon.
1700	The Crown Prince of Bavaria marries Princess Therese von Sachesen-Hildenburghanusen on October 17. The five-day event was the initial Oktoberfest celebration.
1719	Smoking prohibitions are introduced in France.
1729	The first anti-opium law is introduced in China, allowing opium to be imported only under licence. The East India Company of Great Britain immediately begins smuggling opium into China.
	Gin mania among the British poor and working class is reportedly created by an increasing percentage of alcohol by volume and the decreasing price of gin.
1747	French philosopher Condillac refers to inebriety as a disease and calls for state-sponsored treatment.
1761	English physician John Hill warns snuff users that this form of tobacco use increases their risk of developing nasal cancer.
1768	The first Western documentation of khat is made by Swedish botanist Peter Froskal.
1769	Captain James Cook arrives in New Zealand smoking a pipe, and is promptly doused with water by local inhabitants when he steps ashore in case he is a demon.
1772	Benjamin Rush, Surgeon General of the American Revolutionary Army, signer of the Declaration of Independence, and the United States' first professor of medicine, calls for the abandonment of distilled spirits and the substitution of cider, beer, wine, and non-alcoholic drinks in his "Sermons to Gentlemen Upon Temperance and Exercise."

1784	Benjamin Rush writes that pathological drinking is a disease in his article *An Inquiry into the Effects of Ardent Spirits upon the Human Body and Mind*.
1787	The 55 delegates at the American Constitutional Convention, which leads to the signing of the Declaration of Independence, consume 54 bottles of Madeira, 60 bottles of claret, 8 bottles of whisky, 22 bottles of cider, 12 bottles of beer, and seven bowls of alcoholic punch.
1789	On the eve of the French Revolution, wine consumption among Parisians is 120 L per person. The first American temperance society is organized in Litchfield, Connecticut.
1799	Friedrich Serturner discovers the major active ingredient of opium, which he names morphine, beginning the study of opioid pharmacology. Prohibition of opium in China leads to a thriving black market in the product. Nitrous oxide is synthesized.
1806	Morphine is distilled from opium in Germany.
1810	In the United States there are 14,191 legal distilleries, with the average annual adult alcohol intake estimated at about 18 L.
1812	Delirium tremens is recognized and medically described.
1819	The Cherokee Nation passes a law prohibiting white trafficking of liquor on their lands. The law is amended the following year so that African-American slaves are also prohibited from selling their masters' alcohol on Native lands.
1820	China imposes harsher restrictions on the opium trade. Opium smuggling is reported to quadruple. Caffeine is isolated from coffee.
1822	Thomas De Quincey publishes *Confessions of an English Opium-Eater*. This work and Samuel Taylor Coleridge's poem "Xanadu" launch the Romantic image of the aristocratic, bohemian opium user.
1826	The American Temperance Society is formed.
1827	The British East Indian Company has a monopoly on opium production in India. The estimated income derived from "sales" is estimated at £2 million, half the cost of running the British Civil Service.
1836	The American Temperance Movement's membership exceeds 1 million.
1840	Cannabis is imported to Jamaica by Indian labourers. Washingtonians, named after Martha Washington, become the first alcohol-based self-help group, providing moral support for

abusive alcohol drinkers, "rehabilitating" over 100,000 inebriates during the decade, and reaching a membership of over 400,000 by the 1850s.

Great Britain declares war on China after the Chinese emperor attempts to ban England's importation of opium from India. A second opium war is waged from 1856 to 1860. The wars are partly the result of a huge trade deficit run up by England because of the importation of tea. From 1829 to 1840, Chinese exports had brought into the national economy nearly $7 million, but imports, mainly opium, had cost $56 million.

1845 Tea is introduced to Morocco when British merchants, frustrated by their inability to access ports because of the Crimean War, begin to off-load their cargo in Tangier and Mogador. Mint tea has since become a staple of Moroccan culture.

1848 Sigmund Freud writes about the medicinal value of cocaine.

1849 The term "alcoholism" is coined by Swedish public-health physician Dr. Magnus Huss.

1853 Dr. Alexander Wood invents the hypodermic needle.

1854 The Forbes-Mackenzie Act is instituted in Scotland, banning the sale of alcohol on Sunday.

Philip Morris begins making his own cigarettes in England. Old Bond Street soon became the centre of the retail tobacco trade.

1855 Thirteen American states have alcohol prohibition laws in place. The hemp industry is second only to cotton in terms of economic value in the southern United States.

Slave owners in the United States use alcohol to control their slaves. Although prohibited from drinking during the working week, slaves are encouraged to drink heavily on Saturday nights and holidays. This controlled promotion of drunkenness through activities such as drinking contests is viewed by some abolitionists as a means to reduce the threat of slave escapes and revolts.

1858 The Treaty of Tianjin allows both opium and cigarettes to be imported into China duty-free.

1860 Albert Niemann, a German scientist, isolates cocaine from coca leaves.

1861 Morphine use is so regular during the American Civil War that it garners the nickname, "the soldier's disease."

1862 The first federal tobacco tax is introduced in the United States to help finance the Civil War.

1863 Adolph von Baeyer produces a new substance from the condensation of malonic acid and urea, and goes to a local tavern to celebrate his success. He learns from Belgian artillerymen at the establishment that it is the celebration of their patron saint, Saint Barbara, and thus calls the substance barbituric acid. It would be another 42 years before two German chemists would further synthesize barbituric acid into barbital, the first barbiturate.

1864   The New York State Inebriate Asylum in Binghamton, the first medically oriented institution specializing in the treatment of inebriety, is opened.

The first case of morphine addiction involving the use of a hypodermic syringe is reported in the United States.

1871   Despite the majority of testimony indicating no harm with moderate use, the government of Burma (British) bans hemp drugs because one-third of patients in local asylums had regularly used cannabis products.

It is estimated that 20 percent of Americans are using opioid products, primarily in patent medicines.

1873   The Women's Christian Temperance Union is created.

Karl Marx publishes the first volume of *Das Kapital*.

1875   San Francisco becomes the first American jurisdiction to pass an ordinance banning the smoking of opium.

1876   Chocolate is manufactured in Switzerland.

1877   Amphetamines are synthesized.

Strong Drink: The Curse and the Cure is written by American Timothy Shay Arthur. The 675-page book begins with a series of stories on the fall and redemption of "drunkards," followed by a review of rescue asylums for inebriates. The book ends with a description of alcohol abuse as an incurable disease that can only be arrested by the help of God and with total abstinence.

1878   *The New York Times* estimates that there are 200,000 opiate addicts in the United States. It warns of a dangerous fad, especially among society women, of injecting morphine and calls this behaviour a vice.

1879   The Habitual Drunkards Act is introduced in England, which, along with the Inebriates Act of 1898, licences a few retreats for the treatment of psychoactive drug users, though most facilities remain private with minimal public support.

1881   T.S. Arthur's *Saved As By Fire* refers to alcoholism as a spiritual disease requiring spiritual remedies.

1883   James Bonsack of Virginia invents the first machine to automatically roll cigarettes. Until this time, they had to be individually hand-rolled.

Until 1883, hemp is the world's largest agricultural crop, used in the production of fabric, soap, paper, and medicines.

1884	Sigmund Freud publishes "Uber Coca," a review of cocaine and its medicinal uses, including its use in treating addiction to morphine.
1885	The British export 180,000 60 kg boxes of opium to China.
	Merck pharmaceutical ships 83,343 kg of cocaine for medical use.
1886	Dr. J.C. Pemberton of Atlanta, Georgia, creates a temperance beverage composed of cola nuts, caramel, and coca leaves: Coca-Cola. It is advertised as brain tonic and intellectual soda-fountain beverage. Nearly a decade later, pharmacist Caleb Bradham of Bern, North Carolina, begins offering a similar beverage as an elixir for aiding digestion. He names the beverage Pepsi-Cola.
	Scottish author Robert Louis Stevenson writes *The Strange Case of Dr. Jekyll and Mr. Hyde*. During this time he is a regular user of cocaine.
1887	Amphetamines are first synthesized in Germany.
1890	W.C. Brownson publishes *The Disease Theory of Intemperance*.
1891	One of the first facilities devoted exclusively to treating addiction to drugs other than alcohol—Jansen Mattison's Brooklyn Home for Habitues—opens.
1893	The Anti-Saloon League, a temperance society, is formed in the United States.
1895	Heinrich Dreser, working for Germany's Bayer Company, finds that diluting morphine with acetyls produces a drug without the common morphine side effects. Bayer begins production of diacetylmorphine and calls it "heroin."
1896	The psychoactive chemical agent in peyote, mescaline, is isolated.
1898	The Bayer company puts heroin on the market as an antitussive. As a sniffable powder marketed as a cough remedy, it quickly gains favour as a recreational drug.
1900	It is estimated that 3 percent of the American population is dependent on heroin, approximately double the estimated 1992 rate.
	Sigmund Freud publishes *The Interpretation of Dreams*.
	J.M. French publishes *Treatment of Alcoholism as a Disease*.
1901	Marijuana is replaced by Aspirin in a range of pain medications.
1903	Coca-Cola introduces caffeine into its soft drink, replacing the original stimulant, cocaine, though de-cocalized cocaine leaves remain part of the formula.
1906	The American Pure Food and Drug Act is passed, primarily as a result of patent medicines containing heroin and cocaine.
	The Narcotic Drug Importation Act is passed to control the flow of opioids into the United States.
	The Emmanuel Clinic of Boston is among the first to deliver outpatient alcoholism counselling services out of a local community-based clinic.

1908	The Child Act in the United States prohibits giving intoxicating liquors to children under the age of five, and bans those younger than 14 from entering a tavern.
1909	Among Ernest Shackleton's supplies in his quest to reach the South Pole are cocaine tablets to enhance stamina.
	Czechoslovakia (now the Czech Republic and Slovakia) opens its first alcohol treatment facility.
1910	John D. Rockefeller, Jr., is appointed to a grand jury investigating white slavery in New York. He will later found the Bureau of Social Hygiene that will create a Committee on Drug Addictions. The Bureau of Social Hygiene is founded with funds from the Laura Spelman Rockefeller fund for the scientific study of prostitution. In this period, prostitution, venereal diseases (syphilis and gonorrhea), and drug use (including alcohol use) are seen as related problems.
1912	The Hague Opium Convention, also known as the International Opium Convention, formally establishes narcotics control as a fundamental element of international law. The convention enters into force in 1915 to become the first binding international legal instrument governing the shipment of narcotic drugs for medical purposes, establishing the groundwork for the evolving international system of drug control.
1913	R.J. Reynolds introduces the Camel brand of cigarettes.
1914	The Harrison Act is enacted in the United States. It is the first national law aimed at controlling psychoactive drug use, and while it bans cocaine, heroin and cannabis are not prohibited but rather are substantially taxed.
	The Boylan Act in New York State allows for anyone using habit-forming drugs to be committed to an institution licenced by the State Lunacy Board.
1915	The United States Treasury Department Decision 2200 is implemented in response to the Harrison Act. It allows officials of the Treasury Department to prosecute doctors who prescribe narcotic drugs as maintenance to addicts, turning addiction from a medical to a law-enforcement issue in the United States.
1916	A rampage spearheaded by thousands of drunken soldiers who looted saloons and marketplaces leads to a closure of all pubs in Sydney, Australia, at 6:00 p.m. The law will not be repealed until 1955.
1917	Macy's Department stores in New York establish a counselling program to help employees.
1919	The 18th amendment of the United States Constitution is enacted—Prohibition: the Volstead Act. All states except Connecticut and Rhode Island ratify it. The law prohibits the manufacture,

sale, or transportation of intoxicating liquors. However, doctors can still prescribe alcohol, and individuals are still allowed to make homemade wine for personal consumption. During this era, several American wineries bottle grape juice with a label warning that fermentation will occur if yeast and sugar are accidentally added. American President Roosevelt prepares for prohibition by stockpiling enough gin to serve martinis on a regular basis each day at 4:00 p.m. during his entire term of office.

The Bayer pharmaceutical company of Germany loses its patent rights to Aspirin and heroin as a fallout of World War I.

Cigarette smoking becomes prominent globally during World War I as manufacturers provide free cigarettes to Allied troops. Prominent surgeon Alton Ochsner, a medical student, is called in to observe a lung cancer surgery as his professor indicates he might never see another case. Indeed, Ochsner does not actually perform lung cancer surgery until 1936 when he starts seeing tumours arising in men who had begun smoking during the war.

1920	Federal enforcement of Prohibition in the United States begins on January 17 after the formal ratification of the 18th amendement of the United States Constitution. Within the first month, five Prohibition agents are arrested on charges of corruption for aiding bootleggers.
	Legal coca production in Asia by European pharmaceutical companies exceeds that of coca production in South America.
1921	Fourteen American states prohibit the sale of tobacco products. All acts are repealed by 1927.
1922	Cocaine is prohibited in the United States.
1923	A second wave of mandatory sterilization laws in the United States includes alcohol- and drug-dependent persons.
1924	Henry Ford discusses the danger of drinking and driving in an interview appearing in the *Christian Herald*.
	Philip Morris introduces Marlboro as a women's cigarette that is as "mild as May."
1925	The International Opium Convention is passed, extending its scope to cannabis.
	American Public Health Service psychiatrist Lawrence Kolb publishes a landmark set of articles that consolidate the psychopathic view of addicts. He provides a classification of addict types and explains his view that addiction is the result of pre-existing, inherent defects of personality.

| 1926 | From the *International Herald Tribune*, July 13: |

Moscow—The restoration of the sale of Vodka has put money into the Soviet State Treasury. But it is also causing the industrial administrators considerable concern in that the workers are consuming excessive quantities of the fiery liquid. Effects are visible in slack work, especially on the Saturday pay day and on Monday, factory managers state. In some cases factory workers damaged machines with a hope of obtaining a free day while they are repaired.

The Rolleston Act allows British physicians to prescribe heroin for those addicted to heroin. The report calls addiction a disease rather than an indulgence.

1927	The first medical report associating smoking with lung cancer is released.
	Full production of the .38 Colt Detective Special commences in the United States. One of the contributing factors in increasing bullet calibre size from .32 was the fear of the "cocaine crazed Negro" who could not be fully stopped by the smaller-sized bullet.
1928	Lucky Strike cigarettes targets women by associating smoking with thinness in their "Reach for a Lucky instead of a sweet" campaign.
	Solomon Solis-Cohen and Thomas Stotesbury Githens, in *Pharmacotherapeutics, Materia Medica and Drug Action*, characterize addicts as liars who cannot be trusted.
1929	German Fritz Lickint publishes the first formal statistical evidence of a lung cancer–tobacco link.
1930	The Oxford Group is established in the United States. With links to the Washingtonians movement, the Oxford Group is the forerunner of Alcoholics Anonymous, except with an even stronger spiritual and evangelical orientation.
1932	During Prohibition the United States government undertakes a formal poisoning program to replace methyl alcohol in industrial products containing ethyl alcohol, which is being diverted for illegal sales. Over 10,000 people are fatally poisoned by this initiative.
1933	The prohibition of alcohol in the United States is repealed through the enactment of the 21st amendment of the Constitution for a variety of reasons, including the need to create jobs and stimulate the economy.
1934	On November 11, Bill W. is readmitted for the fourth time to Charles Towns Hospital for treatment of his alcoholism. During

this last stay, he has a profound spiritual experience that marks the beginning of his permanent sobriety. During his hospitalization, Dr. William Silkworth presents the allergy concept of alcohol dependency to Bill Wilson, defining alcoholism in terms of physical allergy, obsession, and compulsion.

Drug addiction appears as a diagnostic category for the first time in the American Psychiatric Association's *Standard Classified Nomenclature of Disease.*

1935   On May 11, 1935, Bill Wilson, a former stock broker, demoralized at the end of a failed business trip, found himself in the lobby of the Mayflower Hotel in Akron, Ohio, fearing that he might take a drink and destroy his hard-earned sobriety. His sense of what he needed to prevent his return to drinking was not to reach out to a professional, but to find another alcoholic with whom he could talk. A series of phone calls facilitated by Henrietta Seiberling led him to Dr. Robert Holbrook Smith, who at that time was struggling with his own alcoholism. Their growing friendship, mutual support, and vision of helping other alcoholics marked the formal ignition of AA as a social movement. The date of Dr. Bob Smith's last drink, on June 10, 1935, to steady his nerves before surgery, is celebrated as AA's founding date.

The American Medical Association passes a resolution declaring that "alcoholics are valid patients."

1936   The first AA group forms in Akron, Ohio. AA has 10 successful members enjoying sobriety by the end of the year. By 1937, the number will rise to 40.

Tobacco companies use actual doctors in new advertising campaigns to counter medical claims of health problems produced by smoking. This same practice will be adopted by the Chinese government to market state monopoly tobacco brands to its citizens at the beginning of the 21st century.

1937   Taxation of marijuana sales in the United States is the first step in the prohibition of the drug.

Methadone is synthesized by German scientists Bockmuhl and Ehrhart, who worked for IG Farben.

1938   LSD is synthesized by Swiss physician Albert Hoffman, who was searching for a new blood stimulant.

Judy Garland, 16, receives a regular supply of amphetamines while playing the role of Dorothy in *The Wizard of Oz*. She will die at age 47 from a barbiturate overdose, having battled alcohol and drug issues her entire adult life.

1939   The first edition of the AA *Big Book*, including the 12 steps, is published.

At the encouragement of Dr. Bob Smith, Sister Ignatia, an Irish Catholic nun and member of the Sisters of Charity of Saint Augustine and administrator of St. Thomas Hospital in Akron, Ohio, allows the establishment of a four-bed ward for the treatment of alcohol-dependent men. This is the inaugural alcohol-specific medical in-patient residential treatment facility in North America.

Sigmund Freud dies of cancer of the jaw after 45 years of cigar smoking. Freud advocated the use of cocaine in treating morphine addiction and himself was cocaine-dependent for part of his life, as well as nicotine-dependent.

1940   E.I. Dupont de Neumous and Eastman Kodak Corporation start in-house occupational alcoholism programs, forerunners to contemporary employee assistance programs (EAPs). Maurice Dupont-Lee, the chairman of Dupont, meets with Bill Wilson as a prelude to the program's development.

Psychiatrists now generally consider alcoholism a disease, specifically a psychoneurosis.

1941   Jack Alexander writes an article for the *Saturday Evening Post* entitled "Alcoholics Anonymous." As a result, membership jumps from approximately 2,000 to over 6,000 by the end of the year.

Al-Anon begins with the formation of the first family (wives) groups.

Amphetamines are freely distributed to both Allied and Axis military personnel, a practice that will be maintained by many militaries into the 21st century.

1943   LSD is synthesized in a pharmaceutical research laboratory.

1945   *The Lost Weekend* is released, offering the film industry's first in-depth examination of alcohol abuse. It wins the Oscar for Best Picture, with the girlfriend of the alcoholic protagonist in the film proclaiming, "He's a sick person!"

The Nazis sterilize between 20,000 and 30,000 German alcoholics during their reign, and send as many others to the death camps with "other degenerates" as part of their eugenics movement.

1946   The 12 traditions of Alcoholics Anonymous are formulated and published.

1947   Public Law 80-472 in the United States acknowledges alcoholics as sick individuals who require treatment, allowing the creation of treatment and rehabilitation programs for them.

The international physicians' AA group is established.

1949   The Hazelden Treatment Center opens in Minnesota as a facility to assist priests with their alcohol abuse.

Methadone is recommended as an aid in the detoxification of heroin addicts.

"One Wife's Story" by Lois W. is published in the AA *Grapevine*.

1950	Dr. Bob Smith, co-founder of Alcoholics Anonymous, dies.

British scientist Richard Doll establishes a link between smoking and lung cancer. Three years later a scientist working for R.J. Reynolds confirms the findings. The company report is never officially released.

Wynder and Graham publish a case-control study of 684 lung cancer cases, finding that 96.5 percent have been moderate or heavy smokers, a much higher proportion than found among patients hospitalized for other diseases.

The WHO's Expert Committee on Mental Health publishes a report defining alcoholism as a chronic behaviour disorder, manifested by the repeated drinking of alcoholic beverages in excess of dietary and social uses of the community, and to an extent that interferes with the drinker's health or his social and economic functioning, emphasizing that alcoholism should be considered a disease.

1951   E.M. Jellinek publishes *Disease Concept of Alcoholism*, marking the formal beginnings of the medical model.

Al-Anon is formed as a support to those whose partners are in AA.

Antabuse is introduced.

For at least five years in the 1950s, Kent's Micronite Filter (Lorillard Tobacco Company) contain crocidolite asbestos, one of the deadliest forms of this fibrous mineral. Smokers inhale millions of deadly fibres per year and are never told of the hazard. Filtered brands nonetheless are a huge success, growing in market share from 2 percent in 1950 to 50 percent in 1960.

1952   Al-Anon adopts AA's 12 Steps as their guidelines with one change. In step 12, "alcoholics" is changed to "others."

The first Al-Anon World Directory is published.

The first edition of the American Psychiatric Association's *Diagnostic and Statistical Manual* (DSM-I) is published. Alcoholism and drug addiction is subsumed within the category of sociopathic personality disturbances. This placement reflects the view that alcoholism is an outgrowth of a particular cluster of personality traits.

1953   Sociologist Howard Becker publishes "Becoming a Marihuana User," an examination of the use of cannabis among New York city jazz musicians.

The Opium Protocol is signed, limiting opium production and trade to medical and scientific needs globally.

Narcotics Anonymous (NA) begins in southern California. Initial gatherings are called "rabbit meetings" as no facility will allow the participants to meet regularly as it contravened the existing Rockefeller law, which made it illegal for two known narcotic addicts to meet. To ensure stability, the founding members approach the Los Angeles Police Department to obtain assurances that their meetings will not be raided. By 1960 the group's membership has fallen to four, but struggles forward to the point that on the 50th anniversary, there are over 30,000 weekly meetings in over 100 nations.

1954   The Marlboro cowboy is created for Philip Morris by Chicago ad agency Leo Burnett.

The CIA's Office of Scientific Intelligence publishes "Potential New Agent for Unconventional Warfare: Lysergic Acid Diethyllamine (LSD)." The report's findings will be featured in the 1990 movie *Jacob's Ladder*.

1955   AA grows to 6,000 groups, comprising 150,000 people in 50 countries.

The book *Al-Anon Family Groups* is published.

Methaqualone, more commonly known as Quaalude, is synthesized in India to fight malaria.

1956   The American Medical Association (AMA) recognizes that alcoholics should be allowed admission to general hospitals for treatment, though it will be another 10 years before the association formally recognizes alcoholism as a disease.

The Narcotic Control Act is implemented in the United States, containing a statue allowing for capital punishment for selling heroin to a minor.

Bill Wilson volunteers for LSD trials in the hope that the drug might provide a spiritual awakening for those members of AA who could not achieve this on their own.

Humphry Osmond coins the word "psychedelic" in a letter to Aldous Huxley.

1957   PCP is synthesized for use as an animal tranquilizer.

Alateen and Gamblers Anonymous both begin.

Pope Pius XII suggested that all members of the Jesuit order give up smoking.

Milton Berle becomes spokesman for Miltown, an early benzodiazepine-like drug, leading in part to 5 percent of the American population consuming this early tranquilizer within a year of its initial marketing.

1958   Albert Hoffman isolates psilocybin at the Sandoz pharmaceutical laboratory. He will later discover the hallucinogenic effects of morning glory seeds and LSA (lysergic acid amide). After retiring in the 1970s, he is invited to become a member of the Nobel Prize committee.

1959 Tobacco companies become aware of the dangers of polonium-210, a radioactive substance that causes cancerous growths in the lungs of cigarette smokers, but hide this knowledge from the public. The levels of radiation in cigarettes were responsible for up to 138 deaths per 1,000 smokers over 25 years.

Fentanyl is synthesized.

1960 The beginnings of NA's formal literature are published, with *Who Is an Addict?*, *What Can I Do?*, and *Recovery and Relapse* written by Jimmy K., founding member of NA.

Jellinek's *The Disease Concept of Alcoholism* is published, presenting a typology of alcoholism.

1961 The Single Convention on Narcotic Drugs is adopted, consolidating existing international drug laws into a single convention and formally replacing the 1912 Hague Convention. All nations become signatories with the exception of Afghanistan, Chad, East Timor, Equatorial Guinea, Kiribati, Nauru, Samoa, South Sudan, Tuvalu, and Vanuatu.

1962 Narcotics Anonymous's *White Book* is published.

British troops are given LSD to see how they would react if the hallucinogen were used against them in battle. Enlisted soldiers are asked to volunteer for the experiment. In the same year, the British military eliminates the rum ration for enlisted personnel.

In California, the case of Robinson versus the state concludes with the ruling that addiction is an illness, not a crime.

The California Civil Addict Program begins allowing the courts to order anyone addicted to narcotics, regardless of whether they have been convicted of any offence, into a residential treatment program, followed by up to seven years of supervised parole.

1963 Diet Pepsi is introduced.

Diazepam is granted FDA approval in November 1963, just after American president John F. Kennedy is assassinated.

1964 The US Surgeon General Luther Terry's report, commissioned by President John F. Kennedy, again links tobacco smoking to lung cancer.

Methadone maintenance is introduced as a treatment approach in New York City.

Israeli scientist Dr. Raphael Mechoulame isolates THC.

DOM, a potent hallucinogen, is created by the Dow Chemical company.

Methadone maintenance trials begin in England.

1966 The American Medical Association (AMA) recognizes alcoholism as a disease and it is ratified by the House of Delegates of the

AMA on November 26, 1967, in Houston, Texas.

Mississippi repeals alcohol prohibition.

1967   Narcotics Anonymous begins a General Services Organization to assist the development of new groups, and provide literature and ongoing support.

The possession and use of LSD is prohibited in the United States. New York State's Narcotics Addiction Control Program goes into effect, empowering judges to commit addicts for compulsory treatment for up to five years.

1968   The American Alcoholic Rehabilitation Act passes, stating that "alcoholism is a major health and social problem affecting a significant proportion of the public." Funding is provided by the act to establish facilities across the United States for the prevention of alcoholism and the rehabilitation of alcoholics.

British doctors can no longer prescribe medical heroin to treat heroin addiction.

The second edition of the APA's DSM (DSM-II) follows the precedent of WHO ICD-8 and includes three subcategories of alcohol-related disorders: alcohol addiction, episodic excessive drinking, and habitual excessive drinking. Alcoholism and drug addiction continue to be classified as types of sociopathic personality disturbances.

1969   Blue Cross begins covering in-patient alcoholism programs, formally recognizing alcoholism as a disease.

1970   American president Richard Nixon makes Elvis Presley a federal agent at large for the Bureau of Narcotics and Dangerous Drugs.

1971   President Nixon, dissatisfied with waging war in Southeast Asia, becomes the first American president to call for a global War on Drugs.

Prudential Insurance begins to cover treatment for alcoholism as an employee benefit.

Bill Wilson dies on his 53rd wedding anniversary, having achieved 36 years of sobriety.

1972   Pepsi-Cola becomes the first American consumer product sold in the Soviet Union.

1973   The Drug Enforcement Agency (DEA) is created in the United States by President Nixon.

Fetal Alcohol Syndrome is identified as a pattern of abnormalities occurring in children born to alcohol-abusing women.

Al-Anon publishes Alateen's first book, *Alateen: Hope for Children of Alcoholics*.

1975   Drug gangs kill 40 people in one weekend in the Colombian city of Medellin after police seize 600 kg of cocaine in one of the first major drug seizures in that nation.

Jean Kirkpatrick founds Women For Sobriety, the first secular alcoholism recovery alternative to Alcoholics Anonymous.

1976   AA membership is 1 million in over 90 countries.

Sex and Love Addicts Anonymous and Adult Children of Alcoholics self-help groups begin using an adapted version of the 12 steps of AA.

1977   In England, Project Julia leads to the seizure of 6 million LSD tablets, the arrest of 100 persons who are eventually sentenced to 120 years in jail, and the increase in the cost of an LSD tablet from £1 to £5.

1978   An Asian alternative for heroin growing to the Golden Triangle begins to emerge: the Golden Crescent, comprised of Iran, Afghanistan, and Pakistan.

Valium becomes the all-time leading prescribed medication, averaging 60 million prescriptions per year.

The organization Jewish Alcoholics, Chemically Dependent Persons and Significant Others (JACS) is formed.

1980   MADD (Mothers Against Drunk Driving) is founded by Candy Lightner in Sacramento, California, after her daughter was killed by a drunk driver.

The War on Drugs continues under the Reagan administration in the US with the launch of the "Just Say No" campaign.

The DSM-III concept of alcoholism is shaped by the desirability of specific criteria, the distinction between dependence and drug-related problems that do not involve dependence, and the notion of a continuum of dependence. A shift occurs from a focus on tolerance, craving, withdrawal, and other biological consequences to new dimensions of obsession (preoccupation), compulsion, and relapse.

1981   NA has 1,100 meeting groups around the world, including Australia, Canada, England, Germany, Guam, Ireland, and Scotland.

1982   Colombian drug lord Pablo Escobar wins a seat in Colombia's Congress.

Cocaine Anonymous is launched.

Weldon Angelos, a 24-year-old, is sentenced to 55 years in federal prison for three marijuana sales under mandatory minimum sentencing laws created as part of the ongoing War on Drugs.

1983   Narcotics Anonymous World Service's office opens with one of the original members, Jimmy K., who designed the NA logo, serving as the office manager. The first NA group in India is formed in Bombay (now Mumbai).

1984   The first Narcotics Anonymous group in Israel begins meeting in Tel Aviv.

Hit men kill Colombia's justice minister. Pablo Escobar is indicted for the murder and flees to Panama. The DEA and Colombian police uncover a massive cocaine-production facility deep in the jungle in their pursuit of Escobar.

Nicotine gum is introduced.

1985   Cocaine smuggling shifts into Mexico after American law enforcement cracks down on maritime smuggling into Miami. The godfather of Mexican narcotics trafficking, Miguel Angel Felix Gallardo, pioneers smuggling routes to the United States for the Colombian cartels.

The Secular Organization for Sobriety program begins.

Jack and Lois Trimpey found Rational Recovery (RR).

1986   The first safe injection site facility opens in Switzerland.

The Surgeon General of the United States announces in his annual report that second-hand smoke causes cancer and other smoking-related diseases in non-smokers.

1987   The United States spends 3.9 billion dollars on the War on Drugs.

The first Narcotics Anonymous group in Greece begins meeting in Athens. In 20 years the organization will grow to 27 groups, with 110 meetings per week.

Lois Wilson, founder of Al-Anon and wife of Bill Wilson, dies.

1988   Warning labels appear on alcoholic beverages in some US jurisdictions.

The United Nations Convention against Illicit Traffic in Narcotic Drugs is adopted to control the flow of precursor chemicals in the illicit manufacture of drugs.

Wisconsin adopts the "cocaine mom act", which allows for the forcible confinement of pregnant women who use illegal drugs or alcohol "to a severe degree" and who will not accept treatment.

Alabama uses its "chemical endangerment of a child" law, designed to protect children from meth labs, to prosecute over 100 women whose babies tested positive for drugs.

1989   A new drug, "ice," kills 12 in Honolulu and quickly disappears from the media's radar until it reappears globally as crystal meth.

1990   The first Narcotics Anonymous group in Poland begins meeting in Olsztyn.

Between 1990 and 1996, 1,810 people will die in the United Kingdom due to benzodiazepine overdose, of approximately 110 will be traffic fatalities.

The FBI reports approximately 1 million drug arrests, one-third for trafficking and two-thirds for possession. The international illicit drug market is estimated at $100 billion.

1991	A glass of wine in southern France remains less expensive than a glass of juice.
1992	Jack Trimpey publishes *The Small Book,* an alternative self-help approach to the 12 steps and traditions espoused by Alcoholics Anonymous.
	The first fentanyl patch (Duragesic) is marketed in Canada.
1993	A 36-year-old female British worker, Veronica Bland, is awarded $23,000 in compensation for damage to her health from the effects of passive smoking in her workplace.
	Colombian police, with assistance from the United States, track down Pablo Escobar and kill him. With the Medellin cartel dismantled, a group of traffickers from the Colombian city of Cali rise in power.
1994	Worldwide retail coffee sales are approximately $30 billion.
	Mutual aid group Moderation Management begins focusing on harm reduction rather than abstinence.
1995	The Colombian government estimates that 500 internal security agents were killed in the ongoing War On Drugs.
	Philip Morris, owners of Imperial Tobacco, pay US$35,000 to have Lark cigarettes featured in the James Bond movie *Licence to Kill.*
	"Marlboro Man" David McLean dies of lung cancer.
1996	Proposition 215 is passed, granting seriously ill Californians the right to obtain and use marijuana for medical purposes when that medical use is deemed appropriate and has been recommended by a physician. This is followed by an increase in doctor's visits in California.
1997	A German company introduces Bier Zapfen, a pilsner-flavoured beer popsicle.
	United States District Judge William Osteen rules that the American Food and Drug Administration may regulate tobacco as a drug. The tobacco lobby immediately files an appeal of the ruling as 37 states undertake their own lawsuits against tobacco companies in an attempt to cover smoking-related health care costs. The subsequent agreement between the United States government and tobacco companies sees the distributors of tobacco products agree to pay $3.7 billion in compensation over 25 years.
1998	The National Institute on Drug Addiction and the National Institue on Alcohol Abuse and Alcoholism estimate that alcohol abuse, alcoholism, and other drug addiction costs the United States $245 billion annually in health care, criminal justice, and property damage costs.
1999	Worldwide illicit drug traffic is estimated to be behind only the United States and Japan in terms of economic output.

In Switzerland, a national referendum allows doctors to prescribe heroin to registered drug-dependent persons. An initial Swiss pilot study saw a decrease in new HIV cases, crime rate, prostitution, and homelessness related to heroin addiction.

2000   One-quarter of all crime committed in Sweden is linked to alcohol or other psychoactive drug use.

The United Nations Convention against Transnational Organized Crime is implemented to combat criminal drug trafficking networks.

Between 2000 and 2010, the US spends $7.3 billion on a military and economic aid program called Plan Colombia. While decreasing coca growing in Colombia, it displaces much of it to Bolivia and Peru.

2001   US tobacco giant Philip Morris estimates that the government of the Czech Republic saved $46 million because it did not have to house and care for smokers who died prematurely from tobacco-related illnesses.

Annual coca production is estimated at between 800 and 1,000 tones.

Portugal decriminalizes all psychoactive drug use, including heroin and cocaine, halving the rate of injected drug use to about 0.5 percent of the population, below levels in Britain and Italy.

It is estimated that 2,200 Belgians died from second-hand smoke.

Vietnam becomes the number two world exporter of coffee, behind Brazil but ahead of Colombia, with worldwide retail coffee sales reaching $70 billion, representing over 110 million bags of coffee beans.

2003   New Zealand's remaining residential treatment program closes due to a lack of funding, resulting in the opening of a series of private residential programs across the country.

The Netherlands becomes the first nation to legalize the medical use of cannabis, allowing doctors to prescribe the drug for those who are seriously ill. Pharmacies begin selling the drug at between €40 and €50 ($60 to $80) for a 5 g (0.18 oz.) bag.

2004   In Ireland, alcohol abuse was responsible for 6,584 deaths from 2000 to 2004, as well as more than 3 million hospitalizations (10.3 percent of all hospitalizations), with a cost of over €930 million for the in-patient beds.

Bhutan, a Himalayan kingdom, bans all public smoking and all smoking sales.

2005   The Rand Corporation estimates that the loss to the United States due to methamphetamine use in terms of lost lives, productivity, drug treatment, and law-enforcement expenses is over $23 billion, of which $4.2 billion was spent arresting, prosecuting, and incarcerating methamphetamine users. Other costs included $546 million for drug treatment, $687 million for lost productivity, and $905 million spent removing children from the homes of users.

The United States prison population is approximately 2 million people, of whom one-quarter are imprisoned for drug crimes. In 2005, 113,500 new African-Americans are added to the prison population, compared with 72,000 white inmates and 51,000 Latinos.

A German brewer introduces a nicotine-enhanced beer.

Advertising by China's state-owned tobacco company, responsible for the sale of nearly 2 billion cigarettes a year (approximately one-third of the worldwide output), hails tobacco as a way to prevent ulcers, reduce Parkinson's disease, treat schizophrenia and depression, enhance cognitive abilities, and prevent loneliness. Taxes from cigarette sales account for 10 percent of China's tax revenue.

2006	Supported by the US-financed Mérida Initiative, the Mexican government declares war on the drug cartels responsible for the death or disappearance of 100,000 Mexicans. Since the War on Drugs shifted its focus, the proportion of people consuming illicit drugs in the United States had not changed.
2007	Wales sets a 10-year high with 10,700 drug arrests.

Police in Scotland uncover 143 cannabis grow-ops in rented houses and estimates the annual turnover at around €25 million.

Five thousand people die annually in New Zealand from smoking tobacco.

President Evo Morales, Bolivia's first indigenous president, suspends the operations of the United States Drug Enforcement Administration in Bolivia, accusing the agency of encouraging anti-government protests. President George W. Bush responds by placing the Andean country on an anti-narcotics blacklist that cuts trade preferences.

The Netherlands bans the sale of psychedelic mushrooms in any form after a 17-year-old user, Gaelle Caroff, jumped to her death after ingesting the substance.

2008	In the United Kingdom, methadone prescriptions rise 120 percent in two years, from 70,363 to 146,999.

A report from the Iranian Narcotics Anonymous office reports 155,575 active members, of whom 2,775 (1.8 percent) are female. Nearly 60 percent have been members for less than a year, with 370 (0.2 percent) having been abstinent for seven or more years.

Estimates place the death toll from second-hand cigarette smoke in China at 100,000.

In Mexico, 5,800 people are killed in drug-related violence.

The estimated number of deaths from cocaine use in 14 European nations is 450.

Michigan becomes the 13th state to allow the use of cannabis for medical reasons.

Drug cartel sales are estimated at $300–$500 billion. Pharmaceutical sales are estimated at $300 billion.

2009   The overall number of persons addicted to illicit drugs between the ages of 18 and 39 in Russia is estimated at between 2 and 2.5 million, with more than 140,000 minors registered in rehabilitation centres. In 2008, approximately 30,000 individuals died from drug-related causes, excluding alcohol. One of the major problems is heroin being trafficked out of Afghanistan through the border with Kazakhstan. The average life expectancy of a Russian addicted to illegal opioids is five to seven years, with the primary cause of death being contaminated drugs and needles, along with drug-related crimes.

Iran hangs 44 people for drug smuggling.

Brewing company BrewDog of Fraserburgh, Scotland, releases a limited run of 500 beers with 32 percent alcohol content, dubbed Tactical Nuclear Penguin.

2010   Approximately 6.3 trillion cigarettes are produced globally.

The Chinese government runs the world's biggest tobacco company, collecting an estimated $75 billion in tobacco tax annually.

Paan and gutka chewing substances are used throughout India, with a 400-year-old tradition, consisting of betel, tobacco, areca nut, and spicy fragrances sold for two cents on street corners across the country making it popular among children and young people, making India the world's leader in oral cancer. Sales of these substances is $8–$10 billion per year.

2011   Drug seizures along the US-Mexico border for the years 2005–2011 include 1,400 pounds of heroin, 4,700 pounds of methamphetamine, 2,000 pounds of cocaine, and 13.2 million pounds of marijuana.

A New Zealand coroner testifies at the inquest of Natasha Harris, a mother of eight who suffered a heart attack in 2010, that her death was the result of her dependency on Coca-Cola. Harris, 31, drank more than two gallons of the soft drink every day, ingesting the equivalent of two pounds of sugar and 970 mg of caffeine daily.

2012   Recreational use of cannabis is legalized in Colorado and Washington State to those 21 years of age and older. In the first month of sales, Colorado netted $2 million in taxes. Washington State netted $1 million as only 18 of 40 stores opened on time.

2013   Health Canada licences over a dozen energy drinks containing more than 200 mg of caffeine per serving, approximately half the recommended daily dose, for general sale with no restrictions. In the United States, 13 deaths have been linked to excessive use of the 5-hour Energy drink.

            In England a record 114,920 adults receive specialist alcohol treatment, though less than 40 percent complete treatment free of dependency.

2014   Approximately 3 billion pounds of chocolate are consumed globally.

            In Arizona, California, New York, Virginia, and Washington, the purchase of non-prescription cough medicine containing dextromethorphan (DXM) is restricted to those 18 or older.

            CVS pharmacies in the United States stop selling tobacco products.

            In the United States, more than 10,000 toddlers receive medication for attention-deficit/hyperactivity disorder (ADHD) outside established medical diagnostic guidelines.

            Police in China arrest 60,500 suspects on drug offences and seize more than 11 metric tons of narcotics during a single operation in October. More than 180,000 drug users had been punished by mid-December, including 55,000 who were sent to government-run rehabilitation centres.

2015   Uruguay legalizes cannabis sales to those over 18 years of age. Regulations stipulate that THC content cannot exceed 15 percent. The government oversees the entire supply chain, from growth to sale.

            Dr. David Nutt, former drug czar of the United Kingdom, develops Alcosynth, a supposed non-toxic and non-addictive liquid benzodiazepine that mimics alcohol's effects without producing a hangover.

2030   The World Health Organization reports that an estimated 10 million people will die in 2030 from smoking-related causes, up from 4 million in 2000, the majority in developing nations.

SOURCES FOR APPENDIX A
AND APPENDIX B

Abramson (1995); Addiction Foundation of Manitoba (2013); Addiction Research Foundation (1996); Albert, Boyle, & Ponee (1984); Alberta Alcohol and Drug Abuse Commission (2000); Alcoholics Anonymous (2001); Ames (1989); Ashton (2006); Berridge & Edwards (1981); Black (1988); Brecher (1972); Bureau of National Affairs (1987); Canadian Centre on Substance Abuse (2008); Canadian Press (2001–2014); Chappel & Dupont (1999); Crawshaw (1978); Cunningham (1996); Currie (2003); Davenport-Hines (2001); Dyck & Bradford (2012); El-Seedi, De Smet, Beck, Possnert, & Bruhn (2005); European Monitoring Centre for Drugs and Drug Addiction (2008); Fernandez, Begley, & Marlatt (2006); Fishbein & Pease (1996); Fleming (1975); Foundation for a Drug Free World (2008); Fulton (1978); Giffen, Endicott, & Boorman (1991); Graner (1988); Gray (1995); Hart (1977); Hazelden (2001); Heath (1989); Hector (2001); Henningfield & Ator (1986); Hollister (1972); Inglis (1975); International Narcotics Control Board (2009); Jaffe & Jaffe (1989); Jones & Smith (1973); Karagueuzian, Whitle, Sayre, & Norman (2012); Maxwell (1984); Melinyshyn, Christie, & Shirley (1996); Merlin (2003); Miller & Hunter (1991); Narcotics Anonymous (1987, 2009); National Clearinghouse on Tobacco and Health (1991); Nicosia, Pacula, Kilmer, Lundberg, & Chiesa (2009); Parssinen & Kerner (1980); Peterson, Nisenholz, & Robinson (2003); Ponee (1982); Quinones (1975); Scanlon (1988); Schleichert (1996); Shafey, Eriksen, Ross, & Mackay (2009); Sikorsky (1990); Sinclair (1998); Singer (2006); Sonnenstuhl & Trice (1986); Tice (1992); Timoshenko, Van Truong, & Williams (1996); United Nations Office on Drugs and Crime (2002, 2008, 2009, 2015); Vogt (1989); White (1998); White, Kurtz, & Acker (2001); White, Sanders, & Sanders (2006); Williams, Single, & Mackenzie (1995); World Health Organization (2004); Younger (1991); Zaridze et al. (2009).

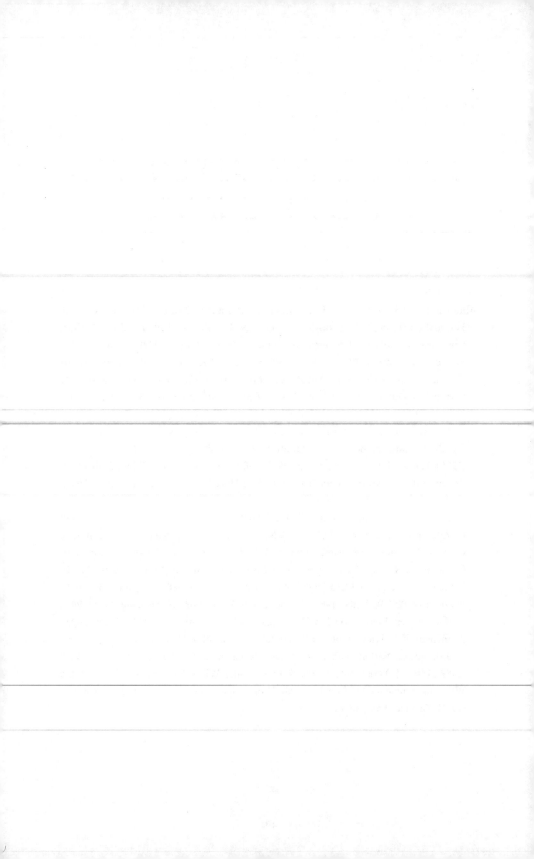

REFERENCES

Abbott, A. (1994). A feminist approach to substance abuse treatment and service delivery. *Social Work in Health Care, 19*(3-4), 67–83.

Abramson, M. (1995). Wine as health elixir. *The Journal, 24*(1), 4.

Acker, C. (2002). *Creating the American junkie: Addiction research in the classic era of narcotic control.* Baltimore, MD: Johns Hopkins University Press.

Adams, R. (1990). *Self-help, social work and empowerment.* London, UK: British Association of Social Workers.

Addiction Foundation of Manitoba. (2013). About AFM. Winnipeg: AFM.

Addiction Research Foundation. (1996). How we rate. *The Journal, 25*(1), 5.

Addiction Studies Institute. (2010). The stages of the Transtheoretical Model of Change. Retrieved from www.utexas.edu/research/cswr/nida/rdpGraphics/rdpConceptArt1.gif

Adoni, H., & Mane, S. (1984). Media and the social construction of reality: Toward an integration of theory and research. *Communication Research, 11*(3), 323–340.

Ahmed, S., & Koob, G. (1997). Cocaine- but not food-seeking behavior is reinstated by stress after extinction. *Psychopharmacology, 132*(3), 289–295.

Ainsworth, M. (1973). The development of infant-mother attachment. In B. Cardwell & H. Ricciuti (Eds.), *Review of child development research* (pp. 1–94). Chicago, IL: University of Chicago Press.

Ainsworth, M. (1991). Attachments and other affectional bonds across the life cycle. In C. Parkes, J. Stevenson-Hinde, & P. Marris (Eds.), *Attachment across the life cycle* (pp. 33–51). London, UK: Routledge.

Ainsworth, M., Blehar, M., Waters, E., & Wall, S. (1978). *Patterns of attachment: A psychological study of the strange situation.* Hillsdale, NJ: Erlbaum.

Alaggia, R., & Csiernik, R. (2010). Coming home: Rediscovering the family in addiction treatment in Canada. In R. Csiernik & W.S. Rowe (Eds.), *Responding to the oppression of addiction: Canadian social work perspectives* (2nd ed.). Toronto, ON: Canadian Scholars' Press.

Albert, W., Boyle, B., & Ponee, C. (1984). *EAP orientation.* Toronto, ON: Addiction Research Foundation.

Alberta Alcohol and Drug Abuse Commission (AADAC). (2000). *Psychiatric drugs.* Edmonton, AB: AADAC.

Alberta Alcohol and Drug Abuse Commission (AADAC). (2001). *Alberta Alcohol and Drug Addiction Commission policy on harm reduction.* Edmonton, AB: AADAC.

Alberta Tobacco Reduction Strategy (ATRS). (2003). *ATRS update.* Edmonton, AB: Alberta Alcohol and Drug Abuse Commission.

Alcoholics Anonymous. (1976). *Alcoholics Anonymous* (3rd ed.). New York: AA World Services.

Alcoholics Anonymous. (2001). *The history of recovery.* New York: AA World Services.

Aldington, S., Harwood, M., Cox, B., Weatherall, M., Beckert, L., Hansell, A., ... Beasely, R. (2008). Cannabis use and risk of lung cancer: A case–control study. *European Respiratory Journal, 31*(2), 280–286.

Aldington, S., Williams, M., Nowitz, M., Weatherall, M., Pritchard, A., McNaughton, A., ... Beasley, R. (2007). The effects of cannabis on pulmonary structure, functions and symptoms. *Thorax, 62*(12), 1058–1063.

Alexander, B. (1985). Drug use, dependence, and addiction at a British Columbia university: Good news and bad news. *Canadian Journal of Higher Education, 15*(1), 77–91.

Alexander, B. (1988). The disease and adaptive models of addiction: A framework evaluation. In S. Peele (Ed.), *Visions of addiction: Major contemporary perspectives on addictions and alcoholism.* Lantham, MD: Lexington Books.

Alexander, B., Beyerstein, B., Hadaway, P., & Coambs, R. (1981). Effects of early and later colony housing on oral ingestion of morphine in rats. *Psychopharmacology Biochemistry and Behavior, 58*(2), 175–179.

Alexander, C., Robinson, P., & Rainforth, M. (1994). Treating alcohol, nicotine and drug abuse through transcendental meditation: A review and statistical meta-analysis. *Alcoholism Treatment Quarterly, 11*(1-2), 11–84.

Alexander, M., & Stockton, G. (2000). Methylphenidate abuse and psychiatric side effects. *Journal of Clinical Psychiatry, 2*(5), 159–164.

Allott, R., Paxton, R., & Leonard, R. (1999). Drug education: A review of British government policy and evidence on effectiveness. *Health Education Research Theory & Practice, 14*(4), 491–505.

Alper, K., Lotsof, H., Frenken, M., Luciano, D., & Bastiaans, J. (1999). Treatment of acute opioid withdrawal with ibogaine. *The American Journal on Addictions, 8*(3), 234–242.

Alper, K., Lotsof, H., & Kaplan, C. (2008). The ibogaine medical subculture. *Journal of Ethnopharmacology, 115*(1), 9–24.

Alwyn, T., John, B., Hodgson, R., & Phillips, C. (2004). The addition of a psychological intervention to a home detoxification programme. *Alcohol & Alcoholism, 39*(6), 536–541.

American Association for the Advancement of Science (AAAS). (2000). Proceedings of the American Association for the Advancement of Science Annual Meeting, "Science in an Uncertain Millennium," February 17–22. Washington, DC: AAAS.

American Cancer Society. (2009). *Deadly in pink: Big tobacco steps up its targeting of women and girls.* Princeton, NJ: Robert Wood Johnson Foundation.

American Council for Drug Education. (1997). *Cocaine and crack.* New York: American Association for the Advancement of Science, American Council for Drug Education.

American Psychiatric Association. (2000). *Diagnostic and statistical manual of mental disorders* (4th ed.). Washington, DC: American Psychiatric Publishing.

American Psychiatric Association. (2013). *Diagnostic and statistical manual of mental disorders* (5th ed.). Washington, DC: American Psychiatric Publishing.

American Society of Addiction Medicine. (2011). *Definition of addiction*. Retrieved from www.asam.org/for-the-public/definition-of-addiction

Ames, G. (1989). Alcohol-related movements and their effects on drinking policies in the American workplace: An historical review. *The Journal of Drug Issues, 19*(4), 489–510.

Ames, G., Duke, M., Moore, R., & Cunradi, C. (2009). The impact of occupational culture on drinking behavior of young adults in the U.S. Navy. *Journal of Mixed Methods Research, 3*(2), 129–150.

Amos, C., Pinney, S., Li, Y., Kupert, E., Lee, J., de Andrade, M., … Anderson, M. (2010). A susceptibility locus on chromosome 6q greatly increases lung cancer risk among light and never smokers. *Cancer Research, 70*(6), 2359–2367.

Anderson, G., & Brown, R. (1984). Real and laboratory gambling, sensation seeking and arousal: Toward a Pavlovian component in general theories of gambling and gambling addictions. *British Journal of Psychology, 75*(3), 401–411.

Anderson, P. (2006). Global use of alcohol, drugs and tobacco. *Drug and Alcohol Review, 25*(6), 489–502.

Andrews, P., Thomson, J., Jr., Amstadter, A., & Neale, M. (2012). *Primum non nocere*: An evolutionary analysis of whether antidepressants do more harm than good. *Frontiers in Psychology, 3*(117). doi:10.3389/fpsyg.2012.00117

Angell, M. (2008). Industry-sponsored clinical research: A broken system. *Journal of the American Medical Association, 300*(9), 1069–1071.

Angst, M., Lazzeroni, L., Nicholas, P., Drover, D., Tingle, M., Ray, A., … Clark, J. (2012). Aversive and reinforcing opioid effects: A pharmacogenomic twin study. *Anesthesiology, 117*(1), 22–37.

Annis, H. (1984). Is inpatient rehabilitation of the alcoholic cost effective? Con position. *Advances in Alcohol and Substance Abuse, 5*(1-2), 175–190.

Antnowicz, J., Metzger, A., & Ramanujam, S. (2011). Paranoid psychosis induced by consumption of methylenedioxypyrovalerone: Two cases. *General Hospital Psychiatry, 33*(6). doi:640.e5-640.e6.

Anton, R. (1994). Medications for treating alcoholism. *Alcohol, Health and Research World, 18*(4), 265–271.

Anton, R. (1999). What is a craving? Models and implications for treatment (alcohol craving). *Alcohol Research & Health, 23*(3), 165–173.

Arendt, M., Mortensen, P., Rosenberg, R., Pedersen, C., & Waltoft, B. (2008). Familial predisposition for psychiatric disorder: Comparison of subjects treated for cannabis-induced psychosis and schizophrenia. *Achieves of General Psychiatry, 65*(11), 1269–1274.

Arminen, I., & Halonen, M. (2007). Laughing with and at patients: The roles of laughter in confrontations in addiction group therapy. *Qualitative Report, 12*(3), 484–513.

Armor, D., Polich, J., & Stambul, H. (1978). *Alcoholism and treatment*. New York: Wiley.

Asay, T., & Lambert, M. (1999). The empirical case for the common factors in therapy: Quantitative findings. In M. Hubble, B. Duncan, & S. Miller (Eds.), *The heart and soul of change: What works in therapy*. Washington, DC: American Psychological Association.

Asbridge, M., Hayden, J., & Cartwright, J. (2012). Acute cannabis consumption and motor vehicle collision risk: Systematic review of observational studies and meta-analysis. *British Journal of Medicine, 344*, e536. doi:10.1136/bmj.e536

Ashton, H. (2002). The benzodiazepines: What they do in the body. *Benzodiazepines: How they work and how to withdraw* (Chapter 1). Retrieved from www.benzo.org.uk/manual/bzcha01.htm

Ashton, H. (2005). The diagnosis and management of benzodiazepine dependence. *Current Opinions in Psychiatry, 18*(2), 249–255.

Ashton, H. (2013). *Benzodiazepines: How they work and how to withdraw: The Ashton Manual supplement*. Retrieved from www.benzo.org.uk/ashsupp11.htm

Ashton, M. (2006). The Rolleston legacy. *Drug and Alcohol Findings, 15*(1), 4–5.

Aubin, H., Farley, A., Lycett, D., Lahmek. P., & Aveyard, P. (2012). Weight gain in smokers after quitting cigarettes: Meta-analysis. *British Medical Journal, 345*, e4439. doi:10.1136/bmj.e4439

Avants, B., Hurt, H., Giannetta, J., Epstein, C., Shera, D., Rao, H., … Gee, J. (2007). Effects of heavy in utero cocaine exposure on adolescent caudate morphology. *Pediatric Neurology, 27*(4), 275–279.

Azodi, O., Orsini, N., Andrén-Sandberg, Å., & Wolk, A. (2011). Effect of type of alcoholic beverage in causing acute pancreatitis. *British Journal of Surgery, 98*(11), 1609–1616.

Azrin, N. (1976). Improvements in the community-reinforcement approach to alcoholism. *Behavioiur Research and Therapy, 14*(4), 339–348.

Babor, T., Caetano, R., Casswell, S., Edwards, G., Giesbrecht, N., Graham, K., … Rossow, I. (2003) *Alcohol: No ordinary commodity—research and public policy*. London, UK: Oxford University Press.

Babor, T., & Del Boca, F. (2002). *Treatment matching in alcoholism*. Rockville, MD: National Institute on Alcohol Abuse and Alcoholism.

Babor, T., Higgins-Biddle, J., Saunders, J., & Monterra, M. (2001). AUDIT—the alcohol use disorders identification test: Guidelines for use in primary care. New York: World Health Organization.

Back, S., Gentilin, S., & Brady, K. (2007). Cognitive-behavioral stress management for individuals with substance use disorders: A pilot study. *The Journal of Nervous and Mental Disease, 195*(8), 662–668.

Bahr, S., & Hoffmann, J. (2010). Parenting style, religiosity, peers, and adolescent heavy drinking. *Journal of Studies on Alcohol and Drugs, 71*(4), 539–543.

Bahr, S., Hoffmann, J., & Yang, X. (2005). Parental and peer influences on the risk of adolescent drug use. *The Journal of Primary Prevention, 26*(6), 529–551.

Baker, P. (2006). Developing a blueprint for evidence-based drug prevention in England. *Drugs: Education, Prevention and Policy, 13*(1), 17–32.

Bales, R. (1946). Cultural differences in rates of alcoholism. *Quarterly Journal of Studies on Alcohol, 35*, 1242–1255.

Balfour, D. (2004). The neurobiology of tobacco dependence: A preclinical perspective on the role of the dopamine projections to the nucleus accumbens. *Nicotine and Tobacco Research, 6*(6), 899–912.

Bandura, A. (1986). *Social foundations of thought and action.* Englewood Cliffs, NJ: Prentice Hall.

Barnes, G. (1979). The alcoholic personality. *Journal of Studies on Alcohol, 40*(7), 571–634.

Barnes, K. (2009). *Drug treatment courts: Basic principles.* Presented at the Canadian Criminal Justice Association Conference, Halifax, Nova Scotia, October 28–31. Retrieved from www.ccja-acjp.ca/cong2009/kofi-barnes.ppt

Barnett, J. (2009). An examination of Western Missouri Correctional Center's therapeutic community. *Journal of Groups in Addiction and Recovery, 4*(1-2), 245–264.

Barnoya, J., & Glantz, S. (2005). Cardiovascular effects of second hand smoke nearly as large as smoking. *Circulation, 111*(20), 2684–2698.

Barr, M.S., Farzan, F., Wing, V.C., George, T.P., Fitzgerald, P.B., & Daskalakis, Z.J. (2011). Repetitive transcranial magnetic stimulation and drug addiction. *International Review of Pyschiatry, 23*(5), 454–466

Barry, H., III. (1988). Psychoanalytic theory of alcoholism. In C. Chaudron & D. Wilkinson (Eds.), *Theories on addiction.* Toronto, ON: Addiction Research Foundation.

Bassin, A. (1975). Different strokes for different folks: A defence of confrontation tactics in psychotherapy. *The Counseling Psychologist, 5*(3), 128–130.

Bauman, K., Ennett, S., Foshee, V., Pemberton, M., King, T., & Koch, G. (2000). Influence of a family-directed program on adolescent cigarette and alcohol cessation. *Prevention Science, 1*(4), 227–237.

Baumann, M., Wang, X., & Rothman, R. (2007). 3,4-Methylenedioxymethamphetamine (MDMA) neurotoxicity in rats: A reappraisal of past and present findings. *Psychopharmacology, 189*(4), 407–424.

Becker, A., Dörter, F., Eckhardt, K., Viniol, A., Baum, E., Kochen, M. … Donner-Banzhoff, N. (2011). The association between a journal's source of revenue and the drug recommendations made in the articles it publishes. *Canadian Medical Journal, 183*(5), 544–548.

Becker, D., Hogue, A. & Liddle, H. (2002). Methods of engagement in family-based preventive intervention. *Child and Adolescent Social Work Journal, 19*(2), 163–179.

Becker, H. (1963). *Outsiders: Studies in the sociology of deviance.* New York: Free Press.

Beier, J., Artel, G., & McClain, C. (2011). Advances in alcoholic liver disease. *Current Gastroenterology Reports, 13*(1), 56–64.

Beirness, D., & Beasley, E. (2009). *Alcohol and drug use among drivers: British Columbia roadside survey 2008.* Ottawa, ON: Canadian Centre on Substance Abuse.

Bennett G., Withers, J., Thomas, P., Higgins, D., Bailey, J., Parry, L., & Davies, E. (2005). A randomised trial of early warning signs relapse prevention training in the treatment of alcohol dependence. *Addictive Behaviors, 30*(6), 1111–1124.

Bennett, T., Holloway, K., & Farrington, D. (2008). The statistical association between drug misuse and crime: A meta-analysis. *Aggression and Violent Behavior: A Review Journal, 13*(2), 107–118.

Benson, A., & Eisenach, D. (2013). Stopping overshopping: An approach to the treatment of compulsive-buying disorder. *Journal of Groups in Addiction & Recovery, 8*(1), 3–24.

Bepko, C. (1991). *Feminism and addiction.* New York: Haworth Press.

Berg, B., Pettinati, H., & Volpicelli, B. (1996). A risk-benefit assessment of naltrexone in the treatment of alcohol dependence. *Drug Safety, 15*(4), 274–282.

Berg, I., & Miller, S. (1992). *Working with the problem drinker: A solution-oriented approach.* New York: Norton.

Berghmans, R., de Jong, J., Tibben, A., & de Wert, G. (2009). On the biomedicalization of alcoholism. *Theoretical Medicine and Bioethics, 30*(4), 311–321.

Bergler, E. (1958). *The psychology of gambling.* New York: Hill and Wang.

Berrettini, W., & Lerman, C. (2005). Pharmacotherapy and pharmacogenetics of nicotine dependence. *American Journal of Psychiatry, 162*(8), 1441–1451.

Berridge, V., & Edwards, G. (1981). *Opium and the people: Opiate use in nineteenth-century England.* New York: St. Martin's Press.

Bertol, E., Fineschi, V., Karch, S., Mari, F., & Riezzo, I. (2004). *Nymphaea* cults in ancient Egypt and the New World: A lesson in empirical pharmacology. *Journal of the Royal Society of Medicine, 97*(2), 84–85.

Beutler, L., Harwood, T., Kimpara, S., Verdirame, D., & Blau, K. (2011). Adapting psychotherapy to the individual patient: Coping style. *Journal of Clinical Psychology, 67*(2), 176–183.

Bewick, B., Trusler, K., Barkham, M., Hill, A., Cahill, J., & Mulhern, B. (2008). The effectiveness of Web-based interventions designed to decrease alcohol consumption: A systematic review. *Preventive Medicine, 47*(1), 17–26.

Bickel, A. (1995). *Family involvement: Strategies for comprehensive alcohol, tobacco, and other drug use prevention programs.* Portland, OR: Northwest Regional Education Laboratory.

Bien, T., Miller, W., & Tonigan, J. (1993). Brief interventions for alcohol problems: A review. *Addiction, 88*(3), 315–336.

Bierut, L. (2011). Genetic vulnerability and susceptibility to substance dependence. *Neuron, 69*(4), 618–627.

Biglan, A., & Metzler, C. (1998). A public health perspective for research on family-focused interventions. In R. Ashery, E. Robertson, & K. Kumpfer (Eds.), *Drug abuse prevention through family interventions.* Rockville, MD: United States Department of Health and Human Services.

Bischof, G., Richmond, C., & Case, A. (2003). Detoxification at home: A brief solution-oriented family system approach. *Contemporary Family Therapy: An International Journal, 25*(1), 17–39.

Black, K. (1988). *Report of the Task Force on Illegal Drug Use in Ontario.* Toronto, ON: Province of Ontario.

Blackwell, T. (2011, November 12). The selling of OxyContin. *National Post.* Retrieved from http://news.nationalpost.com/2011/11/12/the-selling-of-oxycontin/

Blake, S., Amaro, H., Schwartz, P., & Flinchbaugh, L. (2001). A review of substance abuse prevention interventions for young adolescent girls. *Journal of Early Adolescence, 21*(3), 294–324.

Blankers, M., Koeter, M., & Scippers, G. (2011). Internet therapy versus Internet self-help versus no treatment for problematic alcohol use: A randomized controlled trial. *Journal of Consulting and Clinical Psychology, 79*(3), 330–341.

Blaszczynski, A. (2010). *Overcoming compulsive gambling.* London, UK: Constable and Robinson.

Blaszczynski, A., & Nower, L. (2002). A pathways model of problem and pathological gambling. *Addiction, 97*(5), 487–499.

Blaszczynski, A., Winter, S., & McConaghy, N. (1986). Plasma endorphin levels in pathological gamblers. *Journal of Gambling Behavior, 2*(1), 3–14.

Blednov, Y., Cravatt, B., Boehm, S., II, Walker, D., & Harris, R. (2007). Role of endocannabinoids in alcohol consumption and intoxication: Studies of mice lacking fatty acid amide hydrolase. *Neuropsychopharmacology, 32*(7), 1570–1582.

Boak, A., Hamilton, H., Adlaf, E., & Mann, R. (2013). *Drug use among Ontario students: 1977-2013.* Toronto, ON: Centre for Addiction and Mental Health.

Boffetta, P., & Straif, K. (2009). Use of smokeless tobacco and risk of myocardial infarction and stroke: Systematic review and meta-analysis. *British Medical Journal, 339,* b3060. doi:http://dx.doi.org/10.1136/bmj.b3060

Bolla, K., McCann U., & Ricaurte, G. (1998). Memory impairment in abstinent MDMA users. *Neurology, 51*(6), 1532–1557

Bonaparte, M., Freud, A., & Kris, E. (1954). *The origins of psychoanalysis.* New York: Harper Collins.

Borchers, M., Wesselkamper, C., Curull, V., Ramirez-Sarmiento, A., Sánchez-Font, A., Garcia-Aymerich, J., ... Orozco-Levi, M. (2009). Sustained CTL activation by murine pulmonary epithelial cells promotes the development of COPD-like disease. *The Journal of Clinical Investigation, 119*(3), 636–649.

Bornovalova, M., & Daughters, S. (2007). How does dialectical behavior therapy facilitate treatment retention among individuals with comorbid borderline personality disorder and substance use disorders? *Clinical Psychology Review, 27*(8), 923–943.

Bosworth, K. (1998). Assessment of drug abuse prevention curricula developed at the local level. *Journal of Drug Education, 28*(4), 307–325.

Botvin, G. (1990). Substance abuse prevention: Theory, practice and effectiveness. *Crime and Justice, 13,* 461–519.

Botvin, G. (2000). Preventing drug abuse in schools: Social and competence enhancement approaches targeting individual-level etiologic factors. *Addictive Behaviors, 25*(6), 887–897.

Botvin, G., & Griffin, K. (2004). Life skills training: Empirical findings and future directions. *The Journal of Primary Prevention, 25*(2), 211–232.

Boudreau, R. (1997). Addiction and the family. In S. Harrison & V. Carver (Eds.), *Alcohol and drug problems: A practical guide for counsellors* (2nd ed.). Toronto, ON: Addiction Research Foundation.

Bourgeois, F., Kim, J., & Mandl, K. (2014). Premarket safety and efficacy studies for ADHD medications in children. *PLoS ONE, 9*(7), e102249. doi:10.1371/journal.pone.0102249

Bowen, S. (2011). Two serious and challenging medical complications associated with volatile substance misuse: Sudden sniffing death and fetal solvent syndrome. *Substance Use & Misuse, 46*(S1), 68–72.

Bowen, S., Witkiewitz, K., Dillworth, T., Chawla, N., Simpson, T., Ostafin, B., ... Marlatt, G. (2006). Mindfulness meditation and substance use in an incarcerated population. *Psychology of Addictive Behaviors, 20*(3), 343–347.

Bowlby, J. (1958). The nature of the child's tie to his mother. *International Journal of Psychoanalysis, 39*(4), 350–371.

Bowlby, J. (1969). *Attachment: Attachment and loss* (Vol. 1). New York: Basic Books.

Boyatzis, R. (2008). Competencies in the 21st century. *Journal of Management Development, 27*(1), 5–12.

Boyd, N. (1983). The dilemma of Canadian narcotics legislation: The social control of altered states of consciousness. *Contemporary Crises, 7*(3), 257–269.

Boyd, S., Fang, L., Medoff, D., Dixon, L., & Gorelick, D. (2012). Use of a "microecological technique" to study crime incidents around methadone maintenance treatment centers. *Addiction, 107*(9), 1632–1638.

Bozarth, M., Murray, A., & Wise, R. (1989). Influence of housing conditions on the acquisition of intravenous heroin and cocaine self-administration in rats. *Pharmacology, Biochemistry, and Behavior, 33*(4), 903–907.

Brache, K., & Stockwell, T. (2011). Drinking patterns and risk behaviors associated with combined alcohol and energy drink consumption. *Addictive Behaviors, 36*(12), 1133–1140.

Brandon, T., Vidrine, J., & Litvin, E. (2007). Relapse and relapse prevention. *Annual Review of Clinical Psychology, 3*, 257–284.

Brault, M., & Lacourse, E. (2012). Prevalence of prescribed attention-deficit hyperactivity disorder medications and diagnoses among Canadian preschoolers and school-aged children: 1994–2007. *Canadian Journal of Psychiatry, 57*(2), 93–101.

Brautigam, E. (1977). Effects of the transcendental meditation program on drug abusers: A prospective study. In D. Orme-Johnson & J. Farrow (Eds.), *Scientific research on the transcendental meditation program: Collected papers.* New York: M.E.R.U. Press.

Brecher, E. (1972). *Licit and illicit drugs.* Toronto, ON: Little Brown and Company.

Breeding, J., & Baughman, F. (2003). Informed consent and the psychiatric drugging of children. *Journal of Humanistic Psychology, 43*(1), 50–64.

Brennan, R., & Van Hout, M. (2014). Gamma-Hydroxybutyrate (GHB): A scoping review of pharmacology, toxicology, motives for use, and user groups. *Journal of Psychoactive Drugs, 46*(3), 243–251.

Briones, A., Cumsille, F., Henao, A., & Pardo, B. (2013). *The drug problem in the Americas.* Washington, DC: Organization of American States.

British Columbia Ministry of Children and Family Services. (1996). *The workbook on prevention concepts.* Retrieved from www.preventionsource.bc.ca/psbc/guides/workbook/index.html

Britt, E., Hudson, S., & Blampied, N. (2004). Motivational interviewing in health settings: A review. *Patient Education and Counseling, 53*(2), 147–155.

Brooks, J. (2006). Strengthening resilience in children and youths: Maximizing opportunities through the schools. *Children & Schools, 28*(2), 69–76.

Brounstein, P., & Zweig, J. (1999). *Understanding substance abuse prevention—Towards the 21st century: A primer on effective programs.* Rockville, MD: Substance Abuse and Mental Health Administration.

Brown, J. (2001). Youth, drugs and resilience education. *Journal of Drug Education, 31*(1), 83–122.

Brownsberger, W. (2000). Race matters: Disproportionality of incarceration for drug dealings in Massachusetts. *Journal of Drug Issues, 30*(2), 345–374.

Brunette, M., Drake, R., Woods, M., & Harnett, T. (2001). A comparison of long-term and short-term residential treatment programs for dual diagnosis patients. *Psychiatric Services, 52*(4), 526–528.

Bruun, K., Edwards, G., Lummio, M., Makela, K., Pan, L., Popham, R., ... Osterberg, E. (1975). *Alcohol control policies in public health perspective.* Helsinki, FN: Finish Foundation for Alcohol Studies.

Bry, B., Catalano, R., Kumpfer, K., Lochman, J., & Szapocznik, J. (1998). Scientific findings from family prevention intervention research. In R. Ashery, E. Robertson, & K. Kumpfer (Eds.), *Drug abuse prevention through family interventions* (pp. 103–129). Rockville, MD: United States Department of Health and Human Services.

Buchman, D., Illes, J., & Reine, B. (2010). The paradox of addiction neuroscience. *Neuroethics, 4*(1), 65–77.

Buino, S., & Simon, S. (2011). Music interventions in group work with chemically dependent populations. *Social Work with Groups, 34*(3-4), 283–295.

Bunt, G., Muehlbach, B., & Moed, C. (2008). The therapeutic community: An international perspective. *Substance Abuse, 29*(3), 81–87.

Bureau of National Affairs. (1987). *Employee Assistance Programs: Benefits, problems and prospects.* Special Report. Washington, DC: Bureau of National Affairs.

Burnside, L., & Fuchs, D. (2013). Bound by the clock: The experiences of youth with FASD transitioning to adulthood from child welfare care. *First Peoples Child & Family Review, 8*(1), 40–61.

Buscemi, L., & Turchi, C. (2011). An overview of the genetic susceptibility to alcoholism. *Medicine, Science and the Law, 51*(4), S2–S6.

Cade, B., & O'Hanlon, W. (1993). *A brief guide to brief therapy.* New York: Norton.

Cadet, J., Bisagno, V., & Milroy, C. (2014). Neuropathology of substance use disorders. *Acta Neuropathology, 127*(1), 91–107.

Cakic, V., Potkonyak, J., & Marshall, A. (2010). Dimethyltryptamine (DMT): Subjective effects and patterns of use among Australian recreational users. *Drug and Alcohol Dependence, 111*(1), 30–37.

California Department of Health Services. (2005). New data show California military, Korean men and LGBT populations smoke much more than others in the state. Retrieved from www.applications.dhs.ca.gov/pressreleases/store/pressreleases/05-60.html

Callahan, J., & Swift, J. (2009). The impact of client treatment preferences on outcome: A meta-analysis. *Journal of Clinical Psychology, 65*(4), 368–381.

Callahan-Lyon, C. (2014). Electronic cigarettes: Human health effects. *Tobacco Control, 23*(S2), ii36–ii40.

Callow, T., Donaldson, S., & De Ruiter, M. (2008). Effectiveness of home detoxification: A clinical audit. *British Journal of Nursing, 17*(11), 692–695.

Cameron, K., Kolanos, R., Solis, E., Jr., Glennon, R., & Felice, L. (2013). Bath salts components mephedrone and methylenedioxypyrovalerone (MDPV) act synergistically at the human dopamine transporter. *British Journal of Pharmacology, 168*(7), 1750–1757.

Cameron, K., Kolanos, R., Verkariva, R., Felice, L., & Glennon, R. (2013). Mephedrone and methylenedioxypyrovalerone (MDPV), major constituents of "bath salts," produce opposite effects at the human dopamine transporter. *Psychopharmacology, 227*(3), 493–499.

Campbell, A., Nunes, E., Matthews, A., Stitzer, M., Miele, G., Polsky, D., … Ghitza, U. (2014). Internet-delivered treatment for substance abuse: A multisite randomized control trial. *American Journal of Psychiatry, 171*(6), 683–690.

Campbell, C., Hahn, R., Elder, R., Brewer, R., Chattopadhyay, S., Fielding, J., … Middleton, J. (2009). The effectiveness of limiting alcohol outlet density as a means of reducing excessive alcohol consumption and alcohol-related harms. *American Journal of Preventive Medicine, 37*(6), 556–569.

Canadian Addiction Counsellors Certification Federation. (2010). *Canon of ethical principles.* Retrieved from www.caccf.ca/images/pdf/CACCF_Ethics_Eng_Fre.pdf

Canadian Association of Drug Treatment Professionals (CADTP). (n.d.). *DTC program.* Retrieved from www.cadtc.org/DTCProgram.aspx

Canadian Centre on Substance Abuse. (2005). *Methamphetamine fact sheet.* Ottawa, ON: Canadian Centre on Substance Abuse.

Canadian Centre on Substance Abuse. (2006). *Youth volatile solvent abuse.* Ottawa, ON: Canadian Centre on Substance Abuse.

Canadian Centre on Substance Abuse. (2007). *Core competencies for Canada's substance abuse field (version 1).* Ottawa, ON: CCSA.

Canadian Centre on Substance Abuse. (2008). *Common ground.* Ottawa, ON: Canadian Centre on Substance Abuse.

Canadian Centre on Substance Abuse. (2010a). *Stronger together: Canadian standards for community-based youth substance abuse prevention.* Ottawa, ON: Canadian Centre on Substance Abuse.

Canadian Centre on Substance Abuse. (2010b). *Competencies for Canada's substance abuse workforce.* Ottawa, ON: Canadian Centre on Substance Abuse.

Canadian Centre on Substance Abuse. (2014a). *National treatment indicators report.* Ottawa, ON: Canadian Centre on Substance Abuse. Retrieve from www.academia.edu/6537731/National_Treatment_Indicators_Report_2011-2012_Data

Canadian Centre on Substance Abuse. (2014b). *Competencies for Canada's Substance Abuse Workforce.* Ottawa, ON: Canadian Centre on Substance Abuse.

Canadian Medical Association. (2015). *New "Marihuana for Medical Purposes Regulations": What do doctors need to know?* Retrieved from www.cma.ca/En/Pages/medical-marijuana.aspx

Canadian Press. (2001–2014). *The Canadian Press News Service.* Toronto, ON: Canadian Press Enterprises, Inc.

Canadian Society of Addiction Medicine. (2008). *Definition of addiction.* Retrieved from www.csam-smca.org/about/policy-statements/

Carlson, B., & Larkin, H. (2009). Meditation as a coping intervention for treatment of addiction. *Journal of Religion & Spirituality in Social Work: Social Thought, 28*(4), 379–392.

Carlton, P., & Goldstein, L. (1987). Physiological determinants of pathological gambling. In T. Galski (Ed.), *A handbook of pathological gambling* (pp. 111–122). Springfield, IL: Charles C. Thomas.

Carnes, P. (1996). Addiction or compulsion: Politics or illness? *Sexual Addiction and Compulsivity: The Journal of Treatment and Prevention, 3*(2), 127–150.

Carr, A. (1998). Michael White's narrative therapy. *Contemporary Family Therapy, 20*(4), 485–503.

Carroll, K. (1996). Relapse prevention as a psychosocial treatment: A review of controlled clinical trials. *Experimental and Clinical Psychopharmacology, 4*(1), 46–54.

Carroll, K., & Onken, L. (2005). Behavioral therapies for drug abuse. *American Journal of Psychiatry, 162*(8), 1452–1460.

Carroll, M. (1985). *PCP: The dangerous angel.* New York: Chelsea House Publishers.

Carroll, M. (1990). PCP and hallucinogens. *Advances in Alcohol and Substance Abuse, 9*(1-2), 167–190.

Carroll, M., & Gallo, G. (1985). *Quaaludes.* New York: Chelsea House Publishers.

Carter, W., & Barker, R. (2011). Does completion of juvenile drug court deter adult criminality? *Journal of Social Work Practice in the Addictions, 11*(2), 181–193.

Carvalho, F. (2003). The toxicological potential of khat. *Journal of Ethnopharmacology, 87*(1), 1–2.

Case, S., & Haines, K. (2003). Promoting prevention: Preventing youth drug use in Swansea, UK, by targeting risk and protective factors. *Journal of Substance Use, 8*(4), 243–251.

Cassin, S., & von Ranson, K. (2007). Is binge eating experienced as an addiction? *Appetite, 49*(3), 687–690.

Catalano, R., Berglund, M., Ryan, J., Lonczak, H., & Hawkins, J. (2004). Positive youth development in the United States: Research findings on evaluations of positive youth development programs. *The Annals of the American Academy of Political Science, 591*(1), 98–124.

Catalano, R., Hawkins, J., Krenz, C., Gillmore, M., Morrison, D., Wells, E., & Abbott, R. (1993). Using research to guide culturally appropriate drug abuse prevention. *Journal of Consulting and Clinical Psychology, 61*(5), 804–811.

Caulkins, J., Pacula, R., Paddock, S., & Chiesa, J. (2002). *School-based drug prevention: What kind of drug use does it prevent?* Santa Monica, CA: RAND.

Center on Alcohol Marketing and Youth. (2012). *Youth exposure to alcohol advertising on television, 2001-2009.* Baltimore, MD: Johns Hopkins University.

Centre for Addiction and Mental Health (CAMH). (2001). *Ecstasy: Do you know....* Toronto, ON: CAMH.

Centre for Addiction and Mental Health (CAMH). (1999). *Addiction and drug prevention programs for youth: What works?* Toronto, ON: CAMH.

Chaloupka, F., Grossman, M., & Saffer, H. (2002). *The effects of price on alcohol consumption and alcohol-related problems.* Bethesda, MD: National Institute on Alcohol Abuse and Alcoholism.

Chambers, R., Sajdyk, T., Conroy, S., Lafuze, J., Fitz, S., & Shekhar, A. (2007). Neonatal amygdala lesions: Co-occurring impact on social/fear-related behavior and cocaine sensitization in adult rats. *Behavioral Neuroscience, 121*(6), 1316–1327.

Chandler, L. (2003). Ethanol and brain plasticity: Receptors and molecular networks of the postsynaptic density as targets of ethanol. *Pharmacology & Therapeutics, 99*(3), 311–326.

Chappel, J., & DuPont, R. (1999). Twelve-step and mutual-help programs for addictive disorders. *The Psychiatric Clinics of North America, 22*(2), 425–446.

Chaudron, C., & Wilkinson, D. (1988). *Theories on addiction.* Toronto, ON: Addiction Research Foundation.

Chen, H., Huang, X., Guo, X., Mailman, R., Park, Y., Kamel, F., ... Blair, A. (2010). Smoking duration, intensity, and risk of Parkinson disease. *Neurology, 74*(11), 878–884.

Chen, Y., Dales, R., & Lin, M. (2003). The epidemiology of chronic rhinosinusitis in Canadians. *The Laryngoscope, 113*(7), 1199–1205.

Chenier, N. (2001). *Substance abuse and public policy.* Ottawa, ON: Government of Canada.

Cho, S., & Wang, W. (2009). Acupuncture for alcohol dependence: A systematic review. *Alcoholism: Clinical and Experimental, 33*(8), 305–1313.

Christensen, M., & Kohlmeier, K. (2014). Age-related changes in functional postsynaptic nicotinic acetylcholine receptor subunits in neurons of the laterodorsal tegmental nucleus, a nucleus important in drug addiction. *Addiction Biology.* doi:10.1111/adb.12194

Cianci, R., & Gambrel, P. (2003). Maslow's hierarchy of needs: Does it apply in a collectivist culture? *Journal of Applied Management and Entrepreneurship, 8*(2), 143–161.

Clark, C. (1995). Alcoholics Anonymous: Common misconceptions. *American Psychological Association Addiction Newsletter, 2*(3), 9–22.

Clark, H., Ringwalt, L., Hanley, S., Shablen, S., Flewelling, R., & Hano, M. (2010). Project SUCCESS' effects on the substance use of alternative high school students. *Addictive Behaviors, 35*(3), 209–217.

Clarke, D. (2006). Impulsivity as a mediator in the relationship between depression and problem gambling. *Personality and Individual Differences, 40*(1), 5–15.

Cloninger, C. (1987). Neurogenetic adaptive mechanisms in alcoholism. *Science, 236*(4), 410–416.

Coleman Institute. (2014). *Ultra-rapid detoxification.* Retrieved from www.thecolemaninstitute.com/ultra-rapid-detox

Collin, C. (2006). *Substance abuse issues and public policy in Canada: Canada's federal drug strategy.* Ottawa, ON: Parliamentary Information and Research Service.

Collins, L. (2002). Alcohol and drug addiction in women: Phenomenology and prevention. In M. Ballou & L. Brown (Eds.), *Rethinking mental health and disorder: Feminist perspectives.* New York: Guilford Press.

Collins, S., Clifasefi, S., Dana, E., Andrasik, M., Stahl, N., Kirouac, M., & Malone, D. (2012). Where harm reduction meets housing first: Exploring alcohol's role in a project-based housing first setting. *International Journal of Drug Policy, 23*(2), 111–119.

Colorado Department of Revenue. (2015). *Colorado marijuana tax data.* Retrieved from https://www.colorado.gov/pacific/revenue/colorado-marijuana-tax-data

Comings, D., Rosenthal, R., Lesieur, H., & Rugle, L. (1996). A study of the dopamine D2 receptor gene in pathological gambling. *Pharmacogenetics, 6*(3), 223–234.

Connor, J., Kypri, K., Bell, M., & Cousins, K. (2010). Alcohol outlet density, levels of drinking and alcohol-related harm in New Zealand: A national study. *Journal of Epidemiological and Community Health, 65*(10), 841–846.

Conrad, P. (2007). *The medicalization of society.* Baltimore, MD: Johns Hopkins University Press.

Conrad, P., & Barker, K. (2010). The social construction of illness: Key insights and policy implications. *Journal of Health and Social Behavior, 51*(1), S67–S79.

Cook, C. (1988). The Minnesota model in the management of drug and alcohol dependency: Miracle, method or myth? The philosophy and the programme. *British Journal of Addiction, 83*(6), 625–634.

Copeland, J., Frewen, A., & Elkins, K. (2009). *Management of cannabis use disorder and related issues*. Sydney, NSW: National Cannabis Prevention and Information Centre.

Cornelis, M., & El-Sohemy, A. (2007). Coffee, caffeine, and coronary heart disease. *Current Opinion in Lipidology, 18*(1), 13–19.

Corwin, R., & Grigson, P. (2009). Symposium overview—food addiction: Fact or fiction? *Journal of Nutrition, 139*(3), 617–619.

Cosgrove, L., & Krimsky, S. (2012). A comparison of *DSM*-IV and *DSM*-5 panel members' financial associations with industry: A pernicious problem persists. *PLoS Medicine, 9*(3). doi:10.1371/journal.pmed.1001190

Cosgrove, L., Krimsky, S., Vijayaraghavan, M., & Schneider, L. (2006). Financial ties between DSM-IV panel members and the pharmaceutical industry. *Psychotherapy and Psychosomatics, 75*(2), 154–160.

Cowen, K. (1998). The Prozac versus placebo debate. *Journal of Addictions and Mental Health, 1*(1), 5–12.

Cox, W. (1979). The alcoholic personality. In B. Maher (Ed.), *Progress in experimental personality research* (Vol. 9). New York: Academic Press.

Cox, W. (1988). Personality theory. In C. Chaudron & D. Wilkinson (Eds.), *Theories on addiction* (pp. 143–172). Toronto, ON: Addiction Research Foundation.

Cox, W., & Klinger, E. (1988). A motivational model of alcohol use. *Journal of Abnormal Psychology, 97*(2), 168–180.

Crawshaw, P. (1978). *Historical aspects and current developments: Core knowledge in the drug field*. Ottawa, ON: Health and Welfare Canada.

Crean, R., Crane, N., & Mason, B. (2011). An evidence-based review of acute and long-term effects of cannabis use on executive cognitive functions. *Journal of Addiction Medicine, 5*(1), 1–8.

Crumbaugh, J., & Carr, G. (1979). Treatment of alcoholics with logotherapy. *The International Journal of the Addictions, 14*(6), 847–853.

Cruz, F., Rubio, F., & Hope, B. (2014). Using *c-fos* to study neuronal ensembles in corticostriatal circuitry of addiction. *Brain Research*. doi:10.1016/j.brainres.2014.11.005

Cruz, S. (2011). The latest evidence in the neuroscience of solvent misuse. *Substance Use and Misuse, 46*(1), 62–67.

Csiernik, R. (2002). Determining the value of Alcoholics Anonymous. *Canadian Social Work, 4*(1), 14–22.

Csiernik, R. (2010). Maintaining the continuum of care: Arguing for community based residential addiction programs. R. Csiernik & W. Rowe (Eds.), *Responding to the oppression of addiction: Canadian social work responses* (2nd ed., pp. 113–120). Toronto, ON: Canadian Scholars' Press.

Csiernik, R., & Arundel, M.K. (2013). Does counselling format play a role in client retention? *Journal of Groups in Addiction and Recovery, 8*(4), 262–269.

Csiernik, R., & Rowe, W. (2010). Creating a social work understanding of addiction. In R. Csiernik and W. Rowe (Eds.), *Responding to the oppression of addiction: Canadian social work responses* (2nd ed., pp. 3–16). Toronto, ON: Canadian Scholars' Press.

Csiernik, R., & Troller, J. (2002). Evaluating the effectiveness of a relapse prevention group. *Journal of Social Work Practice in the Addictions, 2*(2), 29–38.

Cuijpers, P. (2002). Effective ingredients of school-based prevention programs: A systematic review. *Addictive Behaviors, 27*(6), 1009–1023.

Cuijpers, P. (2003). Three decades of drug prevention research. *Drugs: Education, Prevention and Policy, 10*(1), 7–20.

Cunningham, P., & Henggeler, S. (2001). Implementation of an empirically based drug and violence prevention and intervention program in public school settings. *Journal of Clinical Child Psychology, 30*(1), 221–232.

Cunningham, R. (1996). *Smoke and mirrors: The Canadian tobacco war.* Ottawa, ON: International Development Research Centre.

Curran, H., & Morgan, C. (2000). Cognitive, dissociative and psychotogenic effects of ketamine in recreational users on the night of drug use and 3 days later. *Addiction, 95*(4), 575–590.

Currie, J. (2003). *Manufacturing addiction: The over-prescription of benzodiazepines and sleeping pills to women in Canada.* Vancouver, BC: British Columbia Centre of Excellence for Women's Health.

Daling, J., Doody, D., Sun, X., Trabert, B., Weiss, N., Chen, C., ... Schwartz, S. (2009). Association of marijuana use and the incidence of testicular germ cell tumors. *Cancer, 115*(6), 1215–1223.

Dallas, M. (2011, November 6). Alcohol, asthma and allergies don't mix. *Health.* Retrieved from http://news.health.com/2011/11/06/alcohol-asthma-and-allergies-dont-mix/

Davenport-Hines, R. (2001). *The pursuit of oblivion: A global history of narcotics.* London, UK: Weidenfeld and Nicholson.

Davies, L., Jones, A., Vamvakas, G., Dubourg, R., & Donmall, M. (2009). *The drug treatment outcomes research study: Cost-effectiveness analysis.* London, UK: Home Office.

Davis, C., & Claridge, G. (1998). The eating disorders as addiction: A psychobiological perspective. *Addictive Behaviors, 23*(4), 463–475.

Davis, S., Huebner, A., Piercy, F., Shettler, L., Meszaros, P., & Matheson, J. (2004). Female adolescent smoking: A depth study on best prevention practices. *Journal of Drug Education, 34*(3), 295–311.

Dawe, S., & Loxton, N. (2004). The role of impulsivity in the development of substance use and eating disorders. *Neuroscience & Biobehavioral Reviews, 28*(3), 343–351.

de Haes, W., & Schuurman, J. (1975). Results of an evaluation study of three drug education methods. *International Journal of Health Education, 28*(4), S1–S16.

De Leon, G. (1988). Legal pressures in therapeutic communities. In C. Leukefeld & F. Tims (Eds.), *Compulsory treatment of drug abuse: Research and clinical practice* (NIDA Research Monograph, No. 86). Rockville, MD: US Department of Health and Human Services.

De Leon, G. (1995). Therapeutic communities for addictions: A theoretical framework. *The International Journal of the Addictions, 30*(12), 1603–1645.

De Leon, G. (1997). *Community as method: Therapeutic communities for special populations and special settings.* Westport, CA: Praeger Publishers.

De Leon, G., Melnick, G., & Cleland C. (2008). Client matching: A severity-treatment intensity paradigm. *Journal of Addictive Disorders, 27*(3), 99–113.

De Maeyer, J., Vanderplasschen, W., & Broekaert, E. (2010). Quality of life among opiate-dependent individuals: A review of the literature. *International Journal of Drug Policy, 21*(5), 364–380.

de Shazer, S., & Dolan, Y. (2007). *More than miracles: The state of the art in solution focused brief therapy.* Binghamton, NY: Haworth Press.

de Vocht, F., Sobala, W., Wilczynska, U., Kromhout, H., Szeszenia-Dabrowska, N., & Peplonska, B. (2009). Cancer mortality and occupational exposure to aromatic amines and inhalable aerosols in rubber tire manufacturing in Poland. *Cancer Epidemiology, 33*(2), 94–102.

Degenhardt, L., & Hall, W. (2012). Extent of illicit drug use and dependence, and their contribution to the global burden of disease. *The Lancet, 379*(9810), 55–70.

Dehghani-Arani, F., Rostami, R., & Nadali, H. (2013). Neurofeedback training for opiate addiction: Improvement of mental health and craving. *Applied Psychophysiology and Biofeedback, 38*(2), 133–141.

Delcher, C., Maldaono-Mollina, M., & Wagenaar, A. (2012). Effects of alcohol taxes on alcohol-related disease mortality in New York State from 1969 to 2006. *Addictive Behaviors, 37*(7), 783–789.

Denys, K., Rasmussen, C., & Henneveld, D. (2011). The effectiveness of a community-based intervention for parents with FASD. *Community Mental Health Journal, 47*(2), 209–219.

Derevensky, J., Gupta, R., & Csiernik, R. (2010). Problem gambling: Current knowledge and clinical perspectives. In R. Csiernik & W. Rowe (Eds.), *Responding to the oppression of addiction: Canadian social work perspectives* (2nd ed., pp. 313–333). Toronto, ON: Canadian Scholars' Press.

Derzon, J., Sale, E., Springer, J., & Brounstein, P. (2005). Estimating intervention effectiveness: Synthetic projection of field evaluation results. *The Journal of Primary Prevention, 26*(4), 321–343.

Dick, D., Aliev, F., Latendresse, S., Hickman, M., Heron, J., Macleod, J., ... Kendler, K. (2013). Adolescent alcohol use is predicted by childhood temperament factors before age 5, with mediation through personality and peers. *Alcoholism: Clinical and Experimental Research, 37*(12), 2108–2117.

Dickson-Gomez, J., Convey, M., Hilario, H., Corbett, A., & Weeks, M. (2007). Unofficial policy: Access to housing, housing information and social services among homeless drug users in Hartford, Connecticut. *Substance Abuse Treatment, Prevention, and Policy, 2*(8). doi:10.1186/1747-597X-2-8

DiClemente, C. (2007). The Transtheoretical Model of intentional behaviour change. *Drugs and Alcohol Today, 7*(1), 29–33.

DiLeo, P. (2003). *A message from the Office of the Commissioner: A decent place to live ... a basic right ... an essential for recovery.* Retrieved from www.ct.gov/dmhas/cwp/view.asp?a=2905&q=334404

Dimeff, L., & Linehan, M. (2008). Dialetical behavior therapy for substance abusers. *Addiction Science and Clinical Practice, 4*(2), 39–47.

Dingela, M., Hammer, R., Ostergren, J., McCormick, J., & Koenig, B. (2012). Chronic addiction, compulsion, and the empirical evidence. *American Journal of Bioethics Neuroscience, 3*(2), 58–59.

Dionne, P., Vasiliadis, H., Latimer, E., Berbiche, D., & Preville, M. (2013). *Psychiatric Services, 64*(4), 331–338.

Dishion, T., & McMahon, R. (1998). Parental monitoring and the prevention of child and adolescent problem behavior: A conceptual and empirical formulation. *Clinical Child and Family Psychology Review, 1*(1), 61–75.

Dolan, S., Bechara, A., & Nathan, P. (2007). Executive dysfunction as a risk marker for substance abuse: The role of impulsive personality traits. *Behavioral Sciences and the Law, 26*(6), 799–822.

Dole, V., & Nyswander, M. (1965). A medical treatment for diacetylmorphine (heroin) addiction. *Journal of the American Medical Association, 193*(8), 646–650.

Dom, G., D'Haene, P., Hulstiin, W., & Sabbe, B. (2006). Impulsivity in abstinent early and late-onset alcoholics: Differences in self-report measures and a discounting task. *Addiction, 101*(1), 50–59.

Domino, E., & Luby, E. (2012). Phencyclidine/schizophrenia: One view toward the past, the other to the future. *Schizophrenia Bulletin, 38*(5), 914–919.

Donaldson, S., Graham, J., Piccinin, A., & Hansen, W. (1995). Resistance-skills training and onset of alcohol use: Evidence for beneficial and potentially harmful effects in public schools and in private catholic schools. *Health Psychology, 14*(4), 291–300.

Donegan, N., Rodin, J., O'Brien, C., & Solomon, R. (1983). A learning theory approach to commonalities. In P. Levison, D. Gerstein, & D. Maloff (Eds.), *Commonalities in substance abuse and habitual behavior*. Lexington, MA: Lexington Books.

Donovan, D., & O'Leary, M. (1979). Control orientation among alcoholics: A cognitive social learning perspective. *American Journal of Drug and Alcohol Abuse, 6*(4), 487–499.

Douville, J. (1990). *Active and passive smoking hazards in the workplace*. New York: Van Nostrand Reinhold.

Dowsling, J. (1980). Sex therapy for recovering alcoholics: An essential part of family therapy. *International Journal of the Addictions, 15*(8), 1179–1189.

Doyle, N. (1987). *Involuntary smoking: Health risks for non-smokers*. New York: Public Affairs.

Drabble, L., Jones, S., & Brown, V. (2013). Advancing trauma-informed systems change in a family drug treatment court context. *Journal of Social Work Practice in the Addictions, 13*(1), 91–113.

Dryden, W., & Branch, R. (2012). *The CBT Handbook*. Thousand Oaks, CA: Sage.

Dubey, A. (1997). African plant now a drug in Canada. *The Journal, 26*(5), 3.

Dufur, M., Parcel, T., & McKune, B. (2013). Does capital at home matter more than capital at school? The case of adolescent alcohol and marijuana use. *Journal of Drug Issues, 43*(1), 85–102.

Dultz, L., & Frangos, S. (2013). The impact of alcohol in pedestrian trauma. *Trauma, 15*(1), 64–75.

Dumka, L., Roosa, M., Michaels, M., & Suh, K. (1995). Using research and theory to develop prevention programs for high risk families. *Family Relations, 44*(1), 78–86.

DuPont, R. (1994). The twelve step approach. In N. Miller (Ed.), *Treating coexisting psychiatric and addictive disorders: A practical guide* (pp. 177–197). Center City, MN: Hazelden.

Durlak, J. (1998). Primary prevention mental health programs for children and adolescents are effective. *Journal of Mental Health, 7*(5), 463–469.

Dusenbury, L. (2000). Family-based drug abuse prevention programs: A review. *The Journal of Primary Prevention, 20*(4), 337–352.

Dusenbury, L., Brannigan, R., Falco, M., & Hansen, W. (2003). A review of research on fidelity of implementation: Implications for drug abuse prevention in school settings. *Health Education Research, 18*(2), 237–256.

Dutton-Douglas, M., & Walker, L. (Eds.). (1988). Feminist psychotherapies: Integration of therapeutic and feminist systems. Norwood, NJ: Ablex.

Dyck, E., & Bradford, T. (2012). Peyote on the prairies: Religion, scientists, and Native-newcomer relations in Western Canada. *Journal of Canadian Studies, 46*(1), 28–52.

Dyer, C. (1994). New report criticises Upjohn over Halcion. *British Medical Journal, 3089*(12), 1321–1322.

Dyer, C. (1998). Addict died after rapid opiate detoxification. *British Medical Journal, 316,* 167e. doi:10.1136/bmj.316.7126.167e

Dziegielewski, S. (2005). *Understanding substance addictions.* Chicago, IL: Lyceum Books.

Edens, E., Kasprow, W., Tsai, J., & Rosenheck, R. (2011). Association of substance use and VA service-connected disability benefits with risk of homelessness among veterans. *The American Journal on Addictions, 20*(5), 412–419.

Edwards, G., Babor, T., Darke, S., Hall, W., Marsden, J., Miller, P., & West, R. (2009). Drug trafficking: Time to abolish the death penalty. *Addiction, 104*(8), 1267–1269.

Edwards, G., & Guthrie, S. (1966). A comparison of inpatient and outpatient treatment of alcohol dependence. *The Lancet, 1*(7435), 467–468.

Edwards, G., & Guthrie, S. (1967). A controlled trial of inpatient and outpatient treatment of alcohol dependency. *The Lancet, 1*(7489), 555–559.

Edwards, G., Orford, J., Egert, S., Guthrie, A., Hensman, C., Mitcheson, M., ... Taylor, C. (1977). Alcoholism: A controlled trial of "treatment" and "advice." *Journal of Studies on Alcohol, 38*(5), 1004–1031.

Eisner, M., Klein, J., Hammond, S., Koren, G., Lactao, C., & Iribarren, C. (2005). Directly measured second hand smoke exposure and asthma health outcomes. *Thorax, 60*(10), 814–821.

Ejik, J., Demirakca, T., Frischknecht, U., Hermann, D., Mann, K., & Ende, G. (2012). Rapid partial regeneration of brain volume during the first 14 days of abstinence from alcohol. *Alcoholism: Clinical and Experimental Research, 37*(1), 67–74.

El-Seedi, H., De Smet, P., Beck, O., Possnert, G., & Bruhn, J. (2005). Prehistoric peyote use: Alkaloid analysis and radiocarbon dating of archaeological specimens of Lophophora from Texas. *Journal of Ethnopharmacology, 101*(1-3), 238–242.

Elkashef, A., Vocci, F., Hanson, G., White, J., Wickes, W., & Tiihonen, J. (2008). Pharmacotherapy of methamphetamine addiction: An update. *Substance Abuse, 29*(3), 31–49.

Elkins, R. (1975). Aversion therapy for alcoholism: Chemical, electrical or verbal imaginary? *The International Journal of the Addictions, 10*(2), 157–209.

Ellis, A. (1995). Addictive behaviors and personality disorders. *American Psychological Association Addiction Newsletter, 2*(3), 10–11, 26.

Energy Fiend. (2009). *Caffeine.* Retrieved from www.energyfiend.com

Enoch, M. (2011). The role of early life stress as a predictor for alcohol and drug dependence. *Psychopharmacology, 214*(1), 17–31.

Enoch, M. (2012). The influence of gene-environment interactions on the development of alcoholism and drug dependence. *Current Psychiatry Reports, 14*(2), 150–158.

Erickson, C., & White, W. (2009). The neurobiology of addiction recovery. *Alcoholism Treatment Quarterly, 27*(3), 338–345.

Ersche, K., Jones, P., Williams, G., Robbins, T., & Bullmore, E. (2013). Cocaine dependence: A fast-track for brain ageing? *Molecular Psychiatry, 18*(2), 134–135.

Etter, J. (2010). Electronic cigarettes: A survey of users. *BMC Public Health, 10*(231). doi:10.1186/1471-2458-10-231

Ettner, S., Huang, D., Evans, E., Ash, D., Hardy, M., Jourabchi, M., & Hser, Y. (2006). Benefit–cost in the California treatment outcome project: Does substance abuse treatment "pay for itself"? *Health Services Research, 41*(1), 192–213.

Ettore, E. (1992). *Women and substance abuse.* New Brunswick, NJ: Rutgers University Press.

Etz, K., Robertson, E., & Ashery, R. (1998). Drug abuse prevention through family-based interventions: Future research. In R. Ashery, E. Robertson, & K. Kumpfer (Eds.), *Drug abuse prevention through family interventions* (pp. 1–11). Rockville, MD: US Department of Health and Human Services.

European Monitoring Centre for Drugs and Drug Addiction. (2008). *Monitoring the supply of cocaine to Europe.* Luxembourg: Office for Official Publications of the European Communities.

European Monitoring Centre for Drugs and Drug Addiction (2009a). *Preventing later substance use disorders in at-risk children and adolescents: A review of the theory and evidence base of indicated prevention.* Luxembourg: Office for Official Publications of the European Communities.

European Monitoring Centre for Drugs and Drug Addiction. (2009b). *Understanding the "spice" phenomenon.* Luxembourg: Office for Official Publications of the European Communities.

Everitt, B., & Robbins, T. (2005). Neural systems of reinforcement for drug addiction: From actions to habits to compulsion. *Nature Neuroscience, 8*(10), 1481–1489.

Faggiano, F., Vigna-Taglianti, F., Versino, E., Zambon, A., Borraccino, A., & Lemma, P. (2006). School-based prevention for illicit drugs' use. *Cochrane Database of Systematic Reviews* (Issue 2, Art. No.: CD003020). doi:10.1002/14651858.CD003020.pub2

Fairburn, C., & Harrison, P. (2003). Eating disorders. *The Lancet, 361*(9355), 407–416.

Falco, M. (1976). Methaqualone misuse: Foreign experience and United States drug control policy. *The International Journal of the Addictions, 11*(4), 597–610.

Fals-Stewart, W., & Lam, W. (2010). Computer-assisted cognitive rehabilitation for the treatment of patients with substance use disorders: A randomized clinical trial. *Experimental and Clinical Psychopharmacology, 18*(1), 87–98.

Fals-Stewart, W., & O'Farrell, T. (2003). Behavioral family counseling and naltrexone for male opioid-dependent patients. *Journal of Consulting and Clinical Psychology, 71*(3), 432–442.

Farah, M., Betancourt, L., Shera, D., Savage, J., Giannetta, J., Brodsky, N., … Hurt, H. (2008). Environmental stimulation, parental nurturance and cognitive development in human. *Developmental Science, 11*(5), 793–801.

Faraone, S., Biederman, J., Morley, C., & Spencer, T. (2008). Effects of stimulants on height and weight: A review of the literature. *Journal of the American Academy of Child and Adolescent Psychiatry, 47*(9), 994–1009.

Farber, B., & Doolin, E. (2011). Evidence-based psychotherapy relationships: Positive regard. *Psychotherapy, 48*(1), 58–64.

Fareed, A., Vayalapalli, S., Casarella, J., & Drexler, K. (2012). Effect of buprenorphine dose on treatment outcome. *Journal of Addictive Diseases, 31*(1), 8–18.

Fareed, A., Vayalapalli, S., Stout, S., Casarella, J., Dexler, K., & Bailey, S. (2010). Effect of methadone maintenance treatment on heroin craving: A literature review. *Journal of Addictive Diseases, 30*(1), 27–38.

Fehr, K. (1987). *Pharmacology and drug abuse.* Toronto, ON: Addiction Research Foundation.

Ferguson, D., & Boden, J. (2008). Cannabis use and later life outcome. *Addiction, 103*(6), 969–976.

Fernandez, A., Begley, E., & Marlatt, G. (2006). Family and peer interventions for adults: Past approaches and future directions. *Psychology of Addictive Behaviors, 20*(2), 207–213.

Ferrari, P., Jenab, M., Norat, T., Moskal, A., Slimani, N., Olsen, A., … Jensen, M. (2007). Lifetime and baseline alcohol intake and risk of colon and rectal cancers in the European prospective investigation into cancer and nutrition (EPIC). *International Journal of Cancer, 121*(9), 2065–2072.

Ferri, M., Davoli, M., & Perucci, C. (2011). Heroin maintenance for chronic heroin-dependent individuals. *Cochrane Database of Systematic Reviews* (Issue 12, Art. No.: CD003410). doi:10.1002/14651858.CD003410.pub4

Fillmore, K., Hartka, E., Johnstone, B., Speiglman, R., & Temple, M. (1988). *Spontaneous remission from alcohol problems: A critical review.* Washington, DC: United States Institute of Medicine.

Finckh, A., Dehler, S., Costenbader, K., & Gabay, C. (2007). Cigarette smoking and radiographic progression in rheumatoid arthritis. *Annals of the Rheumatic Diseases, 66*(8), 1066–1071.

Fingarette, H. (1988). *Heavy drinking: The myth of alcoholism as a disease.* Berkley, CA: University of California Press.

Fingarette, H. (1989). The perils of Powell: In search of a factual foundation for the "disease concept of alcoholism." *Drugs and Society, 3*(3-4), 1–27.

Finney, J., Hahn, A., & Moos, R. (1996). The effectiveness of inpatient and outpatient treatment for alcohol abuse: The need to focus on mediators and moderators of setting effect. *Addiction, 91*(12), 1773–1796.

Fishbein, D., & Pease, S. (1996). *The dynamics of drug abuse.* Boston, MA: Allyn & Bacon.

Fisher, G., & Harrison, T. (1997). *Substance abuse: Information for school counsellors, social workers, therapists and counsellors.* Toronto, ON: Allyn & Bacon.

Fisher, S. (1995). Group therapy protocols for persons with personality disorders who abuse substances: Effective treatment alternatives. *Social Work with Groups, 18*(4), 71–89.

Flammer, E., & Bongartz, W. (2003). On the efficacy of hypnosis: A meta-analytic study. *Contemporary Hypnosis, 20*(2), 179–197.

Fleming, A. (1975). *Alcohol: The delightful poison.* New York: Delacorte Press.

Floraa, M., Mascie-Taylorb, C., & Rahmanc, M. (2012). Betel quid chewing and its risk factors in Bangladeshi adults. *South-East Asia Journal of Public Health, 1*(2), 169–181.

Flores, P. (1983). *Group therapy for alcoholics.* New York: Haworth Press.

Flores, P. (2001). Addiction as an attachment disorder: Implications for group therapy. *International Journal of Group Psychotherapy, 51*(1), 63–81.

Flores, P. (2006). Conflict and repair in addiction treatment: An attachment disorder perspective. *Journal of Groups in Addiction and Recovery, 1*(1), 5–26.

Foucault, M. (1965). *Madness and civilization: A history of insanity in the age of reason.* New York: Random House.

Foundation for a DrugFree World. (2008). *The truth about drugs.* Los Angeles: Foundation for a Drug Free World.

Fowler, T., Lifford, K., Shelton, K., Rice, F., Thapar, A., Neale, M., ... van den Bree, M. (2007). Exploring the relationship between genetic and environmental influences on initiation and progression of substance use. *Addiction, 102*(3), 413–422.

Foxcroft, D., Ireland, D., Lister-Sharp, D., Lowe, G., & Breen, R. (2002). Long-term primary prevention for alcohol misuse in young people: A systematic review. *Addiction, 98*(4), 397–411.

Foxcroft, D., Ireland, D., Lowe, G., & Breen, R. (2002). Primary prevention for alcohol misuse in young people. *Cochrane Database Systems Review* (Issue 3, Art. No.: CD003024). doi:10.1002/14651858.CD003024

Foxcroft, D., Lister-Sharp, D., & Lowe, G. (1997). Alcohol misuse prevention for young people: A systematic review reveals methodological concerns and lack of reliable evidence of effectiveness. *Addiction, 92*(5), 531–537.

Freedman, N., Abnet, C., Leitzmann, M., Mouw, T., Subar, A., Hollenbeck, A., & Schatzkin, A. (2007). A prospective study of tobacco, alcohol, and the risk of esophageal and gastric cancer subtypes. *American Journal of Epidemiology, 165*(12), 1424–1433.

Freeman, S., & Alder, J. (2002). Arylethylamine psychotropic recreational drugs: A chemical perspective. *European Journal of Medicinal Chemistry, 37*(7), 527–539.

Freud, S. (1905). Three essays on the theory of sexuality. In J. Strachey (Ed.), *The complete psychological works of Sigmund Freud Volume VII (1901-1905).* New York: W. W. Norton.

Friedlander, M., Escudero, V., Heatherington, L., & Diamond, G. (2011). Alliance in couple and family therapy. *Psychotherapy, 48*(1), 25–33.

Friesen, C., Roscher, M., Alt, A., & Miltner, E. (2008). Methadone, commonly used as maintenance medication for outpatient treatment of opioid dependence, kills leukemia cells and overcomes chemoresistance. *Cancer Research, 68*(15), 6059–6064.

Frost, R., & Steketee, G. (2014). *The Oxford handbook of hoarding and acquiring.* New York: Oxford University Press.

Fuentes Salgado, M., Sutor, B., Albright, R., Jr., & Frye, M. (2014). Every reason to discontinue lithium. *International Journal of Bipolar Disorders, 2*(1), 12.

Fulton, H., Barrett, S., Stewart, S., & MacIsaac, C. (2012). Prescription opioid misuse: Characteristics of earliest and most recent memory of hydromorphone use. *Journal of Addiction Medicine, 6*(2), 137–144.

Fulton, M. (1978). *A chronology of substances of abuse.* Washington, DC: University Press of America.

Fusar-Poli, P., Rubia, K., Rossi, G., Sartori, G., & Balottin, U. (2012). Striatal dopamine transporter alterations in ADHD: Pathophysiology or adaptation to psychostimulants? A meta-analysis. *American Journal of Psychiatry, 169*(3), 264–72.

Gabour, P., & Ing, C. (1991). Stop and think: The application of cognitive-behavioural approaches in work with young people. *Journal of Child and Youth Care, 6*(1), 43–53.

Gadalla, T., & Piran, N. (2009). Eating disorders, substance use disorders and major depression in the Canadian population. *Journal of Mental Health, 18*(6), 486–494.

Gainsbury, S., & Blaszcynski, A. (2011). A systematic review of Internet-based therapy for the treatment of addictions. *Clinical Psychology Review, 31*(3), 490–498.

Gardner, E. (2011). Addiction and brain reward and anti-reward pathways. *Advances in Psychosomatic Medicine, 30*(1), 22–60.

Gardner, S., Green, P., & Marcus, C. (1994). *Signs of effectiveness II: Preventing alcohol, tobacco and other drug use; A risk factor/resiliency-based approach.* Rockville, MD: Center for Substance Abuse Prevention.

Garland, E. (2004). Facing the evidence: Antidepressant treatment in children and adolescents. *Canadian Medical Journal, 170*(4), 489–491.

Garland, E., Schwarz, N., Kelly, A., Whitt, A., & Howard, M. (2012). Mindfulness-orientated recovery enhancement for alcohol dependence: Therapeutic mechanism and intervention acceptability. *Journal of Social Work Practice in the Addictions, 12*(4), 242–263.

Garnier, H., & Stein, J. (2002). An 18 year model of family and peer effects on adolescent drug use and delinquency. *Journal of Youth and Adolescence, 31*(1), 45–56.

Gartner, A., & Riessman, F. (1977). *Self-help in the human services.* San Francisco, CA: Jossey-Bass.

Gately, I. (2001). *Tobacco: A cultural history of how an exotic plant seduced civilization.* New York: Grove Press.

Gaume, J., Gmel, G., Faouzi, M., & Daeppen, J. (2009). Counselor skill influences outcomes of brief motivational interventions. *Journal of Substance Abuse Treatment, 37*(2), 151–159.

Gearhardt, A., White, M., & Potenza, M. (2011). Binge eating disorder and food addiction. *Current Drug Abuse Reviews, 4*(3), 201–207.

Gehrke, R. (2011, August 1). Utah tobacco sales drop nearly 10 million packs. *The Salt Lake Tribune.* Retrieved from www.sltrib.com/sltrib/politics/52273720-90/tax-sales-million-tobacco.html.csp

Geller, L. (1982). The failure of self-actualization theory: A critique of Carl Rogers and Abraham Maslow. *Journal of Humanistic Psychology, 22*(2), 56–73.

Gevirtz, C., Frost, E., & Kaye, A. (2011). Ultra-rapid opiate detoxification. In R. Urman, W. Gross, & B. Philip (Eds.), *Anesthesia outside of the operating room* (pp. 309–315). New York: Oxford University Press.

Giffen, P., Endicott, S., & Boorman, S.C. (1991). *Panic and indifference: The politics of Canada's dry laws; A study in the sociology of law.* Ottawa, ON: Canadian Centre on Substance Abuse.

Gifford, E., & Humphreys, K. (2007). The psychological science of addiction. *Addiction, 102*(3), 352–361.

Gilligan, C., Kypri, K., & Lubman, D. (2012). Changing parental behaviour to reduce risky drinking among adolescents: Current evidence and future directions. *Alcohol and Alcoholism, 47*(3), 349–354.

Glatt, M. (1958). Group therapy in alcoholism. *British Journal of Addiction, 54*(2), 133–148.

Glatt, M. (1980). The alcoholic: Controlled drinking. *British Journal of Alcohol and Alcoholism, 15*(2), 48–55.

Glover, E. (1928). The aetiology of alcoholism. *Journal of the Royal Society of Medicine, 21*, 1351–1355.

Goldstein, A. (1976). Opioid peptides (endorphins) in pituitary and brain. *Science, 193*(4528), 1081–1086.

Goldstein, A. (1979). Heroin maintenance: A medical view. A conversation between a physician and a politician. *Journal of Drug Issues, 9*(4), 341–347.

Gomes, T., Mamdani, M., Paterson, J., Dhalla, I., & Juurlink, D. (2014). Trends in high-dose opioid prescribing in Canada. *Canadian Family Physician, 60*(9), 826–832.

González-Maeso, J., Weisstaub, N., Zhou, M., Chan, P., Ivic, L., Ang, R., ... Bradley, M. (2007). Hallucinogens recruit specific cortical 5-HT$_{2A}$ receptor-mediated signalling pathways to affect behavior. *Neuron, 53*(3), 439–452.

González-Pinto, A., Vega, P., Ibáñez, B., Mosquera, F., Barbeito, S., Gutiérrez, M., ... Vieta, E. (2008). Impact of cannabis and other drugs on age at onset of psychosis. *Journal of Clinical Psychiatry, 69*(8), 1210–1216.

Goode, E., & Ben-Yehuda, N. (1994). Moral panics: Culture politics, and social constructions. *Annual Review of Sociology, 20*, 149–171.

Goodman, A. (1990). Addiction: Definition and implications. *British Journal of Addictions, 85*(11), 1403–1408.

Goodman, D. (2013). Opioid dose and risk of road trauma in Canada: A population-based study. *Journal of the American Medical Association, 173*(3), 196–201.

Goodwin, D., Schulsinger, E., Hermansen, L., Guze, S., & Winokur, G. (1973). Alcohol problems in adoptees raised apart from biological parents. *Archives of General Psychiatry, 28*(2), 238–243.

Gorman, D. (1997). The failure of drug education. *Public Interest, 129*(Fall), 50–60.

Gorman, D. (2002). Defining and operationalizing "research-based" prevention: A critique (with case studies) of the US Department of Education's safe, disciplined and drug-free schools exemplary programs. *Evaluation and Program Planning, 25*(3), 295–302.

Gorman, D. (2003). The best of practices, the worst of practices: The making of science-based primary prevention programs. *Psychiatric Services, 54*(8), 1087–1089.

Gottfredson, D., & Wilson, D. (2003). Characteristics of effective school-based substance abuse prevention. *Prevention Science, 4*(1), 27–38.

Gottheil, E., Thornton, C., & Weinstein, S. (2002). Effectiveness of high versus low structure individual counseling for substance abuse. *American Journal on Addictions, 11*(4), 279–290.

Goulart, F. (1984). *The caffeine book*. New York: Dodd, Mead & Company.

Government of Canada. (2015). Controlled Drugs and Substances Act [S. C. 1996, c. 19]. Retreved from http://laws-lois.justice.gc.ca/eng/acts/c-38.8/

Graham, A., & Adams, J. (2014). Alcohol marketing in televised English professional football: A frequency analysis. *Alcohol and Alcoholism, 49*(3), 343–348.

Graner, N. (1988). *The encyclopedia of psychoactive drugs: Drugs and the law.* New York: Chelsea House Publishers.

Grant, J. (2009). Profile of substance abuse, gender, crime, and drug policy in the United States and Canada. *Journal of Offender Rehabilitation, 48*(8), 654–668.

Grant, J., Schreiber, L., & Odlaug, B. (2013). Phenomenology and treatment of behavioural addictions. *Canadian Journal of Psychiatry, 58*(5), 252–259.

Grape, S., Schug, B., & Schug, S. (2010). Formulations of fentanyl for the management of pain. *Drugs, 70*(1), 57–72.

Gray, J. (1995). *Booze: When whisky ruled the west.* Toronto, ON: MacMillan of Canada.

Green, J., Lynn, S., & Montgomery, G. (2006). A meta-analysis of gender, smoking cessation, and hypnosis: A brief communication. *International Journal of Clinical and Experimental Hypnosis, 54*(2), 224–233.

Green, M. (1980). *Components of the treatment system for clients with drug and/or alcohol problems.* Toronto, ON: Addiction Research Foundation.

Greenberg, G. (2010). *Manufacturing depression: The secret history of modern disease.* New York: Simon & Schuster.

Greenberg, M., Domitrovich, C., & Bumbarger, B. (2000). *Preventing mental disorders in school-aged children: A review of the effectiveness of prevention programs.* Rockville, MD: Substance Abuse Mental Health Services Administration.

Grella, C., & Lovinger, K. (2011). 30-year trajectories of heroin and other drug use among men and women sampled from methadone treatment in California. *Drug and Alcohol Dependency, 118*(2-3), 251–258.

Griffin, K., Botvin, G., Scheier, L., Diaz, T., & Miller, N. (2000). Parenting practices of predictors of substance use, delinquency, and aggression among urban minority youth: Moderating effects of family structure and gender. *Psychology of Addictive Behaviors, 14*(2), 174–184.

Griffin, T., & Svendsen, R. (1992). *Promising prevention strategies for the 90s.* Piscataway, NJ: Center of Alcohol Studies.

Grizenko, N., Cai, E., Jolicoeur, C., & Ter-Stepanian, M. (2013). Effects of methylphenidate on acute math performance in children with attention-deficit hyperactivity disorder. *Canadian Journal of Psychiatry, 58*(11), 632–639.

Grob, C., Danforth, A., Chopra, G., Hagerty, M., McKay, C., Halberstadt, A., & Greer, G. (2011). Pilot study of psilocybin treatment for anxiety in patients with advanced-stage cancer. *Archives of General Psychiatry, 68*(1), 71–78.

Grogan, S. (1999). *Body image: Understanding body dissatisfaction in men, women, and children.* New York: Routledge.

Guerino, P., Harrison, P., & Sabol, W. (2010). *Prisoners in 2010* (Rev. ed.). Washington, DC: United States Bureau of Justice Statistics.

Gupta, B., & Gupta, U. (1999). *Caffeine and behavior: Current views and research trends.* New York: CRC Press.

Gupta, M., & Knapp, K. (2013). Lithium carbonate decreases acute suicidality in posttraumatic stress disorder. *Australia & New Zealand Journal of Psychiatry, 47*(12), 1217.

Gupta, P., & Ray, C. (2004). Epidemiology of betel quid usage. *Annals of the Academy of Medicine, Singapore, 33*(S), 31S–36S.

Guthrie, B., & Flinchbaugh, L. (2001). Gender-specific substance prevention programming: Going beyond just focusing on girls. *Journal of Early Adolescence, 21*(3), 354–372.

Hackshaw, A., Rodeck, C., & Boniface, S. (2011). Maternal smoking in pregnancy and birth defects: A systematic review based on 173,687 malformed cases and 11.7 million controls. *Human Reproduction Update, 15*(5), 589–604.

Haden, M. (2006). *Economic fact sheet: Facts and figures relating to illegal drugs.* Vancouver, BC: Addiction Services, Vancouver Coastal Authority.

Hafez, N., & Ling, P. (2005). How Philip Morris built Marlboro into a global brand for young adults: Implications for international tobacco control. *Tobacco Control, 14*(2), 262–271.

Hagan, G. (1999). *HIV/AIDS and the drug culture.* New York: Haworth Press.

Hagele, C., Friedel, E., Kienast, T., & Kiefer, F. (2014). How do we "learn" addiction? Risk factors and mechanisms getting addicted to alcohol. *Neuropsychobiology, 70*(1), 67–70.

Hall, J., & Huber, D. (2000). Telephone management in substance abuse treatment. *Telemedicine Journal and e-Health, 6*(4), 401–407.

Hall, M., & Vander Bilt, J. (2000). *Facing the odds: The mathematics of gambling and other risks.* Boston, MA: Harvard University Press.

Hallfors, D., & Godette, D. (2002). Will the "principles of effectiveness" improve prevention practice? Early findings from a diffusion study. *Health Education Research, 17*(4), 461–470.

Halpern, J., Sherwood, A., Hudson, J., Yurgelun-Todd, D., & Pope, Jr. (2005). Psychological and cognitive effects of long-term peyote use among Native Americans. *Biological Psychiatry, 58*(8), 624–631.

Hamilton, R., Olmedo, R., Shah, S., Hung, O., Howland, M., Perrone, J., … Hoffman, R. (2002). Complications of ultrarapid opioid detoxification with subcutaneous naltexone pellets. *Academic Emergency Medicine, 9*(1), 63–68.

Hankins, C. (1998). Syringe exchange in Canada: Good but not enough to stem the HIV tide. *Substance Use and Misuse, 33*(5), 1129–1146.

Hans, M. (2010). Chemistry, pharmacology, and metabolism of emerging drugs of abuse. *Therapeutic Drug Monitoring, 32*(5), 544–549.

Harding, S. (1987). *Feminism and methodology.* Bloomington, IL: University of Indiana Press.

Harkin, A., Connor, T., Mulrooney, J., Kelly, J., & Leonard, B. (2001). Prior exposure to methylenedioxyamphetamine (MDA) induces serotonergic loss and changes in spontaneous exploratory and amphetamine-induced behaviors in rats. *Life Sciences, 68*(12), 1367–1382.

Harrow, M., Jobe, T., & Faull, R. (2012). Do all schizophrenia patients need antipsychotic treatment continuously throughout their lifetime? A 20-year longitudinal study. *Psychological Medicine, 42*(10), 1–11.

Hart, K., & Singh, T. (2009). An existential model of flourishing subsequent to treatment for addiction: The importance of living a meaningful and spiritual life. *Illness, Crisis, and Loss, 17*(2), 125–147.

Hart, L. (1977). A review of treatment and rehabilitation legislation regarding alcohol abusers and alcoholics in the United States: 1920–1971. *The International Journal of the Addictions, 12*(5), 667–678.

Hasler, B., Smith, L., Cousins, J., & Bootzins, R. (2012). Circadian rhythms, sleep, and substance abuse. *Sleep Medicine Reviews, 16*(1), 67–81.

Hawkins, E., Cummins, L., & Marlatt, G. (2004). Preventing substance abuse in American Indian and Alaska native youth: Promising strategies for healthier communities. *Psychological Bulletin, 130*(2), 304–323.

Hawthorne, G. (2001). Drug education: Myth and reality. *Drug and Alcohol Review, 20*(1), 111–119.

Hayashida, M. (1998). An overview of outpatient and inpatient detoxification. *Alcohol Health and Research World, 22*(1), 44–46.

Hayashida, M., Alterman, A., McLellan, A., O'Brien, C., Purtill, J., Volpicelli, J., ... Hall, C. (1989). Comparative effectiveness and costs of inpatient and outpatient detoxification of patients with mild-to-moderate alcohol withdrawal syndrome. *New England Journal of Medicine, 320*(6), 358–364.

Hayen, B., Canuel, N., & Shanse, J. (2013). What was brewing in the Natufian? An archaeological assessment of brewing technology in the Epipaleolithic. *Journal of Archaeological Method and Theory, 20*(1), 102–150.

Hayes, S., Masuda, A., Bissett, R., Luoma, J., & Guerrero, L. (2004). DBT, FAP, and ACT: How empirically oriented are the new behavior therapy technologies? *Journal of Behavior Therapy, 35*(1), 35–54.

Hays, S., Hays, C., & Mulhall, P. (2003). Community risk and protective factors and adolescent substance use. *The Journal of Primary Prevention, 24*(2), 125–142.

Hayward, B., Cook, R., & Thorne, J. (1994). *Community-based prevention services for high risk youth: A study of the Governor's DFSCA program*. Research Triangle Park, NC: Research Triangle Institute.

Hazan, C., & Shaver, P. (1987). Romantic love conceptualized as an attachment process. *Journal of Personality and Social Psychology, 52*(6), 511–524.

Hazelden. (2001). *The history of recovery*. Centre City, MN: Hazelden.

Health Canada. (2001). *Reducing the harm associated with injection drug use in Canada*. Ottawa, ON: Health Canada.

Health Canada. (2007). *Healthy living: Rewards of quitting*. Ottawa, ON: Health Canada.

Health Canada. (2008). *Methadone maintenance treatment*. Retrieved from www.hc-sc.gc.ca/hc-ps/pubs/adp-apd/methadone-treatment-traitement/index-eng.php#fnb20

Health Canada. (2009). *Straight facts about drugs and drug abuse*. Ottawa, ON: Health Canada.

Health Canada. (2013a). Health Canada's review recommends codeine only be used in patients aged 12 and over. Retrieved from http://healthycanadians.gc.ca/recall-alert-rappel-avis/hc-sc/2013/33915a-eng.php

Health Canada. (2013b). *Are you eligible?* Retrieved from www.hc-sc.gc.ca/dhpmps/marihuana/how-comment/eligible-admissible-eng.php#a1

Health Canada. (2014a). *Canadian alcohol and drug monitoring survey*. Ottawa, ON: Health Canada.

Health Canada. (2014b). *Medical use of marijuana.* Retrieved from www.hc-sc.gc.ca/dhp-mps/marihuana/index-eng.php

Healy, B., Ali, E., Guttmann, C., Chitnis, T., Glanz, B., Buckle, G., … Ascherio, A. (2009). Smoking and disease progression in multiple sclerosis. *Archives of Neurology, 66*(7), 858–864.

Heath, A., Jardine, R., & Martin, N. (1989). Interactive effects of genotype and social environment on alcohol consumption and female twins. *Journal of Studies on Alcohol, 50*(1), 38–48.

Heath, D. (1989). The new temperance movement: Through the looking glass. *Drugs and Society, 3*(3-4), 143–168.

Heather, N., Hönekopp, J., & Smailes, D. (2009). Progressive stage transition does mean getting better: A further test of the Transtheoretical Model in recovery from alcohol problems. *Addiction, 104*(6), 949–958.

Hecht, M., & Raup-Krieger, J. (2006). The principle of cultural grounding in school-based substance abuse programs: The drug resistance strategies project. *Journal of Language and Social Psychology, 25*(3), 301–319.

Hector, I. (2001). Changing funding patterns and the effect on mental health care in Canada. In Q. Rae-Grant (Ed.), *Psychiatry in Canada: 50 years (1951-2001)* (pp. 59–76). Ottawa, ON: Canadian Psychiatric Association.

Heinen, M., Verhage, B., Ambergen, T., Goldbohm, R., & van den Brandt, P. (2009). Alcohol consumption and risk of pancreatic cancer in the Netherlands cohort study. *American Journal of Epidemiology, 169*(10), 1233–1242.

Heller, T. (2003). *Eating disorders: A handbook for teens, families, and teachers.* Jefferson, NC: McFarland & Company.

Hellman, M., Schoenmakers, T., Nordstrom, B., & Van Holst, R. (2013). *Addiction Research and Theory, 21*(2), 102–112.

Hendershot, C., Witkiewitz, K., George, W., & Marlatt, G. (2011). Relapse prevention for addictive behaviors. *Substance Abuse Treatment, Prevention, and Policy, 6*(1). Retrieved from www.substanceabusepolicy.com/content/6/1/17

Henningfield, J., & Ator, N. (1986). *Barbiturates.* New York: Chelsea House.

Hepworth, D., & Larsen, J. (2012). *Direct social work practice* (9th ed.). Pacific Grove, CA: American Psychiatric Publishing Company.

Herbert, J., & Foreman, E. (2011). Acceptance and mindfulness in cognitive behavior therapy. In J. Herbert & E. Foreman (Eds.), *The evolution of cognitive behavior therapy* (pp. 3–25). Hoboken, NJ: John Wiley and Sons.

Hesselbrock, M., Hesselbrock, V., & Chartier, K. (2013). Genetics of alcohol dependence and social work research: Do they mix? *Social Work in Public Health, 28*(3-4), 178–193.

Hester, R., & Miller, W. (Eds.). (1995). *Handbook of alcoholism treatment approaches: Effective alternatives* (2nd ed.). Needham Heights, MA: Allyn & Bacon.

Hester, R., Nirenberg, T., & Begin, A. (1990). Behavioral treatment of alcohol and drug abuse. In M. Galanter (Ed.), *Recent developments in alcoholism* (Vol. 8, pp. 305–327). New York: Plenum Press.

Hickert, A., & Taylor, M. (2011). Supportive housing for addicted, incarcerated homeless adults. *Journal of Social Service Research, 37*(2), 136–151.

Hiebert-Murphy, D., & Woytkiw, L. (2010). A model for working with women dealing with child sexual abuse and addiction: The Laurel Centre, Winnipeg, Manitoba. In R. Csiernik & W. Rowe (Eds.), *Responding to the oppression of addiction: Canadian social work perspectives* (2nd ed., pp. 91–108). Toronto, ON: Canadian Scholars' Press.

Hill, K. (1983). *Helping you helps me.* Ottawa, ON: Canadian Council on Social Development.

Hirayama, T. (1981). Non-smoking wives of heavy smokers have a higher risk of lung cancer: A study from Japan. *British Medical Journal, 282*(6259), 183–185.

Hiroi, N., & Agatsuma, S. (2005). Genetic susceptibility to substance dependence. *Molecular Psychiatry, 10*(4), 336–344.

Hoehne, D. (1988). Self-help and social change. *Social movements/social change.* Toronto, ON: Between the Lines.

Hofstede, G. (1984). The cultural relativity of the quality of life concept. *Academy of Management Review, 9*(3), 389–398.

Hofstee, W., De Raad, B., & Goldberg, L. (1992). Integration of the big five and circumplex approaches to trait structures. *Journal of Personality and Social Psychology, 63*(1), 146–163.

Hogue, A., Liddle, H., Becker, D., & Johnson-Leckrone, J. (2002). Family-based prevention counseling for high-risk young adolescents: Immediate outcome. *Journal of Community Psychology, 30*(1), 1–22.

Holbrook, T., Galarneau, M., Dye, J., Quinn, K., & Dougherty, A. (2010). Morphine use after combat injury in Iraq and post-traumatic stress disorder. *New England Journal of Medicine, 362*(2), 110–117.

Holder, J., & Shriner, B. (2012). Subluxation based chiropractic care in the management of cocaine addiction: A case report. *Annals of Vertebral Subluxation Research, 14*(1), 8–17.

Holderness, C., Brooks-Gunn, J., & Warren, M. (1994). Co-morbidity of eating disorders and substance abuse: Review of the literature. *International Journal of Eating Disorders, 16*(1), 1–34.

Hollister, L. (1972). Psychoactive drugs in historical perspective. *Journal of Drug Issues,* (Winter), 1–8.

Holmes, A., Fitzgerald, P., De Brouse, L., Colacicco, G., Flynn, S., Masneuf, S., ... Camp, M. (2012). *Nature Neuroscience, 15*(10), 1359–1361.

Holt, J. (2015). A Latter-Day Saint approach to addiction: Aetiology, consequences and treatment in a theological context. *Religions, 6*(1), 1–13.

Horton, D. (1943). The functions of alcohol in primitive societies: A cross cultural study. *Quarterly Journal of Studies on Alcohol, 4,* 199–320.

Hubbard, J., Franco, S., & Onaivi, E. (1999). Marijuana: Medical implications. *American Family Physician, 60*(12), 2583–2593.

Hubble, M., Duncan, B., Miller, S., & Wampold, B. (2010). Introduction. In B. Duncan, S. Miller, B. Wampold, & M. Hubble (Eds.), *The heart and soul of change: Delivering what works in therapy* (2nd ed., pp. 23–46). Washington, DC: American Psychological Association.

Hundley, J., Woodrum, D., Saunders, B., Doherty, G., & Gauger, P. (2005). Revisiting lithium-associated hyperparathyroidism in the era of intraoperative parathyroid hormone monitoring. *Surgery, 138*(6), 1027–1031.

Hunt, G., & Azrin, N. (1973). A community-reinforcement approach to alcoholism. *Behaviour Research and Therapy, 11*(1), 91–104.

Hunt, J., van der Hel, O., McMillan, G., Boffetta, P., & Brennan, P. (2005). Renal cell carcinoma in relation to cigarette smoking: Meta-analysis of 24 studies. *International Journal of Cancer, 114*(1), 101–108.

Hurt, H., Brodsky, N., Roth, H., Malmud, E., & Giannetta, J. (2005). School performance of children with gestational cocaine exposure. *Neurotoxiology and Teratology, 27*(2), 203–211.

Hurt, H., Giannetta, J., Korczkowski, M., Hoang, A., Tang, K., Beancourt, L., … Detre, J. (2008). Functional magnetic resonance imaging and working memory in adolescents with gestational cocaine exposure. *The Journal of Pediatrics, 152*(3), 371–377.

Hurt, H., Malmud, E., Betancourt, L., Braitman, L., Brodsky, N., & Giannetta, J. (1997). Children with in utero cocaine exposure do not differ from control subjects on intelligence testing. *Archives of Pediatrics and Adolescent Medicine, 151*(12), 1237–1241.

Hurt, H., Malmud, E., Betancourt, L., Brodsky, N., & Giannetta, J. (2001). A prospective comparison of developmental outcome of children with in utero cocaine exposure and controls using the Battelle Developmental Inventory. *Journal of Developmental & Behavioral Pediatrics, 22*(1), 27–34.

Hyshka, E., Strathdee, S., Wood, E., & Kerr, T. (2012). Needle exchange and the HIV epidemic in Vancouver: Lessons learned from 15 years of research. *International Journal of Drug Policy, 23*(4), 261–270.

Ilgen, M., & Moos, R. (2005). Deterioration following alcohol use disorder treatment in Project Match. *Journal of Studies in Alcohol, 66*(4), 517–525.

Imel, Z., Wampold, B., Miller, S., & Fleming, R. (2008). Distinctions with a difference: Direct comparisons of psychotherapies for alcohol use disorders. *Psychology of Addictive Behaviors, 22*(4), 533–543.

Inglis, B. (1975). *The forbidden game: A social history of drugs.* New York: Scribner.

Inner City Health. (2010). *Programs and services.* Retrieved from http://ottawainnercityhealth. ca/FCKeditor/editor/fileCabinet/OICH_Alcohol_FAQ_Read_More_Document1.pdf

International Blue Cross. (2002). New party drugs. *IFBC Information Bulletin, 1,* 6.

International Drug Policy Consortium. (2010). *Drug policy guide.* London, UK: International Drug Policy Consortium.

International Drug Policy Consortium. (2012). *Drug policy guide* (2nd ed.). London, UK: International Drug Policy Consortium.

International Monetary Fund. (2008). *World economic outlook database.* Washington, DC: International Monetary Fund.

International Narcotics Control Board. (2009). *Report of the International Narcotics Control Board, 2008.* New York: United Nations.

International Narcotics Control Board. (2014). *Report of the International Narcotics Control Board, 2013.* New York: United Nations.

Iovieno, N., Tedeschini, K., Bentley, H., Evins, E., & Papakostas, G. (2011). Antidepressants for major depressive disorder and dysthymic disorder in patients with comorbid alcohol use disorders: A meta-analysis of placebo-controlled randomized trials. *The Journal of Clinical Psychiatry, 72*(8), 1144–1151.

Jabbar, S., & Hanly, M. (2013). Fatal caffeine overdose: A case report and review of literature. *American Journal of Forensic Medicine & Pathology, 34*(4), 321–324.

Jackson, T., & Smith, J. (1978). A comparison of two aversion treatment methods for alcoholism. *Journal of Studies on Alcohol, 39*(1), 187–191.

Jaffe, J., & Jaffe, F. (1989). Historical perspectives of subjective effects measures in assessing the abuse potential of drugs. In M. Fischman & N. Mello (Eds.), *Testing for abuse liability of drugs in humans* (pp. 43–69). Rockville, MD: National Institute on Drug Abuse.

Jansen, K. (2000). A review of the nonmedical use of ketamine: Use, users and consequences. *Journal of Psychoactive Drugs, 32*(4), 419–432.

Janssen, P., Demorest, L., Kelly, A., Thiessen, P., & Abrahams, R. (2012). Auricular acupuncture for chemically dependent pregnant women: A randomized controlled trial of the NADA protocol. *Substance Abuse Treatment, Prevention and Policy, 7*(48). doi:10.1186/1747-597X-7-48

Jansson, L., & Velez, M. (2012). Neonatal abstinence syndrome. *Current Opinion in Pediatrics, 24*(2), 252–258.

Jarvik, S. (1967). Psychopharmacological revolution. *Psychology Today, 59*(1), 18–24.

Jellinek, E. (1952). Phases of alcohol addiction. *Quarterly Journal of Studies on Alcohol, 13*(4), 673–684.

Jellinek, E. (1960). *The disease concept of alcoholism.* New Haven, CN: Hillhouse Press.

Jensen, C., Cushing, C., Aylward, B., Craig, J., Sorell, D., & Steele, R. (2011). Effectiveness of motivational interviewing interventions for adolescent substance use behavior change: A meta-analytic review. *Journal of Consulting and Clinical Psychology, 79*(4), 433–440.

Jerome, L., Schuster, S., & Yazar-Klosinski, B. (2013). Can MDMA play a role in the treatment of substance abuse? *Current Drug Abuse Reviews, 6*(1), 54–62.

Jit, M., Aveyard, P., Barton, P., & Meads, C. (2010). Predicting the life-time benefit of school-based smoking prevention programmes. *Addiction, 105*(6), 1109–1116.

Johnson, V. (1973). *I'll quit tomorrow.* San Francisco, CA: Harper & Row.

Johnston Counsulting. (2014). *Clients' outcome report: Addiction supportive housing review (phase two).* Toronto, ON: Addictions & Mental Health Ontario.

Jones, K. (1986). Fetal alcohol syndrome. *Pediatrics in Review, 8*(1), 122–126.

Jones, K., & Smith, D. (1973). Recognition of the fetal alcohol syndrome in early infancy. *The Lancet, 302*(7836), 999–1001.

Jones-Smith, E. (2012). *Theories of counselling and psychotherapy.* Los Angeles, CA: Sage.

Join Together. (2012). *Kerlikowske: Addiction is a disease, not a moral failure.* Retrieved from www.drugfree.org/join-together/kerlikowske-addiction-is-a-disease-not-a-moral-failure/

Jourard. R. (2014). *Criminal offence penalty chart: Drug offence.* Retrieved from www.defencelaw.com/penalties-drugs.html

Julien, R., Advokat, C., & Comaty, J. (2008). *A primer of drug action: A comprehensive guide to the actions, uses, and side effects of psychoactive drugs* (11th ed.). New York: Worth Publishers.

Jung, J. (1994). *Under the influence: Alcohol and human behavior.* Pacific Grove, CA: Brooks/Cole Publishing.

Kahan, M., Srivastava, A., Ordean, A., & Cirone, S. (2011). Buprenorphine: New treatment of opioid addiction in primary care. *Canadian Family Physician, 57*(3), 281–289.

Kallant, H. (2009). What neurobiology cannot tell us about addiction. *Addiction, 105*(5), 780–789.

Kalsched, D. (2014). *The inner world of trauma: Archetypal defences of the personal spirit*. New York: Routledge.

Karagueuzian, H., Whitle, C., Sayre, J., & Norman, A. (2012). Cigarette smoke radioactivity and lung cancer risk. *Nicotine and Tobacco Research, 14*(1), 79–90.

Karaiskos, D., Tzavellas, E., Balta, G., & Paparrigopoulos, T. (2010). Social network addiction: A new clinical disorder? *European Psychiatry, 25*(S1), 855.

Kaskutas, L. (1989). Women for sobriety: A qualitative analysis. *Contemporary Drug Problems*, (Summer), 177–199.

Katz, A., & Bender, E. (1976). *The strength in us*. New York: New Viewpoints.

Kay, G. (2000). The effects of antihistamines on cognition and performance. *Journal of Allergy and Clinical Immunology, 105*(6), S622–S627.

Kellen, A., & Powers, L. (2010). Drug use, addiction and the criminal justice system. In R. Csiernik & W. Rowe (Eds.), *Responding to the oppression of addiction* (2nd ed., pp. 215–234). Toronto, ON: Canadian Scholars' Press.

Kelly, A. (2004). Memory and addiction: Shared neural circuitry and molecular mechanisms. *Neuron, 44*(1), 161–179.

Kempf-Leonard, K., Tracy, P., & Howell, J. (2001). Serious, violent, and chronic juvenile offenders: The relationship of delinquency career types to adult criminality. *Justice Quarterly, 18*(3), 449–478.

Kendler, K., Heath, A., Neale, M., Kessler, R., & Eaves, L. (1992). A population-based twin study of alcoholism in women. *Journal of the American Medical Association, 268*(14), 1877–1882.

Kendler, K., Sundquist, K., Ohlsson, H., Palmér, K., Maes, H., Winkleby, M., & Sundquist, J. (2012). Genetic and familial environmental influences on the risk for drug abuse: A national Swedish adoption study. *Archives of General Psychiatry, 69*(7), 690–697.

Kennedy, S., & Cooke, R. (2000). Recent advances in the treatment of depression. Retrieved from wwl.cpa-pc.org:8080/French_Site/Publications/Archives/Bulletin/2000/Aug/Recent.asp

Kent, H. (2002). New "daytox" centre opens for subgroup of Vancouver drug/alcohol addicts. *Canadian Medical Association Journal, 166*(5), 643.

Kerr, T., Small, W., Hyshkal, E., Maher, L., & Shannon, K. (2013). "It's more about the heroin": Injection drug users' response to an overdose warning campaign in a Canadian setting. *Addiction, 108*(7), 1270–1276.

Kerrigan, S., & Lindsey, T. (2005). Fatal caffeine overdose: Two case studies. *Forensic Science International, 153*(1), 67–69.

Kesselheim, A. (2011). Covert pharmaceutical promotion in free medical journals. *Canadian Medical Journal, 183*(5), 534–535.

Khantzian, E. (2003). Understanding addictive vulnerability: An evolving psychodynamic perspective. *Neuro-Psychoanalysis, 5*(1), 5–21.

Khatib, M., Jarrar, Z., Bizrah, M., & Checinski, K. (2013). Khat: Social habit or cultural burden? A survey and review. *Journal of Ethnicity in Substance Abuse, 12*(2), 140–153.

Kimberly, M., & Osmond, M. (2010). Concurrent disorders and social work intervention. In R. Csiernik and W. Rowe (Eds.), *Responding to the oppression of addiction: Canadian social work responses* (2nd ed., pp. 227–248). Toronto, ON: Canadian Scholars' Press.

Kimura, M., & Higuchi, S. (2011). Genetics of alcohol dependence. *Psychiatry and Clinical Neurosciences, 65*(3), 213–225.

King, A., de Wit, H., McNamara, P., & Cao, D. (2011). Stimulant, and sedative alcohol responses and relationship to future binge drinking. *Archives of General Psychiatry, 68*(4), 389–399.

King, V., Brooner, R., Peirce, J., Kolodner, K., & Kidorf, M. (2014). A randomized trial of Web-based videoconferencing for substance abuse counselling. *Journal of Substance Abuse Treatment, 46*(1), 36–42.

King, V., Stoller, K., Kidorf, M., Kindbom, K., Hursh, S., Brady, T., & Brooner, R. (2009). Assessing the effectiveness of an Internet-based videoconferencing platform for delivering intensified substance abuse counseling. *Journal of Substance Abuse Treatment, 36*(3), 331–338.

Kirby, M. (2004). *Mental health, mental illness and addiction: Overview of policies and programs in Canada.* Ottawa, ON: The Senate Standing Committee on Social Affairs, Science and Technology.

Kirchmayer, U., Davoli, M., & Verster, A. (2003). Naltrexone maintenance treatment for opioid dependence. *The Cochrane Database of Systematic Reviews* (Issue 4, Art. No.: CD001333). doi:10.1002/14651858.CD001333

Kishline, A. (1994). *Moderate drinking: The new option for problem drinkers.* Tucson, AZ.: See Sharp Press.

Kitchener, K. (1984). Intuition, critical evaluation and ethical principles: The foundations for ethical decisions in counseling psychology. *Counseling Psychologist, 12*(1), 43–56.

Kliem, S., Kröger, C., & Kossfelder, J. (2010). Dialectical behavior therapy for borderline personality disorder: A meta-analysis using mixed-effects modeling. *Journal of Consulting and Clinical Psychology, 78*(6), 936–951.

Koehn, C., O'Neill, L., & Sherry, J. (2012). Hope-focused interventions in substance abuse counselling. *International Journal of Mental Health and Addiction, 10*(4), 441–452.

Kolden, G., Klein, M., Wang, C., & Austin, S. (2011). *Psychotherapy, 48*(1), 65–71.

Koltko-Rivera, M. (2006). Rediscovering the later version of Maslow's hierarchy of needs: Self-transcendence and opportunities for theory, research, and unification. *Review of General Psychology, 10*(4), 302–317.

Komro, K., Maldonado-Molina, M., Tobler, A., Bonds, J., & Muller, K. (2007). Effects of home access and availability of alcohol on young adolescents' alcohol use. *Addiction, 102*(10), 1597–1608.

Konova, A., Moeller, S., Tomasi, D., Volkow, N., & Goldstein, R. (2013). Effects of methylphenidate on resting-state functional connectivity of the mesocorticolimbic dopamine pathways in cocaine addiction. *JAMA Psychiatry, 70*(8), 857–868.

Koob, G., & Roberts, H. (1999). Brain reward circuits in alcoholism. *CNS Spectrums, 4*(1), 23–38.

Koski, A., Sirén, R., Vuori, E., & Poikolainen, K. (2007). Alcohol tax cuts and increase in alcohol-positive sudden deaths—a time-series intervention analysis. *Addiction, 102*(3), 362–368.

Kottler, J., & Montgomery, M. (2010). *Theories of counselling and therapy.* Thousand Oaks, CA: Sage.

Kozlowski, L., Wilkinson, A., Skinner, W., Kent, C., Franklin, T., & Pope, M. (1989). Comparing tobacco cigarette dependence with other drug dependencies greater or equal "difficulty quitting" and "urges to use," but less "pleasure" from cigarettes. *Journal of the American Medical Association, 261*(6), 898–901.

Kozor, R., Grieve, S., Buchholz, S., Kaye, S., Darke, S., Bhindi, R., & Figtree, G. (2014). Regular cocaine use is associated with increased systolic blood pressure, aortic stiffness and left ventricular mass in young otherwise healthy individuals. *PLoS One, 9*(4), e89710. doi:10.1371/journal.pone.0089710

Krabbe, P., Koning, J., Heinen, N., Laheij, R., Van Cauter, R., & De Jong, C. (2003). Rapid detoxification from opioid dependence under general anaesthesia versus standard methadone tapering: Abstinence rates and withdrawal distress experiences. *Addiction Biology, 8*(3), 351–358.

Kramer, P. (1993). *Listening to Prozac.* New York: Penguin Books.

Kranzler, H., & Van Kirk, J. (2006). Efficacy of naltrexone and acamprosate for alcoholism treatment: A meta-analysis. *Alcoholism: Clinical and Experimental Research, 25*(9), 1335–1341.

Kraus, D., Castonguay, L., Boswell, J., Nordberg, S., & Hayes, J. (2011). Therapist effectiveness: Implications for accountability and patient care. *Psychotherapy Research, 21*(3), 267–276.

Krebs, T., & Johansen, P. (2012). Lysergic acid diethylamide (LSD) for alcoholism: Meta-analysis. *Journal of Psychopharmacology, 26*(7), 994–1002.

Krogh, C. (1995). *Compendium of pharmaceuticals and specialties.* Ottawa, ON: Canadian Pharmaceutical Association.

Krystal, J., Cramer, J., Krol, W., Kirk, G., & Rosenheck, R. (2001). Naltrexone in the treatment of alcohol dependence. *New England Journal of Medicine, 345*(24), 1734-1739.

Ksaanetz, F., Deroche-Gamonet, V., Beerson, N., Balado, E., Lafourcade, M., Manzoni, O., & Piazza, P. (2010). Transition to addiction is associated with a persistent impairment in synaptic plasticity. *Science, 328*(5986), 1709–1712.

Kubiliene, A., Marksiene, R., Kazlauskas, S., Sadauskiene, I., Razukas, A., & Ivanov, L. (2008). Acute toxicity of ibogaine and noribogaine. *Medicina, 44*(12), 984–988.

Kuhar, M. (2002). Social rank and vulnerability to drug abuse. *Nature Neuroscience, 5*(2), 169–180.

Kulis, S., Marsiglia, F., Elek, E., Dustman, P., Wagstaff, D., & Hecht, M. (2005). Mexican/Mexican-American adolescents and keepin' it REAL: An evidence-based substance use prevention program. *Children and Schools, 27*(3), 133–145.

Kully-Martens, K., Treit, S., Pei, J., & Rasmussen, C. (2013). Affective decision-making on the Iowa Gambling Task in children and adolescents with fetal alcohol spectrum disorders. *Journal of the International Neuropsychological Society, 19*(2), 137–144.

Kumpfer, K., Alexander, J., McDonald, L., & Olds, D. (1998). Family-focused substance abuse prevention: What has been learned from other fields. In R. Ashery, E. Robertson, & K. Kumpfer (Eds.), *Drug abuse prevention through family interventions* (pp. 78–102). Rockville, MD: United States Department of Health and Human Services.

Kumpfer, K., & Alvarado, R. (2003). Family-strengthening approaches for the prevention of youth problem behaviors. *American Psychologist, 58*(6), 457–465.

Kumpfer, K., & Kaftarian, S. (2000). Bridging the gaps between family-focused research and substance abuse prevention practice: Preface. *The Journal of Primary Prevention, 21*(2), 169–183.

Kung, E., & Farrell, A. (2000). The roles of parents and peers in early adolescent substance use: An examination of mediating and moderating effects. *Journal of Child and Family Studies, 9*(4), 509–528.

Kurtz, L., & Powell, T. (1987). Three approaches to understanding self-help groups. *Social Work with Groups, 10*(3), 69–80.

Kus, R. (1995). Prayer and meditation in addiction recovery. *Journal of Chemical Dependency Treatment, 5*(2), 101–115.

Kyle, P., Iverson, R., Gajaogowni, R., & Spencer, L. (2011). Illicit bath salts: Not for bathing. *Journal of the Mississippi State Medical Association, 52*(12), 375–377.

Kypri, K., Dean, J., & Stojanovski, E. (2007). Parent attitudes on the supply of alcohol to minors. *Drug and Alcohol Review, 26*(1), 41–47.

Kypri, K., Voas, R., Langley, J., Stephenson, S., Begg, D., Tippets, A., & Davie, G. (2006). Minimum purchasing age for alcohol and traffic crash injuries among 15–19 year-olds in New Zealand. *American Journal of Public Health, 96*(1), 126–131.

LaBrie, J., Hummer, J., & Pedersen, E. (2007). Reasons for drinking in the college student context: The differential role and risk of the social motivator. *Journal of Studies on Alcohol and Drugs, 68*(3), 393–398.

Lachenmeier, D., Kanteres, F., & Rehm, J. (2009). Carcinogenicity of acetaldehyde in alcoholic beverages: Risk assessment outside ethanol metabolism. *Addiction, 104*(4), 533–550.

Ladouceur, R., & Walker, M. (1996). A cognitive perspective on gambling. In P. Salkovskies (Ed.), *Trends in cognitive and behavioural therapies* (pp. 89–120). Chichester, UK: John Wiley and Sons.

Lalazaryan, A., & Zare-Farashbandi, F. (2014). A review of models and theories of health information seeking behavior. *International Journal of Health System & Disaster Management, 2*(4), 193–203. Retrieved from www.ijhsdm.org/text.asp?2014/2/4/193/144371

Land, T., Keithly, L., Kane, K., Chen, L., Paskowsky, M., Cullen, D., ... Li, W. (2014). Recent increases in efficiency in cigarette nicotine delivery: Implications for tobacco control. *Nicotine & Tobacco Research, 16*(6), 753–758.

Lander, L., Howsare, J., & Byrne, M. (2013). The impact of substance use disorders on families and children: From theory to practice. *Social Work in Public Health, 28*(3-4), 194–205.

Landolfi, E. (2013). Exercise addiction. *Sports Medicine, 43*(2), 111–119.

Larimer, M. (2012). *From controlled drinking to housing first: Marlatt's impact on harm reduction research and practice*. Presented at the 120th American Psychological Association Annual Convention, Orlando, Florida, August 2–5.

Larimer, M., Malone, D., Garner, M., Atkins, D., Burlingham, B., Lonczak, H., ... & Marlatt, G. (2009). Health care and public service use and costs before and after provision of housing for chronically homeless persons with severe alcohol problems. *Journal of the American Medical Association, 301*(13), 1349–1357.

Latino-Martel, P., Chan, D., Druesne-Pecollo, N., Barrandon, E., Hercberg, S., & Norat, T. (2010). Maternal alcohol consumption during pregnancy and risk of childhood leukemia: Systematic review and meta-analysis. *Cancer Epidemiology Biomarkers and Prevention, 19*(5), 1238–1260.

Lawrence, A., Luty, J., Bogdan, N., Sahakian, B., & Clark, L. (2009). Impulsivity and response inhibition in alcohol dependence and problem gambling. *Psychopharmacology, 207*(1), 163–172.

Lawson, G. (1992). Twelve-step programs and the treatment of adolescent substance abusers. In G. Lawson & A. Lawson (Eds.), *Adolescent substance abuse: Etiology, treatment and prevention* (pp. 165–186). Gaithersberg, MD: Aspen Publications.

Lawson, G., Peterson, J., & Lawson, A. (1983). *Alcoholism and the family: A guide to treatment and prevention.* Gaithersberg, MD: Aspen Publications.

Lawson, P. (2005). Intervention in the workplace. In R. Csiernik (Ed.), *Wellness and work: Employee assistance programming in Canada* (pp. 203–208). Toronto, ON: Canadian Scholars' Press.

Le Dain Commission. (1973). *Final report of the Commission of Inquiry into the Non-Medical Use of Drugs.* Ottawa, ON: Information Canada.

Ledermann, S. (1956). *Alcohol, alcoholisme, alcoholisation* (Vol. 1). Paris: Presses Universitaires de France.

Lee, S., Humphreys, K., Flory, K., Liu, R., & Glass, K. (2011). Prospective association of childhood attention-deficit/hyperactivity disorder (ADHD) and substance use and abuse/dependence: A meta-analytic review. *Clinical Psychology Review, 31*(3), 328–341.

Leonardi-Bee, J., Britton, J., & Venn, A. (2011). Second hand smoke and adverse fetal outcomes in non-smoking pregnant women: A meta-analysis. *Pediatrics, 127*(4), 734–741.

Leshner, A. (1997). Addiction is a brain disease, and it matters. *Science, 278*(5335), 45–47.

Lesieur, H., & Rosenthal, R. (1991). Pathological gambling: A review of the literature. *Journal of Gambling Studies, 7*(1), 5–39.

Lethem, J. (2002). Brief solution focused therapy. *Child and Adolescent Mental Health, 7*(4), 189–192.

Lev-Rana, S., Le Foll, B., McKenzie, K., George, T., & Rehme, J. (2013). Cannabis use and cannabis use disorders among individuals with mental illness. *Comprehensive Psychiatry, 54*(6), 589–598.

Lev-Rana, S., Le Foll, B., McKenzie, K., & Rehme, J. (2012). Cannabis use and mental health-related quality of life among individuals with anxiety disorders. *Journal of Anxiety Disorders, 26*(8), 799–810.

Levinthal, C. (2012). *Drugs, behavior, and modern society* (7th ed.). Boston, MA: Allyn and Bacon.

Levy, J., Meek, P., & Rosenberg, M. (2014). US-based drug cost parameter estimation for economic evaluations. *Medical Decision Making.* doi:10.1177/0272989X14563987

Lewis, J., Dana, R., & Belevins, G. (1988). *Substance abuse counselling: An individualized approach.* Pacific Grove, CA.: Brooks/Cole Publishing.

Lewis, M., & Lockmuller, J. (1990). Alcohol reinforcement. *Alcohol Health and Research World, 14*(2), 98–103.

Li, H., Lu, Q., Xiao, E., Li, Q., He, Z., & Mei, X. (2014). Methamphetamine enhances the development of schizophrenia in first-degree relatives of patients with schizophrenia. *Canadian Journal of Psychiatry, 59*(2), 107–113.

Li, M., & Burmeister, M. (2009). New insights into the genetics of addiction. *Nature Reviews Genetics, 10*(4), 225–231.

Li, X., & Wolf, M. (2015). Multiple faces of BDNF in cocaine addiction. *Behavioural Brain Research, 279*(3), 240–254.

Licht, R. (2011). Lithium: Still a major option in the management of bipolar disorder. *CNS Neuroscience & Therapeutics, 18*(3), 219–226.

Liddle, H., & Hogue, A. (2000). A family-based development-ecological preventive intervention for high-risk adolescents. *Journal of Marital and Family Therapy, 26*(3), 265–279.

Lin, W., Jiang, R., Wu, H., Chen, F., & Liu, S. (2011). Smoking, alcohol, and betel quid and oral cancer: A prospective cohort study. *Journal of Oncology.* doi:10.1155/2011/525976

Linehan, M. (1993). *Cognitive behavioral treatment of borderline personality disorder.* New York: Guilford Press.

Linehan, M., Armstrong, H., Suarez, A., Allmon, D., & Heard, H. (1991). Cognitive-behavioral treatment of chronically parasuicidal borderline patients. *Archives of General Psychiatry, 48*(12), 1060–1064.

Linehan, M., Heard, H., & Armstrong, H. (1993). Naturalistic follow-up of a behavioral treatment of chronically parasuicidal borderline patients. *Archives of General Psychiatry, 50*(12), 971–974.

Lines, R. (2007). *The death penalty for drug offences: A violation of international human rights law.* London, UK: International Harm Reduction Association.

Linn, E. (1975). Clinical manifestation of psychiatric disorders. In A. Freedman, H. Kaplan, & B. Sadock (Eds.), *Comprehensive textbook of psychiatry* (pp. 990–1034). Baltimore, MD: Williams & Wilkins.

Lipton, D. (1995). *The effectiveness of treatment for drug abusers under criminal justice supervision.* Washington, DC: United States Department of Justice.

Litten, R., & Allen, J. (1998). Advances in the development of medications for alcoholism treatment. *Psychopharmacology, 139*(1-2), 20–33.

Llewellyn, D., Lang, I., Langa, K., Naughton, F., & Matthews, F. (2009). Exposure to second hand smoke and cognitive impairment in non-smokers: National cross sectional study with cotinine measurement. *British Medical Journal, 338.* doi:10.1136/bmj.b462

Lochman, J., & van den Steenhoven, A. (2002). Family-based approaches to substance abuse prevention. *The Journal of Primary Prevention, 23*(1), 49–114.

Loewenberg, F., & Dolgoff, R. (2008). *Ethical decision making for social work practice.* Itasca, IL: F.E. Peacock Publishers.

Longabaugh, R., & Morgenstern, J. (1999). Cognitive-behavioral coping-skills therapy for alcohol dependence: Current status and future directions. Alcohol Research and Health, 23(1), 78–85.

Lopez, G. (2014, September 10). The White House's plan to reform the war on drugs. *Vox Media.* Retrieved from www.vox.com/2014/9/10/6126541/the-white-houses-plan-to-reform-the-war-on-drugs

López-Muñoz, F., Ucha-Udabe, R., & Alamo, C. (2005). The history of barbiturates a century after their clinical introduction. *Journal of Neuropsychiatric Disease and Treatment, 1*(4), 329–343.

Loughran, H. (2009). Group work in the context of alcohol treatment. *Journal of Teaching in the Addictions, 9*(1-2), 125–141.

Lu, L., Liu, Y., Zhu, W., Shi, J., Liu, Y., Ling, W., & Kosten, T. (2009). Traditional medicine in the treatment of drug addiction. *American Journal of Drug and Alcohol Abuse, 35*(1), 1–11.

Ludwig, A. (1975). The psychiatrist as physician. *Journal of the American Medical Association, 234*(6), 603–604.

Lum, K., Polansky, J., Jackler, R., & Glantz, S. (2008). Signed, sealed and delivered: "Big tobacco" in Hollywood, 1927–1995. *Tobacco Control, 17*(4), 313–323.

Lundahl, B., Kunz, C., Brownell, C., Tollefson, D., & Burke, B. (2010). A meta-analysis of motivational interviewing: Twenty-five years of empirical studies. *Research on Social Work Practice, 20*(2), 137–160.

Lundborg, P. (2007). Parents' willingness to provide alcohol and adolescents' alcohol use: Evidence from Swedish data. *Vulnerable Children and Youth Studies, 2*(1), 60–70.

Lurie, Y., Gopher, A., Lavon, O., Almog, S., Sulimani, L., & Bentur, Y. (2012). Severe paramethoxymethamphetamine (PMMA) and paramethoxyamphetamine (PMA) outbreak in Israel. *Clinical Toxicology, 50*(1), 39–43.

Lynam, D., Milich, R., Zimmerman, R., Novak, S., Logan, T., Martin, C., ... Clayton, R. (1999). Project DARE: No effects at 10-year follow up. *Journal of Consulting and Clinical Psychology, 67*(4), 590–593.

Ma, G., & Thompson, B. (1999). Needs for youth substance abuse and violence prevention in schools and communities. *The Journal of Primary Prevention, 20*(2), 93–105.

Maas, U., & Strubelt, S. (2006). Fatalities after taking ibogaine in addiction treatment could be related to sudden cardiac death caused by autonomic dysfunction. *Medical Hypotheses, 67*(4), 960–964.

MacGregor, S., & Herring, R. (2010). *The Alcohol Concern SMART Recovery pilot project final evaluation report.* London, UK: Middlesex University.

MacKinnon, D., & Lockwood, C. (2003). Advances in statistical methods for substance abuse prevention research. *Prevention Science, 4*(3), 155–171.

MacMaster, S. (2004). Harm reduction: A new perspective on substance abuse services. *Journal of Social Work, 49*(3), 356–363.

Maertens, R., White, P., Rickert, W., Levasseur, G., Douglas, G., Bellier, P., ... Desjardins, S. (2009). The genotoxicity of mainstream and sidestream marijuana and tobacco smoke condensates. *Chemical Research in Toxicology, 22*(8), 1406–1414.

Magill, M. (2015). Branding addiction therapies and reified specific factors. *Addiction, 110*(3), 415–416.

Magill, M., & Ray, L. (2009). Cognitive-behavioral treatment with adult alcohol and illicit drug users: A meta-analysis of randomized controlled trials. *Journal of Studies on Alcohol and Drugs, 70*(4), 516–527.

Mahabee-Gittens, E., Xiao, Y., Gordon, J., & Khoury, J. (2013). The dynamic role of parental influences in preventing adolescent smoking initiation. *Addictive Behaviors, 38*(4), 1905–1911.

Main, M., & Solomon, J. (1986). Discovery of an insecure-disorganized/disoriented attachment pattern: Procedures, findings and implications for the classification of behavior. In T. Brazelton & M. Yogman (Eds.), *Affective development in infancy* (pp. 95–124). Norwood, NJ: Ablex.

Main, T. (1946). The hospital as a therapeutic institution. *Bulletin of the Menninger Clinic, 10*(1), 66–70.

Maisto, S., Galizio, M., & Connors, G. (1995). *Drug use and abuse.* Toronto, ON: Harcourt Press.

Malik, P., Gasser, R., Kemmler, G., Moncayo, R., Finkenstedt, G., Kurz, M., & Fleischhacker, W. (2008). Low bone mineral density and impaired bone metabolism in young alcoholic patients without liver cirrhosis: A cross-sectional study. *Alcoholism: Clinical and Experimental Research, 33*(2), 375–381.

Mandell, W., Olden, M., Wenzel, S., Dahl, J., & Ebener, P. (2008). Do dimensions of TC treatment predict retention and outcomes? *Journal of Substance Abuse Treatment, 35*(3), 223–231.

Manning, N. (1989). *The therapeutic community movement: Charisma and routinization.* London, UK: Routledge.

Manzardo, A., Stein, L., & Belluzzi, J. (2002). Rats prefer cocaine over nicotine in a two-lever self-administration choice test. *Brain Research, 924*(1), 10–19.

Marlatt, G. (1973). A comparison of aversive conditioning procedures in the treatment of alcoholism. Anaheim, CA: Western Psychological Association.

Marlatt, G. (1985). Relapse prevention: Theoretical rationale and overview of the model. In G. Marlatt & J. Gordon (Eds.), *Relapse prevention* (pp. 3–70). New York: Guilford Press.

Marlatt, G., & George, W. (1984). Relapse prevention: Introduction and overview of the model. *British Journal of Addiction, 79*(3), 261–273.

Marlatt, G., & Gordon, J. (Eds.). (1985). *Relapse prevention.* New York: Guilford Press.

Marovino, T. (1994). Laser auriculotherapy as part of the nicotine detoxification process: Evaluation of 1280 subjects and theoretical considerations of a developing model. *American Journal of Acupuncture, 22*(2), 129–135.

Marrelli, A. (2001). *Introduction to competency modeling.* New York: American Express.

Marsiglia, F., Holleran, L., & Jackson, K. (2000). Assessing the effects of external resources on school-based substance abuse prevention programs. *Social Work in Education, 22*(3), 145–161.

Martin, W., Minatrea, N., & Watson, J. (2009). Animal-assisted therapy in the treatment of substance dependence. *Anthrozoos: A Multidisciplinary Journal of the Interactions of People and Animals, 22*(2), 137–148.

Martins, S., & Alexandre, P. (2009). The association of ecstasy use and academic achievement among adolescents in two U.S. national surveys. *Addictive Behaviors, 34*(1), 1–124.

Marx, K. (2004). *Capital: A critique of political economy* (Vol. 1). London, UK: Penguin Books.

Maslow, A. (1970). *Motivation and personality.* New York: Harper & Row.

Matt, G., Quintana, P., Zakarina, J., Fortmann, A., Chatfield, D., Hoh, E., ... Hovell, M. (2011). When smokers move out and non-smokers move in: Residential thirdhand smoke pollution and exposure. *Tobacco Control, 20*(1), e1. doi:10.1136/tc.2010.037382

Maurel, D., Boisseau, N., Benhamou, C., & Jaffe, C. (2011). Alcohol and bone: Review of dose effects and mechanisms. *Osteoporosis International, 13*(1), 56–64.

Maxwell, M. (1984). *The Alcoholics Anonymous experience.* Toronto, ON: McGraw-Hill Books.

May, C. (1997). Habitual drunkards and the invention of alcoholism: Susceptibility and culpability in nineteenth century medicine. *Addiction Research, 5*(2), 169–187.

May, C. (2001). Pathology, identity and the social construction of alcohol dependence. *Sociology, 35*(2), 385–401.

McCarthy, D., Mycyk, M., & DesLauriers, C. (2006). Hospitalization for caffeine abuse is associated with concomitant abuse of other pharmaceutical products. *Annals of Emergency Medicine, 48*(4), 101.

McCarty, D. (2008). *Substance abuse treatment benefits and costs knowledge asset.* Robert Wood Johnson Foundation's Substance Abuse Policy Research Program. Retrieved from http://saprp.org/knowledgeassets/knowledge_detail.cfm?KAID=1

McClelland, D., Davis, W., Kalin, R., & Wanner, E. (1972). *The drinking man.* New York: Free Press.

McCollister, K., & French, M. (2003). The relative contribution of outcome domains in the total economic benefit of addiction interventions: A review of first findings. *Addiction, 98*(12), 1647–1659.

McConaghy, N., Armstrong, M., Blaszczynski, A., & Allcock, C. (1983). Controlled comparison of aversive therapy and imaginal desensitisation in compulsive gambling. *British Journal of Psychiatry, 142*(4), 366–372.

McConnell, H. (1989). Sick behaviours. *The Journal, 16*(1), 14.

McCrady, B., Epstein, E., Cook, S., Jensen, N., & Hildebrandt, T. (2009). A randomized trial of individual and couple behavioral alcohol treatment for women. *Journal of Consulting and Clinical Psychology, 77*(2), 243–256.

McElrath, D. (1997). The Minnesota model. *Journal of Psychoactive Drugs, 29*(2), 141–144.

McElroy, S., Keck, P., Pope, H., Smith, J., & Strakowski, S. (1994). Compulsive buying: A report of 20 cases. *Journal of Clinical Psychiatry, 55*(6), 242–248.

McGraw, M. (2012). Is your patient high on bath salts? *Nursing, 42*(1), 26–32.

McGregor, C., Ali, R., White, J., Thomas, P., & Gowing, L. (2002). A comparison of antagonist-precipitated withdrawal under anesthesia to standard inpatient withdrawal as a precursor to maintenance naltrexone treatment in heroin users: Outcomes at 6 and 12 months. *Drug and Alcohol Dependence, 68*(1), 5–14.

McGue, M., Iacono, W., & Krueger, R. (2006). The association of early adolescent problem behavior and adult psychopathology: A multivariate behavioral genetic perspective. *Behavior Genetics, 36*(4), 591–602.

McKay, J. (2005). Is there a case for extended interventions for alcohol and drug use disorders? *Addiction, 100*(11), 1594–1610.

McKay, J., Van Horn, D., Oslin, D., Ivey, M., Drapkin, M., Coviello, D., … Lynch, K. (2011). Extended telephone-based continuing care for alcohol dependence: 24-month outcomes and subgroup analyses. *Addiction, 106*(10), 1760–1769.

McKim, W., & Hancock, H. (2013). *Drugs and behavior* (7th ed.). Englewood Cliffs, NJ: Prentice Hall.

McLellan, A., Arndt, I., Metzger, D., Woody, G., & O'Brien, C. (1993). The effects of psychosocial services in substance abuse treatment. *Journal of the American Medical Association, 269*(15), 1953–1959.

McLellan, A., Hagan, T., Levine, M., Gould, F., Meyers, K., Bencivengo, M., & Durell, J. (1998). Supplemental social services improve outcomes in public addiction treatment. *Addiction, 93*(10), 1489–1499.

McLellan, A., Luborsky, L., Woody, G., O'Brien, C., & Druley, K. (1983). Increased effectiveness of substance abuse treatment: A prospective study of patient-treatment "matching." *Journal of Nervous and Mental Disorders, 171*(10), 597–605.

McMorris, B., Catalano, R., Kim, M., Toumbourou, J., & Hemphill, S. (2011). Influence of family factors and supervised alcohol use on adolescent alcohol use and harms: Similarities between youth in different alcohol policy contexts. *Journal of Studies on Alcohol and Drugs, 72*(3), 418–428.

Mehra, R., Moore, B., Crothers, K., Tetrault, J., & Fiellin, D. (2006). The association between marijuana smoking and lung cancer. *Archives of Internal Medicine, 166*(13), 1359–1367.

Meier, P. (2008). *Independent review of the effects of alcohol pricing and promotion.* Sheffield, UK: University of Sheffield.

Meissner, W., Schmidt, U., Hartmann, M., Kah, R., & Reinhart, K. (2000). Oral naloxone reverses opioid-associated constipation. *Pain, 84*(1), 105–109.

Melinyshyn, M., Christie, R., & Shirley, M. (1996). *Travelling the same road: A report on concurrent disorders in Ontario.* Toronto, ON: Addiction Research Foundation.

Merikle, P. (1988). Subliminal auditory messages: An evaluation. *Psychology and Marketing, 5*(4), 355–372.

Merlin, M. (2003). Archaeological evidence for the tradition of psychoactive plant use in the Old World. *Economic Botany, 57*(3), 295–323.

Messinis, L., Kyprianidou, A., Malefaki, S., & Papathanasopoulos, P. (2006). Neuropsychological deficits in long-term frequent cannabis users. *Neurology, 66*(5), 737–739.

Methadone Strategy Working Group. (2001). *Countering the crisis: Ontario's prescription for opioid dependence.* Toronto, ON: Methadone Strategy Working Group.

Meyer, R. (1989). Prospects for a rational pharmacotherapy of alcoholism. *Journal of Clinical Psychiatry, 50*(11), 403–412.

Middlemiss, P. (2002). Home detox gains support. *GP: General Practitioner, 32.* Retrieved from www.accessmylibrary.com/article-1G1-87784108/gp-business-home-detox.html

Midford, R., Munro, G., McBride, N., Snow, P., & Ladzinski, U. (2002). Principles that underpin effective school-based drug education. *Journal of Drug Education, 32*(4), 363–386.

Millati Islami World Services. (2010a). 12 steps. Retrieved from www.millatiislami.org/Welcome/12-steps

Millati Islami World Services. (2010b). 12 traditions. Retrieved from www.millatiislami. org/Welcome/12-traditions

Miller, M., Swanson, S., Azrael, D., Pate, V., & Stürmer, T. (2014). Antidepressant dose, age, and the risk of deliberate self-harm. *JAMA Internal Medicine, 174*(6), 899–909.

Miller, N. (1999). Mortality risks in alcoholism and effects of abstinence and addiction treatment. *Addictive Disorders, 22*(2), 371–383.

Miller, N., & Gold, M. (1990). The disease and adaptive models of addiction: A re-evaluation. *Journal of Drug Issues, 20*(1), 29–35.

Miller, P., Book, S., & Stewart, S. (2011). Medical treatment of alcohol dependence: A systematic review. *The International Journal of Psychiatry in Medicine, 42*(3), 227–266.

Miller, S., & Berg, I. (1995). *The miracle method: A radically new approach to problem drinking.* New York: W.W. Norton.

Miller, W. (1983a). Controlled drinking: A history and a critical review. *Journal of Studies on Alcohol, 44*(1), 68–82.

Miller, W. (1983b). Motivational interviewing with problem drinkers. *Behavioural Psychotherapy, 11*(2), 147–172.

Miller, W. (1995). Increasing motivation for change. In R. Hester & W. Miller (Eds.), *Handbook of alcoholism treatment approaches: Effective alternatives,* (2nd ed., pp. 89–104). Boston, MA: Allyn & Bacon.

Miller, W., Forcehimes, A., & Zweben, A. (2011). *Treating addiction: A guide for professionals.* New York: Guilford Press.

Miller, W., & Hester, R. (1986a). The effectiveness of alcoholism treatment: What research reveals. In W. Miller & N. Heather (Eds.)., *Treating addictive behaviors: Processes of change* (pp. 121–174). New York: Plenaum Press.

Miller, W., & Hester, R. (1986b). Inpatient alcoholism treatment: Who benefits? *American Psychologist, 41*(7), 794–805.

Miller, W., & Hunter, L. (1991). Household context and youth smoking behaviour. *Canadian Journal of Public Health, 82*(1), 83–85.

Miller, W., & Rollnick, S. (1991). *Motivational interviewing: Preparing people to change addictive behaviour.* New York: Guilford Press.

Miller, W., & Rollnick, S. (2002). *Motivational interviewing: Preparing people for change. 2nd ed.* New York: Guilford Press.

Miller, W., & Rollnick, S. (2009). Ten things that motivational interviewing is not. *Behavioural and Cognitive Psychotherapy, 37*(2), 129–140.

Miller, W., & Rose, G. (2009). Toward a theory of motivational interviewing. *American Psychologist, 64*(6), 527–537.

Miller-Day, M. (2002). Parent-adolescent communication about alcohol, tobacco, and other drug use. *Journal of Adolescent Research, 17*(6), 604–616.

Minkoff, K., Zweben, J., Rosenthal, R., & Ries, R. (2004). Development of service intensity criteria and program categories for individuals with co-occurring disorders. *Journal of Addictive Diseases, 22*(S1), 113–129.

Minnesota Department of Education. (1992). *Promising prevention strategies: A look at what works*. St. Paul, MN: Minnesota Department of Education.

Mirabile, R. (1997). Everything you wanted to know about competency modeling. *Training and Development, 51*(8), 73–78.

Mirin, S. (1984). Behavioral factors in drug dependency and withdrawal: A discussion. In G. Serban (Ed.), *The social and medical aspects of drug abuse* (pp. 205–213). New York: Spectrum Publishing.

Mirmiran, M., Scholtens, J., van de Poll, N., Uylings, H., van der Gugten, J., & Boer, G. (1983). Effects of experimental suppression of active REM sleep during early development upon adult brain and behavior in the rat. *Brain Research, 283*(2-3), 277–286.

Miron, J. (1999). *Violence and the U.S. prohibitions of drugs and alcohol. American Law and Economics Review, 1*(1), 78-114.

Miron, J. (2005). *The budgetary implications of marijuana prohibition*. Retrieved from http://chanvreinfo.ch/info/en/IMG/pdf/The_Budgetary_Implications_of_Marijuana_Prohibition_MironReport_2005.pdf

Miron, J. (2008). *The budgetary implications of drug prohibition*. Retrieved from http://leap.cc/dia/miron-economic-report.pdf

Miron, J., & Waldock, K. (2010). *The budgetary impact of ending drug prohibition*. Boston, MA: Cato Institute.

Moderation Management. (2014). *What is Moderation Management?* Retrieved from www.moderation.org/whatisMM.shtml

Mohai, C. (1991). *Are school-based drug prevention programs working?* Retrieved from http://eric.ed.gov/?q=Mohai%2c+&id=ED341886

Monahan, R. (1977). Secondary prevention of drug dependence through the transcendental meditation program in metropolitan Philadelphia. *The International Journal of the Addictions, 12*(6), 729–754.

Montgomery, S., & Ekbom, A. (2002). Smoking during pregnancy and children's risk of diabetes. *British Medical Journal, 324*(7328), 26–27.

Montoya, I., Atkinson, J., & McFaden, W. (2003). Best characteristics of adolescent gateway drug prevention programs. *Journal of Addictions Nursing, 14*(2), 75–83.

Moore, B., Fazzino, T., Garnet, B., Cutter, C., & Barry, D. (2011). Computer-based interventions for drug use disorders: A systematic review. *Journal of Substance Abuse Treatment, 40*(3), 215–223.

Moos, R. (2005). Iatrogenic effects of psychosocial interventions for substance use disorders: Prevalence, predictors, prevention. *Addiction, 100*(5), 595–604.

Moran, M. (2009). Psychiatrists write fewer than 1 in 4 psychoactive prescriptions. *Psychiatric News, 44*(20), 10.

Morgan, C., Muetzelfeldt, L., & Curran, H. (2008). Ketamine use, cognition and psychological well-being: A comparison of frequent, infrequent and ex-users with polydrug and non-using controls. *Addiction, 104*(1), 77–87.

Morgan, S., Smolina, K., Mooney, D., Raymond, C., Bowen, M., Gorczynski, C., & Rutherford, K. (2013). *The Canadian Rx atlas* (3rd ed.). Vancouver, BC: UBC Centre for Health Services and Policy Research.

Morzorati, L., Ramchandani, V., Fleury, L., Li, T., & O'Connor, S. (2002). Self-reported subjective perception of intoxication reflects family history of alcoholism when breath alcohol levels are constant. *Alcoholism, Clinical and Experimental Research, 26*(8), 1299–1306.

Motiuk, L., & Vuong, B. (2002). *Homicide, sex, robbery and drug offenders in federal corrections: An end-of-2001 review.* Ottawa, ON: Correctional Service of Canada Research Branch.

Moussas, G., Christodoulou, C., & Douzenis, A. (2009). A short review on the aetiology and pathophysiology of alcoholism. *Annals of General Psychiatry, 8*(1). doi:10.1186/1744-859X-8-10

Moyers, T., Martin, T., Manuel, J., Hendrickson, S., & Miller, W. (2005). Assessing competence in the use of motivational interviewing. *Journal of Substance Abuse Treatment, 28*(1), 19–26.

Mukamal, K. (2012). Understanding the mechanisms that link alcohol and lower risk of coronary heart disease. *Clinical Chemistry, 58*(4), 664–666.

Muller, A., & Clausen, T. (2014). Group exercise to improve quality of life among substance use disorder patients. *Scandinavian Journal of Public Health.* doi:10.1177/1403494814561819

Munafo, M., & Johnstone, E. (2008). Genes and cigarette smoking. *Addiction, 103*(6), 893–904.

Murphy, E. (1922). *The black candle.* Toronto, ON: Thomas Allen.

Myers, R., & Miller, W. (2001). *A community reinforcement approach to addiction treatment.* Cambridge, UK: Cambridge University Press.

Myers, R., Villanueva, M., & Smith J. (2005). The community reinforcement approach: History and new directions. *Journal of Cognitive Psychotherapy: An International Quarterly, 19*(3), 251–264.

Nadler, A., Holder, J., & Talsky, M. (1998). Torque release technique: A technique model for chiropractic's second century. *Canadian Chiropractor, 3*(1), 1–6.

Nair, U., Bartsch, H., & Nair, J. (2004). Alert for an epidemic of oral cancer due to use of the betel quid substitutes gutkha and pan masala: A review of agents and causative mechanisms. *Mutagenesi, 19*(9), 251–262.

Nakken, C. (1996). *The addictive personality: Understanding the addictive process and compulsive behavior.* Center City, MN: Hazelden.

Nance, E. (1992). Inpatient treatment of alcoholism: A necessary part of the therapeutic armamentarium. *Psychiatric Hospital, 21*(1), 9–12.

Naqvi, N., Rudrauf, D., Damasio, H., & Antoine Bechara, A. (2007). Damage to the insula disrupts addiction to cigarette smoking. *Science, 315*(5811), 531–534.

Narcotics Anonymous. (1987). *Narcotics Anonymous* (4th ed.). Van Nuys, CA: Narcotics Anonymous World Services.

Narcotics Anonymous. (2009). *History.* Retrieved from www.na12.org/index.php/history.html

Nasrulla, A. (2000). Khat: Harmless stimulant or addictive drug? *Journal of Addiction and Mental Health, 3*(3), 5–7.

Nation, J., Cardon, A., Heard, H., Valles, R., & Bratton, G. (2003). Perinatal lead exposure and relapse to drug-seeking behavior in the rat: A cocaine reinstatement study. *Psychopharmacology, 168*(1-2), 236–243.

Nation, J., Livermore, C., & Bratton, G. (1995). Cadmium exposure attenuates the initiation of behavioral sensitization to cocaine. *Brain Research, 70*(1-2), 223–232.

Nation, M., Crusto, C., Wandersman, A., Kumpfer, K., Seybolt, D., Morrissey-Kane, E., & Davino, K. (2003). What works in prevention: Principles of effective prevention programs. *American Psychologist, 58*(6), 449–456.

National Center on Addiction and Substance Abuse. (2009). *The importance of family dinners V.* New York: Columbia University.

National Center on Addiction and Substance Abuse. (2012). *The importance of family dinners VIII.* New York: Columbia University.

National Clearinghouse on Tobacco and Health (1991). *Fact sheet series.* Ottawa, ON: National Clearinghouse on Tobacco and Health.

National Institute on Alcohol Abuse and Alcoholism. (1996). *How to cut down on your drinking.* Washington, DC: US Department of Health and Human Services, National Institutes of Health.

National Institute on Alcohol Abuse and Alcoholism. (2000). *Alcohol alert 48.* Washington, DC: US Department of Health and Human Services, National Institutes of Health.

National Institute on Alcohol Abuse and Alcoholism. (2005). *Helping patients who drink too much: A clinician's guide* (NIH Publication No. 07-3769). Washington, DC: US Department of Health and Human Services, National Institutes of Health. Retrieved from http:// pubs.niaaa.nih.gov/publications/Practitioner/CliniciansGuide2005/guide.pdf

National Institute on Drug Abuse. (1988). *A cognitive behavioral approach: Treating cocaine addiction.* Washington, DC: US Department of Health and Human Services, National Institutes of Health.

National Institute on Drug Abuse. (2007). *The science of addiction: Drugs, brains and behavior.* Washington, DC: US Department of Health and Human Services, National Institutes of Health.

National Institute on Drug Abuse. (2010). *Research report series: Inhalant abuse* (NIH Publication No. 10-3818). Washington, DC: US Department of Health and Human Services, National Institutes of Health.

National Institute on Drug Abuse. (2012). *The science of drug abuse and addiction.* Retrieved from www.drugabuse.gov/publications/media-guide/science-drug-abuse-addiction

National Treatment Agency. (2012). *Estimating the crime reduction benefits of drug treatment and recovery.* London, UK: National Health Service.

National Treatment Strategy Working Group. (2008). *A systemic approach to substance use in Canada.* Ottawa, ON: National Framework for Action to Reduce the Harms Associated with Alcohol and Other Drugs and Substances in Canada.

Neher, A. (1991). Maslow's theory of motivation: A critique. *Journal of Humanistic Psychology, 31*(3), 89–112.

Nencini, P., Ahmed, A., & Elmi, A. (1986). Subjective effects of khat chewing in humans. *Drug and Alcohol Dependence, 18*(1), 97–105.

Nestler, E. (2005). The neurobiology of cocaine addiction. *Science and Practice Perspectives, 3*(1), 3–4.

Neuberger, K. (2012). The status of horticultural therapy around the world: Practice, research, education. *Acta Horticulture, 954*(2), 187–189.

Nicosia, N., Pacula, R., Kilmer, B., Lundberg, R., & Chiesa, J. (2009). *The economic cost of methamphetamine use in the United States, 2005.* Santa Monica, CA: RAND Corporation.

Nidecker, M., DiClemente, C., Bennett, M., & Bellack, A. (2008). Application of the Transtheoretical Model of Change: Psychometric properties of leading measures in patients with co-occurring drug abuse and severe mental illness. *Addictive Behaviors, 33*(8), 1021–1030.

Nilsen, P. (2010). Brief alcohol intervention—where to from here? Challenges remain for research and practice. *Addiction, 105*(6), 954–959.

Nixon, S., Tivis, R., & Parsons, O. (1992). Interpersonal problem-solving in male and female alcoholics. *Alcoholism: Clinical and Experimental Research, 16*(4), 684–687.

Noone, M., Dua, J., & Markham, R. (1999). Stress, cognitive factors, and coping resources as predictors of relapse in alcoholics. *Addictive Behaviors, 24*(5), 687–693.

Norström, T., & Pape, H. (2012). Associations between adolescent heavy drinking and problem drinking in early adulthood: Implications for prevention. *Journal of Studies on Alcohol and Drugs, 73*(4), 542–548.

Nosyk, B., Geller, J., Guh, D., Oviedo-Joekes, E., Brissette, S., Marsh, D., ... Anis, A. (2010). The effect of motivational status on treatment outcome in the North American Opiate Medication Initiative (NAOMI) study. *Drug and Alcohol Dependence, 111*(1-2), 161–165.

Nosyk, B., Marshall, B., Fischer, B., Montaner, J., Wood, E., & Kerr, T. (2012). Increases in the availability of prescribed opioids in a Canadian setting. *Drug and Alcohol Dependence, 126*(1), 7–12.

Nutt, D., King, L., Saulbury, W., & Blakemore, C. (2007). Development of a rational scale to assess the harm of drugs of potential misuse. *The Lancet, 369*(9566), 1047–1053.

Oberg, M., Jaakkola, M., Woodward, A., Peruga, A., & Pruss-Ustun, A. (2011). Worldwide burden of disease from exposure to second-hand smoke: A retrospective analysis of data from 192 countries. *The Lancet, 377*(9760), 139–146.

Ocean, G., & Smith, G. (1993). Social reward, conflict and commitment: A theoretical model of gambling behavior. *Journal of Gambling Studies, 9*(4), 321–339.

O'Connell, D. (2002). Managing psychiatric comorbidity in inpatient addictions treatment. In D. O'Connell & E. Beyer (Eds.), *Managing the dually diagnosed patient: Current issues and clinical approaches* (pp. 3–28). New York: Haworth Press.

O'Connell, M., Kasprow, W., & Rosenheck, R. (2013). The impact of current alcohol and drug use on outcomes among homeless veterans entering supported housing. *Psychological Services, 10*(2), 241–249.

Odjers, C., Caspi, A., Nagin, D., Piquero, A., Slutske, W., Milne, B., ... Moffitt, T. (2008). Is it important to prevent early exposure to drugs and alcohol among adolescents? *Psychological Science, 19*(10), 1037–1044.

Office of the Auditor General of Ontario. (2008). *2008 Annual Report.* Toronto, ON: Queen's Printer for Ontario.

Ogborne, A., Annis, H., & Sanchez-Craig, M. (1978). *Report of the task force on halfway houses.* Toronto, ON: Addiction Research Foundation.

Ogborne, A., & Graves, G. (2005). Optimizing Canada's addiction treatment workforce: Results of a national survey of service providers. Ottawa, ON: Canadian Centre on Substance Abuse.

O'Hanlon, W., & Weiner-Davis, M. (1989). *In search of solutions: A new direction in psychotherapy.* New York: W. W. Norton.

O'Hare, T. (2005). *Evidence-based practices for social workers.* Chicago, IL: Lyceum.

Ohlendorf-Moffat, P. (1993). Addictions as allergies. *Pathways, 2*(1), 6–8.

Oksanen, A. (2013). Deleuze and the theory of addiction. *Journal of Psychoactive Drugs, 45*(1), 57–67.

O'Malley, S., Jaffe, A., Chang, G., Schottenfeld, R., Meyer, R., & Rounsaville, B. (1992). Naltrexone and coping skills therapy for alcohol dependence. *Archives of General Psychiatry, 49*(11), 881–887.

Ontario Ministry of Health and Long Term Care. (2010). *Methylphenidate extended release.* Toronto, ON: Province of Ontario.

Orford, J., Velleman, R., Natera, G., Templeton, L., & Copello, A. (2013). Addiction in the family is a major but neglected contributor to the global burden of adult ill-health. *Social Science and Medicine, 78*(1), 70–77.

Osmond, M., & Kimberley, M. (2010). Patterns of intimacy and sexual expression in interaction with addictions. In R. Csiernik & W. Rowe (Eds.), *Responding to the oppression of addiction: Canadian social work responses* (2nd ed., pp. 149–168). Toronto, ON: Canadian Scholars' Press.

Oster, R. (1983). Peer counseling: Drug and alcohol abuse prevention. *Journal of Primary Prevention, 3*(3), 188–199.

Ota, A., Akimaru, K., Suzuki, S., & Ono, Y. (2008). Depictions of smoking in recent high-grossing Japanese movies. *Tobacco Control, 17*(2), 143–144.

Overstreet, D., Miller, C., Janowksy, D., & Russell, R. (1996). Potential animal model of multiple chemical sensitivity with cholinergic supersensitivity. *Toxicology, 111*(1-3), 119–134.

Paglia, A., & Room, R. (1999). Preventing substance use problems among youth: A literature review and recommendations. *The Journal of Primary Prevention, 20*(1), 3–50.

Pandey, G., Fawcett, J., Gibbons, R., Clark, C., & Davis, J. (1988). Platelet monoamine oxidase in alcoholism. *Biological Psychiatry, 24*(1), 15–24.

Pape, B. (1990). *Self-help/mutual aid.* Toronto, ON: Canadian Mental Health Association.

Paris, J. (2005). *The fall of an icon: Psychoanalysis and academic psychiatry.* Toronto, ON: University of Toronto Press.

Parrott, A. (2014). The potential dangers of using MDMA for psychotherapy. *Journal of Psychoactive Drugs, 46*(1), 37–43.

Parssinen, T., & Kerner, K. (1980). Development of the disease model of drug addiction in Britain, 1870–1926. *Medical History, 24*(3), 275–296.

Patra, J., Giesbrecht, N., Rehm, J., & Bekmuradov, D. (2012). Are alcohol prices and taxes an evidence-based approach to reducing alcohol-related harm and promoting public health and safety: A literature review. *Contemporary Drug Problems, 39*(1), 7–48.

Pattison, E., Sobell, M., & Sobell, L. (1977). *Emerging concepts of alcohol dependence.* New York: Springer.

Paul, S. (2006). Alcohol-sensitive GABA receptors and alcohol antagonists. *Proceedings of the National Academy of Science, 103*(22), 8307–8308.

Pauly, B., Reist, D., Belle-Isle, L., & Schactman, C. (2013). Housing and harm reduction: What is the role of harm reduction in addressing homelessness? *International Journal of Drug Policy, 24*(4), 284–290.

Peachy, J. (1986). The role of drugs in the treatment of opioid addicts. *The Medical Journal of Australia, 145*(4), 395–399.

Peele, S. (1983). *The science of experience.* Lexington, MA: Lexington Books.

Peele, S. (1985). What treatment for addiction can do and what it can't; what treatment for addiction should do and what it shouldn't. *Journal of Substance Abuse Treatment, 2*(3), 225–228.

Peele, S. (1989). Ain't misbehavin'—addiction has become an all-purpose excuse. *The Sciences,* (July/August), 1–10.

Peele, S., & Brodsky, A. (1992). *Truth about addiction and recovery.* New York: Simon & Schuster.

Pelchat, M. (2002). Of human bondage: Food craving, obsession, compulsion, and addiction. *Physiology and Behavior, 76*(3), 347–352.

Pendery, M., Maltzman, I., & West, L. (1982). Controlled drinking by alcoholics? New findings and a re-evaluation of a major affirmative study. *Science, 217*(4555), 169–175.

Peralta, R., & Steele, J. (2010). Nonmedical prescription drug use among US college students at a midwest university: A partial test of social learning theory. *Substance Use and Misuse, 45*(6), 865–887.

Pernell-Arnold, A., & Finley, L. (2012). Training mental health providers in cultural competence: A transformative learning process. *Journal of Psychiatric Rehabilitation, 15*(4), 334–356.

Perrino, T., Coatsworth, J., Briones, I., Pantin, H., & Szapocznic, J. (2001). Initial engagement in parent-centered preventive interventions: A family systems perspective. *The Journal of Primary Prevention, 22*(1), 21–44.

Perry, C., Komro, K., Veblen-Mortenson, S., Bosma, L., Farbakhsh, K., Munson, K., … Lytle, L. (2003). A randomized controlled trial of middle and junior high school D.A.R.E. and D.A.R.E. plus programs. *Archives of Pediatric Medicine, 157*(2), 178–184.

Pescosolido, B., Martin, J., Long, S., Medina, T., Phelan, J., & Link, B. (2010). "A disease like any other"? A decade of change in public reactions to schizophrenia, depression, and alcohol dependence. *American Journal of Psychiatry, 167*(11), 1321–1330.

Petersen, K. (1987). *Company town: Potlatch, Idaho, and the Potlatch Lumber Company.* Pullman, WA: Washington State University Press.

Peterson, J., Nisenholz, B., & Robinson, G. (2003). *A nation under the influence: America's addiction to alcohol.* New York: A and B.

Petroff, O. (2002). GABA and glutamate in the human brain. *Neuroscientist, 8*(6), 562–573.

Petry, N. (2005). *Pathological gambling: Etiology, comorbidity, and treatment.* Washington, DC: American Psychological Association.

Petry, N. (2012). *Contingency management for substance abuse treatment: A guide to implementing this evidence-based practice.* New York: Taylor & Francis.

Pettit, B. (2012). *Invisible men: Mass incarceration and the myth of black progress.* New York: Russell Sage Foundation.

Pickard, H. (2012). The purpose in chronic addiction. *American Journal of Behavioral Neuroscience, 3*(2), 40–49.

Piper, D., Moberg, D., & King, M. (2000). The Healthy for Life project: Behavioral outcomes. *The Journal of Primary Prevention, 21*(1), 47–73.

Plomin, R., Haworth, C., & Davis, O. (2009). Common disorders are quantitative traits. *Nature Reviews Genetics, 10*(12), 872–878.

Podymow, T., Turnbull, J., Coyle, D., Yetisir, E., & Wells, G. (2006). Shelter-based managed alcohol administration to chronically homeless people addicted to alcohol. *Canadian Medical Association Journal, 174*(1), 45–49.

Polcin, D. (2009). Communal-living settings for adults recovering from substance abuse. *Journal of Groups in Addiction and Recovery, 4*(1-2), 7–22.

Polcin, D., Mericle, A., Howell, J., Sheridan, D., & Christensen, J. (2014). Maximizing social model principles in residential recovery settings. *Journal of Psychoactive Drugs, 46*(5), 436–443.

Pollack, M., Penava, S., Bolton, E., Worthington, J., Allen, G., Farach, F., & Otto, M. (2002). A novel cognitive-behavioral approach for treatment-resistant drug dependence. *Journal of Substance Abuse Treatment, 23*(2), 133–142.

Ponee, C. (1982). *The historical development of employee assistance programs.* Toronto, ON: Addiction Research Foundation.

Popova, S., Mohapatra, S., Patra, J., Duhig, A., & Rehm, J. (2011). A literature review of cost-benefit analyses for the treatment of alcohol dependence. *International Journal of Environmental Research and Public Health, 8*(8), 3351–3364.

Porath-Waller, A. (2009). *Maternal cannabis use during pregnancy.* Ottawa, ON: Canadian Centre on Substance Abuse.

Poulin, C., & Nicholson, J. (2005). Should harm minimization as an approach to adolescent substance use be embraced by junior and senior high schools? *International Journal of Drug Policy, 16*(6), 403–414.

Powell, C., Stevens, S., Lo Dolce, B., Sinclair, K., & Swenson-Smith, C. (2012). Outcomes of a trauma-informed Arizona family drug court. *Journal of Social Work Practice in the Addictions, 12*(3), 219–241.

Pratt, O., Rooprai, H., Shaw, G., & Thomson, A. (1990). The genesis of alcoholic brain tissue injury. *Alcohol and Alcoholism, 25*(2-3), 217–230.

Price, R., Hilchey, C., Darredeau, C., Fulton, H., & Barrett, S. (2010). Brief communication: Energy drink co-administration is associated with increased reported alcohol ingestion. *Drug & Alcohol Review, 29*(3), 331–333.

Price, R., Nock, M., Charney, D., & Mathew, S. (2009). Effects of intravenous ketamine on explicit and implicit measures of suicidality in treatment-resistant depression. *Biological Psychiatry, 66*(5), 522–526.

PRIDE Canada. (2001). *Parent's guide to prevention.* Saskatoon, SK: University of Saskatchewan.

Primack, B., Douglas, E., & Kraemer, K. (2009). Exposure to cannabis in popular music and cannabis use among adolescents. *Addiction, 105*(3), 515–523.

Pringsheim, T., Lam, D., & Patten, S. (2011). The pharmacoepidemiology of antipsychotic medications for Canadian children and adolescents: 2005–2009. *Journal of Child and Adolescent Psychopharmacology, 21*(6), 537–543.

Prior, V., & Glaser, D. (2006). *Understanding attachment and attachment disorders: Theory, evidence and practice.* London, UK: Jessica Kingsley Publishers.

Prochaska, J. (2008). Decision making in the Transtheoretical Model of behavior change. *Medical Decision Making, 28*(6), 845–849.

Prochaska, J., & DiClemente, C. (1982). Stages and process of self-change in smoking: Towards an integrative model of change. *Psychotherapy, 20*(2), 161–173.

Prochaska, J., DiClemente, C., & Norcross, J. (1992). In search of how people change: Applications to addictive behaviors. *American Psychologist, 47*(9), 1102–1114.

Prochaska, J., & Velicer, W. (1997). The Transtheoretical Model of health behavior change. *American Journal of Health Promotion, 12*(1), 38–48.

Propel Centre for Population Health Impact. (2014). *2012/2013 youth smoking survey: Results profile.* Waterloo, ON: University of Waterloo.

Pruett, J., Nishimura, N., & Priest, R. (2007). The role of meditation in addiction recovery. *Counseling and Values, 52*(1), 71–84.

Psychoyos, D., & Vinod, K. (2013). Marijuana, spice "herbal high," and early neural development: Implications for rescheduling and legalization. *Drug Test Analysis, 5*(1), 27–45.

Ptaszik, A. (2007). The courage to laugh: Comedy program fights stigma, boosts self-esteem. *Crosscurrents, 10*(3), 4–5.

Pugh, A. (2004). Harnessing the benefits of animal assisted therapy. *Crosscurrents, 8*(2), 5.

Purdue Pharma. (2004). *Palladone.* Stamford, CN: Purdue Pharma.

Quinones, M. (1975). Drug abuse during the Civil War (1861–1865). *The International Journal of the Addictions, 10*(6), 1007–1020.

Quirion, B. (2014). Modalités et enjeux du traitement sous contrainte auprès des toxicomanes. *Santé mentale au Québec, 39*(2), 39–56.

Rabasseda, X. (2011). A report from the 2011 annual meeting of the American Academy of Allergy, Asthma and Immunology (March 18–22, 2011, San Francisco). *Drugs of Today, 47*(4), 313–323.

Rahula, W. (2006). *What the Buddha taught.* Colombo, Sri Lanka: Buddhist Cultural Centre.

Ramchandani, V., Umhau, J., Pavon, F., Ruiz-Velasco, V., Margas, W., Sun, H., ... Heilig, M. (2011). A genetic determinant of the striatal dopamine response to alcohol in men. *Molecular Psychiatry, 16*(6), 809–817.

Randolph, T. (1956). The descriptive features of food addiction: Addictive eating and drinking. *Quarterly Journal of Studies on Alcohol, 17*(2), 198–224.

Rankin, J. (1978). Etiology. In L. Phillips, G. Ramsey, L. Blumenthal, & P. Crawshaw (Eds.), *Core knowledge in the drug field.* Ottawa, ON: Health and Welfare Canada.

Rapp, C., & Goscha, R. (2006). *The strengths model: Case management with people with psychiatric disabilities.* New York: Oxford University Press.

Rasmussen, N. (2014). Stigma and the addiction paradigm for obesity: Lessons from 1950s America. *Addiction, 110*(2), 217–225.

Ray, W., Taylor, J., Meador, K., Lichtenstein, M., Griffin, M., Fought, R., ... Blazer, D. (1993). Reducing antipyschotic drug use in nursing homes: *A controlled trial of provider education. Archives of Internal Medicine, 153*(6), 713–721.

Redmond, C., Spoth, R., Shin, C., & Lepper, H. (1999). Modeling long-term parent outcomes of two universal family-focused preventive interventions: One year follow-up results. *Journal of Consulting and Clinical Psychology, 67*(6), 975–984.

Reed, D. (2015). Ultra-violet indoor tanning addiction: A reinforcer pathologies interpretation. *Addictive Behaviors, 41*(4), 247–251.

Rehm, J., Baliunas, D., Brochu, S., Fischer, B., Gnam, W., Patra, J., … Single E. (2006). *The costs of substance abuse in Canada, 2002.* Ottawa, ON: Canadian Centre on Substance Abuse.

Rehm, J., Mathers, C., Popova, S., Thavorncharoensap, M., Teerawattananon, Y., & Patra, J. (2009). Global burden of disease and injury and economic cost attributable to alcohol use and alcohol-use disorders. *The Lancet, 373*(9682), 2223–2233.

Reich, T. (1988). Beyond the gene. *Alcohol Health and Research World, 12*(4), 104–108.

Reid, J., Hammond, D., Rynard, V., & Burkhalter, R. (2014). *Tobacco use in Canada: Patterns and trends.* Waterloo, ON: Propel Centre for Population Health Impact, University of Waterloo.

Reinarman, C. (2005). Addiction as accomplishment: The discursive construction of disease. *Addiction Research and Theory, 13*(4), 307–320.

Resnicow, K., & Botvin, G. (1993). School-based substance use prevention programs: Why do effects decay? *Preventive Medicine, 22*(4), 484–490.

Resnicow, K., Soler, R., Braithwaite, R., Ahluwalia, J., & Butler, J. (2000). Cultural sensitivity in substance use prevention. *Journal of Community Psychology, 28*(3), 271–290.

Riba, J., Valle, M., Urbana, M., Yritia, M., Morteand, M., & Barbonoj, M. (2011). Human pharmacology of ayahuasca: Subjective and cardiovascular effects, monoamine metabolite excretion and pharmacokinetics. *The Journal of Pharmacology and Therapeutics, 306*(1), 73–83.

Richards, J., & Rodgers, T. (2001). *Approaches to methods in language and teaching* (2nd ed.). Cambridge, UK: Cambridge University Press.

Richards, M., Jarvis, M., Thompson, N., & Wadsworth, M. (2003). Cigarette smoking and cognitive decline in midlife: Evidence from a prospective birth cohort study. *American Journal of Public Health, 93*(6), 994–998.

Rickards, L., McGraw, S., Araki, L., Casey, R., High, C., Hombs, M., & Raysor, R. (2010). Collaborative initiative to help end chronic homelessness: Introduction. *Journal of Behavioral Health Services & Research, 37*(2), 149–166.

Riley, D. (1998). *Drugs and drug policy in Canada: A brief review and commentary.* Ottawa, ON: Canadian Foundation for Drug Policy & International Harm Reduction Association.

Riley, D., Sobell, L., Leo, G., Sobell, M., & Klajner, F. (1985) *Behavioural treatment of alcohol problems: A review and a comparison of behavioural studies.* Toronto, ON: Addiction Research Foundation.

Ritz, B., Ascherio, A., Checkoway, H., Marder, K., Nelson, L., Rocca, W., … Gorell, J. (2007). Pooled analysis of tobacco use and risk of Parkinson disease. *Archives of Neurology, 64*(7), 990–997.

Roberto, M., Cruz, M., Gilpin, N., Sabino, V., Schweitzer, P., Baio, M., … Parsons, L. (2010). Corticotropin releasing factor-induced amygdala gamma-aminobutyric acid release plays a key role in alcohol dependence. *Biological Psychiatry, 67*(9), 831–839.

Roberts, G., McCall, D., Stevens-Lavigne, A., Anderson, J., Paglia, A., Bollenbach, S., … Gliksman, L. (2001). *Preventing substance use problems among young people: A compendium of best practices.* Ottawa, ON: Health Canada.

Roberts, G., Ogborne, A., Leigh, G., & Adam, L. (1999). *Profile of substance abuse treatment and rehabilitation in Canada.* Ottawa, ON: Health Canada.

Roberts, L., Shaner, A., & Eckman, T. (1999). *Overcoming addictions: Skills training for people with schizophrenia.* New York: W.W. Norton.

Robins, L., Helzer, J., Hesselbrock, M., & Wish, E. (2010). Vietnam veterans three years after Vietnam: How our study changed our view of heroin. *American Journal on Addictions, 19*(3), 203–211.

Robinson, D., & Henry, S. (1977). *Self-help and health.* Bungay, UK: Chaucer Press.

Roche, A., Watt, K., & Fischer, J. (2001). General practitioners' views of home detoxification. *Drug & Alcohol Review, 20*(4), 395–406.

Rodu, B., & Jansson, C. (2004). Smokeless tobacco and oral cancer: A review of the risks and determinants. *Critical Reviews in Oral Biology and Medicine, 15*(5), 252–263.

Roffman, R. (1976). Addiction concepts and the Vietnam experience. *Urban and Social Change Review, 9*(2), 16–18.

Rogers, C. (1959). *Psychology: A study of a science.* Toronto, ON: McGraw-Hill.

Rogers, G., Elston, J., Garside, R., Roome, C., Taylor, R., Younger, P., … Somerville, M. (2009). The harmful health effects of recreational ecstasy: A systematic review of observational evidence. *Health Technology Assessment, 13*(6), 1–315.

Rojas, M. (2015). Suffering ailments and addiction problems in the family. *World Suffering and Quality of Life: Social Indicators Research Series, 56,* 203–216.

Rollnick, S., & Miller, W. (1995). What is motivational interviewing? *Behavioural and Cognitive Psychotherapy, 23*(4), 325–334.

Rollnick, S., Miller, W., & Butler, C. (2008). *Motivational interviewing in health care: Helping patients change behavior.* New York: Guilford Press.

Romeder, J. (1990). *The self-help way: Mutual aid and health.* Ottawa, ON: Canadian Council on Social Development.

Ronsley, R., Scott, D., Warburton, W., Hamdi, R., Louie, D., Davidson, J., & Panagiotopoulos, C. (2013). A population-based study of antipsychotic prescription trends in children and adolescents in British Columbia from 1996–2011. *Canadian Journal of Psychiatry, 58*(6), 361–369.

Room, R., Stoduto, G., Demers, A., Ogborne, A., & Giesbrecht, N. (2006). Alcohol in the Canadian context. In N. Giesbrecht, A. Demers, & E. Lindquist (Eds.), *Sober reflections: Commerce, public health, and the evolution of alcohol policy in Canada, 1980-2000* (pp. 14–42). Montreal, QC: McGill-Queen's University Press.

Roozen, H., Waart, R., & Van Der Kroft, P. (2010). Community reinforcement and family training: An effective option to engage treatment-resistant substance-abusing individuals in treatment. *Addiction, 105*(10), 1729–1738.

Rose, J., Behm, F., Salley, A., Bates, J., Coleman, R., Hawk, T., & Turkington, T. (2007). Regional brain activity correlates of nicotine dependence. *Neuropsychopharmacology, 32*(12), 2441–2452.

Rose, R., Dick, D., Viken, R., Pulkkinen, L., & Kaprio, J. (2001). Drinking or abstaining at age 14? A genetic epidemiological study. *Alcoholism, Clinical and Experimental Research, 25*(11), 1594–1604.

Rosecrance, J. (1985). Compulsive gambling and the medicalization of deviance. *Social Problems, 32*(3), 275–284.

Rosengren, D., & Wagner, C. (2001). Motivational interviewing: Dancing, not wrestling. In R. Coombs (Ed.), *Addiction recovery tools: A practice handbook*. London, UK: Safe Publications.

Rosenthal, R. (1992). Pathological gambling. *Psychiatric Annals, 22*(2), 72–78.

Rösner S., Hackl-Herrwerth, A., Leucht, S., Lehert, P., Vecchi, S., & Soyka, M. (2010). Acamprosate for alcohol dependence. *Cochrane Database of Systematic Reviews* (Issue 9, Art. No.: CD004332). doi:10.1002/14651858.CD004332.pub2

Ross, E., Reisfield, G., Watson, M., Chronister, C., & Goldberger, B. (2012). Psychoactive "bath salts" intoxication with methylenedioxypyrovalerone. *The Amercian Journal of Medicine, 125*(9), 854–858.

Rossow, I., & Norström, T. (2012). The impact of small changes in bar closing hours on violence: The Norwegian experience from 18 cities. *Addiction, 107*(3), 530–537.

Roth, A., & Fonagy, P. (2005). *What works for whom? A critical review of psychotherapy research.* New York: Guilford Press.

Rothenberg, J., Sullivan, M., Church, S., Seracini, A., Collins, E., Kleber, H., & Nunes, E. (2002). Behavioral naltrexone therapy: An integrated treatment for opiate dependence. *Journal of Substance Abuse Treatment, 23*(4), 351–360.

Rowe, W., & Gonzalez, C. (2010). Supervised injection sites: Harm reduction and health promotion. In R. Csiernik & W. Rowe (Eds.), *Responding to the oppression of addiction: Canadian social work perspectives* (2nd ed., pp. 35–46). Toronto, ON: Canadian Scholars' Press.

Royal Canadian Mounted Police. (2006). *Drug situation in Canada*. Ottawa, ON: RCMP

Royal Canadian Mounted Police. (2010). *Drug situation in Canada*. Ottawa, ON: RCMP

Rugle, L. (1993). Initial thought on viewing pathological gambling from a physiological and intrapsychic structural perspective. *Journal of Gambling Studies, 9*(1), 3–16.

Rush, B., & Ogborne, S. (1992). Alcoholism treatment in Canada: History, current status, and emerging issues. In H. Klingemann, J.-P. Takala, & G. Hunt (Eds.), *Cure, care, or control: Alcoholism treatment in sixteen countries* (pp. 253–267). Albany, NY: SUNY Press.

Russell, M. (1984). *Handbook of feminist therapy.* New York: Springer Publishing.

Rutman, D., & Van Bibber, M. (2010). Parenting with fetal alcohol spectrum disorder. *International Journal of Mental Health and Addiction, 8*(3), 351–361.

Rychtarik, R., Foy, D., Scott, T., Lokey, L., & Prue, D. (1987). Five-six year follow-up of broad spectrum behavioral treatment for alcoholism: Effects of training controlled drinking skills. *Journal of Consulting and Clinical Psychology, 55*(2), 106–108.

Rydell, C., Caulkins, J., & Everingham, S. (1996). Enforcement or treatment? Modeling the relative efficacy of alternatives for controlling cocaine. *Operations Research, 44*(1), 1–9.

Saal, D., Dong, Y., Bonci, A., & Malenka, R. (2003). Drugs of abuse and stress trigger: A common synaptic adaptation in dopamine neurons. *Neuron, 37*(4), 577–582.

Sachs, D. (2009). A psychological analysis of the 12 Steps of Alcoholics Anonymous. *Alcoholism Treatment Quarterly, 27*(2), 199–212.

Sacks, S., Skinner, D., Sacks, J., & Peck, A. (2002). *Manual for engaging homeless mentally ill chemical abusers in a modified TC shelter program.* New York: National Development and Research Institutes.

St. Pierre, T., & Kaltreider, D. (1997). Strategies for involving parents of high-risk youth in drug prevention: A three-year longitudinal study in boys & girls clubs. *Journal of Community Psychology, 25*(5), 473–485.

Sale, E., Sambrano, S., Springer, J., & Turner, C. (2003). Risk protection and substance use in adolescents: A multi-site model. *Journal of Drug Education, 33*(1), 91–105.

Saleh, S., Vaughn, T., Levey, S., Fuortes, L., Uden-Holmen, T., & Hall, J. (2006). Cost-effectiveness of case management in substance abuse treatment. *Research on Social Work Practice, 16*(1), 38–47.

Salmon, R., & Salmon, S. (1977). The causes of heroin addiction: A review of the literature. *The International Journal of the Addictions, 12*(5), 679–696.

Samaan, Z. (2014). Testosterone suppression and methadone treatment in men and women treated for opoid dependence with methadone. *Journal of Child Psychology and Psychiatry, 38*(4), 457–469.

Santamarina-Rubio, E., Perez, K., Ricart, I., Rodriguez-Sanz, A., Rodriguez-Martos, M., Brugal, T., ... Suelves, J. (2009). Substance use among road traffic casualties admitted to emergency departments. *Injury Prevention, 15*(1), 87–94.

Santos, K., Palmini, A., Radziuk A., Rotert, R., & Bastos, F. (2013). The impact of methylphenidate on seizure frequency and severity in children with attention-deficit–hyperactivity disorder and difficult-to-treat epilepsies. *Developmental Medicine & Child Neurology, 55*(7), 654–660.

Sargent, J., Beach, M., Adachi-Mejia, A., Gibson, J., Titus-Ernstoff, L., Carusi, C., ... Dalton, M. (2005). Exposure to movie smoking: Its relation to smoking initiation among US adolescents. *Pediatrics, 116*(5), 1183–1191.

Sartor, C., Grant, J., Bucholz, K., Madden, P., Heath, A., Agrawal A., ... Lynskey, M. (2009). Common genetic contributions to alcohol and cannabis use and dependence symptomatology. *Alcoholism: Clinical and Experimental Research, 34*(3), 545–554.

Saucier, G., & Goldberg, L. (1996). Evidence for the big five in analyses of familiar English personality adjectives. *European Journal of Personality, 10*(1), 61–77.

Scanlon, W. (1988). *Alcoholism and drug abuse in the workplace: Employee assistance programs.* Toronto, ON: Praeger.

Schaps, E., DiBartolo, R., Moskowitz, J., Palley, C., & Churgin, S. (1981). A review of 127 drug abuse prevention program evaluations. *Journal of Drug Issues, 11*(1), 17–43.

Schenk, S., Hunt, T., Klukowski, G., & Amit, Z. (1987). Isolation housing decreases the effectiveness of morphine in the conditioned taste aversion paradigm. *Psychopharmacology, 92*(1), 48–51.

Schenk, S., Lacelle, G., Gorman, K., & Amit, Z. (1987). Cocaine self-administration in rats influenced by environmental conditions: Implication for the etiology of drug abuse. *Neuroscience Letters, 81*(3), 227–231.

Schiff, P., Jr. (2006). Ergot and its alkaloids. *American Journal of Pharmaceutical Education, 70*(5), 98.

Schilder, P. (1941). The psychogenesis of alcoholism. *Quarterly Journal of Studies on Alcoholism, 2*(3), 277–292.

Schiller, L. (1997). Rethinking stages of development in women's groups: Implications for practice. *Journal of Social Work with Groups, 20*(3), 3–19.

Schindler, A., Thomasius, R., Ack, P., Gemeinhardt, B., Kustner, U., & Echert, J. (2005). Attachment and substance use disorders: A review of the literature and a study of drug dependent adolescents. *Attachment and Human Development, 7*(3), 207–228.

Schinke, S., Di Noia, J., & Glassman, J. (2004). Computer-mediated intervention to prevent drug abuse and violence among high-risk youth. *Addictive Behaviors, 29*(1), 225–229.

Schinke, S., Orlandi, M., Botvin, G., Gilchrist, L., Trimble, J., & Locklear, V. (1988). Preventing substance abuse among American-Indian adolescents: A bicultural competence skills approach. *Journal of Counseling Psychology, 35*(1), 87–90.

Schinke, S., & Schwinn, T. (2005). Gender-specific computer-based interventions for preventing drug abuse among girls. *The American Journal of Drug and Alcohol Abuse, 31*(4), 609–616.

Schleichert, E. (1996). *Marijuana.* Springfield, IL: Enslow Publisher Inc.

Schlosser, S., Black, D., Repertinger, S., & Freet, D. (1994). Compulsive buying: Demography, phenomenology, and comorbidity in 46 subjects. *General Hospital Psychiatry, 16*(3), 205–212.

Schmidt, W., & Popham, R. (1978). The single distribution theory of alcohol consumption. *Journal of Studies on Alcohol, 39*(3), 400–419.

Schottenfeld, R., Pascale, R., & Sokolowski, S. (1992). Matching services to needs: Vocational services for substance abusers. *Journal of Substance Abuse Treatment, 9*(1), 3–8.

Schuckit, M., Wilhelmsen, K., Smith, T., Feiler, H., Lind, P., Lange, L., & Kalmijn, J. (2005). Autosomal linkage analysis for the level of response to alcohol. *Alcoholism: Clinical and Experimental Research, 29*(11), 1976–1982.

Schutten, M., & Eijnden, R. (2003). *Alcohol and the workplace: A European comparative study on preventive and supportive measures for problem drinkers in their working environment.* Brussels, BE: European Commission on Employment and Social Affairs.

Schwarz, A. (2013, February 2). Drowned in a stream of prescriptions. *The New York Times.* Retreived from http://www.nytimes.com/2013/02/03/us/concerns-about-adhd-practices-and-amphetamine-addiction.html?_r=0

Scott, W., Kaiser, D., Othmer, S., & Sideroff, S. (2005). Effects of an EEG biofeedback protocol on a mixed substance abusing population. *American Journal of Drug and Alcohol Abuse, 31*(3), 455–469.

Secular Organization for Sobriety. (2014). *Who we are.* Retrieved from http://sossobriety. org/about.html

Segal, B., & Stewart, J. (1996). Substance use and abuse in adolescence: An overview. *Child Psychiatry and Human Development, 26*(4), 193–210.

Self-Help Canada. (1992). *Self-help groups in Canada.* Ottawa, ON: Self-Help Canada.

Self-Help Clearinghouse of Toronto. (1991). *Directory of self-help/mutual aid groups in Metropolitan Toronto.* Toronto, ON: Self-Help Clearinghouse of Toronto.

Seto, A., Einarson, T., & Koren, G. (1997). Pregnancy outcome following first trimester exposure to antihistamines: Meta-analysis. *American Journal of Perinatology, 14*(3), 119–124.

Sewell, R., Halpern, J., & Pope, H., Jr. (2006). Response of cluster headache to psilocybin and LSD. *Neurology, 66*(12), 1920–1922.

Seymour, R., & Smith, D. (2011). The physician's guide to psychoactive drugs. New York: Routledge.

Shafey, O., Eriksen, M., Ross, H., & Mackay, J. (2009). *The tobacco atlas* (3rd ed.). Atlanta, GA: American Cancer Society.

Shaham, Y., Alvares, K., Nespor, S., & Grunberg, N. (1992). Effect of stress on oral morphine and fenatyl self-administration in rats. *Pharmacology, Biochemistry, and Behavior, 41*(3), 615–619.

Sharpe, L., & Tarrier, N. (1993). Towards a cognitive-behavioural theory of problem gambling. *British Journal of Psychiatry, 162*(3), 407–412.

Shenassa, E. (2002). Delivering the goods: The importance of screening accuracy for effective community intervention and prevention. *Journal of Community Psychology, 30*(2), 197–210.

Shepard, J., & Carlson, J. (2003). An empirical evaluation of school-based prevention programs that involve parents. *Psychology in Schools, 40*(6), 641–656.

Shope, J., Elliot, M., Raghunathan, T., & Waller, P. (2001). Long-term follow-up of a high school alcohol misuse prevention program's effect on students' subsequent driving. *Alcoholism: Clinical and Experimental Research, 25*(3), 403–410.

Short, M., Black, L., Smith, A., Wetterneck, C., & Wells, D. (2012). A review of Internet pornography use research: Methodology and content from the past 10 years. *Cyberpsychology, Behavior, and Social Networking, 15*(1), 13–23.

Shuckit, M. (1999). New findings on the genetics of alcoholism. *Journal of the American Medical Association, 281*(20), 1875–1876.

Shumway, S., Bradshaw, S., Harris, K., & Baker, A. (2013). Important factors of early addiction recovery and inpatient treatment. *Alcoholism Treatment Quarterly, 31*(1), 3–24.

Siegal, H., Lane, D., Falck, R., Wang, J., Carlson, R., Rahman, A., & Chambers, D. (2001). Constructing a consensus-based prevention outcome measurement instrument. *Journal of Drug Education, 31*(2), 139–152.

Sikorsky, I., Jr. (1990). *AA's godparents*. Minneapolis, MN: CompCare Publishers.

Silverman, P. (1980). *Mutual aid groups*. Beverly Hills, CA: Sage.

Simons, F., & Simons, K. (2011). Histamine and H_1-antihistamines: Celebrating a century of progress. *Journal of Allergy and Clinical Immunology, 128*(6), 1139–1150.

Sinclair, K. (1998). *The drinker's handbook*. London, ON: ADSTV.

Singer, M. (2006). *Something dangerous: Emergent and changing illicit drug use and community health*. Long Grove, IL: Wavelength Press.

Single, E., Brewster, J., MacNeil, P., Hatcher, J., & Trainor, C. (1995). *Alcohol and drug use: Results from the 1993 General Social Survey*. Ottawa, ON: Canadian Centre on Substance Abuse.

Single, E., Robson, L., Xie, X., & Rehm, J. (1996). *The cost of substance abuse in Canada*. Ottawa, ON: Canadian Centre on Substance Abuse.

Sisson, R., & Azrin, N. (1986). Family-member involvement to initiate and promote treatment of problem drinking. *Journal of Behavior Therapy and Experimental Psychiatry, 17*(1), 15–21.

Skara, S., & Sussman, S. (2003). A review of 25 long-term adolescent tobacco and other drug use prevention program evaluations. *Preventive Medicine, 37*(5), 451–474.

Skog, O. (1980). Total alcohol consumption: Rates of excessive use. *British Journal of Addictions, 75*(3), 133–145.

Smart, R., Gray, G., Finley, J., & Carpen, R. (1977). A comparison of recidivism rates for alcohol detox residents referred to hospitals, halfway houses, and outpatient facilities. *The American Journal of Drug and Alcohol Abuse, 4*(2), 223–232.

Smart, R., Storm, T., Baker, E., & Solursh, L. (1967). *Lysergic acid dietyhlamine in the treatment of alcoholism.* Toronto, ON: Addiction Research Foundation.

SMART Recovery. (2015). *Self management for addiction recovery.* Retrieved from www.smartrecovery.org/

Smedslund, G., Berg, R., Hammerstrøm, K., Steiro, A., Leiknes, K., Dahl, H., & Karlsen, K. (2011). Motivational interviewing for substance abuse. *Cochrane Database of Systematic Reviews* (Issue 5, Art. No.: CD008063). doi:10.1002/14651858.CD008063.pub2

Smith, J., Mansfield, E., & Herrick, H. (1959). The treatment of chronic alcoholics with citrated calcium carbimide (Temposil). *American Journal of Psychiatry, 115*(9), 822–824.

Smith, K., Conroy, C., & Ehler, B. (1984). Lethality of suicide attempt rating scale. *Suicide and Life-Threatening Behavior, 14*(4), 215–242.

Smith, R., & Feigenbaum, K. (2012). Maslow's intellectual betrayal of Ruth Benedict? *Journal of Humanistic Psychology, 53*(3), 307–321.

Snyder, L., Milici, F., Slater, M., Sun, H., & Strizhakova, Y. (2006). Effects of alcohol advertising exposure on drinking among youth. *Archives of Pediatrics & Adolescent Medicine, 160*(1), 18–24.

Snyder, S. (1977). Opiate receptors and internal opiates. *Scientific American, 236*(3), 44–56.

So, M., Bozzo, P., & Inoue, M. (2010). Safety of antihistamines during pregnancy and lactation. *Canadian Family Physician, 56*(5), 427–429.

Sobeck, J., Abbey, A., & Agius, E. (2006). Lessons learned from implementing school-based substance abuse prevention curriculum. *Children and Schools, 28*(2), 77–85.

Sobell, M., & Sobell, L. (1973). Individualized behavior therapy for alcoholics. *Behavior Therapy, 4*(1), 49–72.

Sobell, M., & Sobell, L. (1974). Alternatives to abstinence: Time to acknowledge reality. *Addictions, 2*(1), 2–29.

Solomon, R., Richmond, J., & Usprich, S. (1989). *Overview of alcohol and drug law.* Toronto, ON: Addiction Research Foundation.

Sonnenstuhl, W., & Trice, H. (1986). *Strategies for employee assistance programs: The crucial balance.* Cornell, NY: IRL Press.

Spaderna, M., Addy, P., & D'Souza, D. (2013). Spicing things up: Synthetic cannabinoids. *Psychopharmacology, 228*(4), 525–540.

Specht, H., & Courtney, M. (1994). *Unfaithful angels: How social work has abandoned its mission.* Toronto, ON: Maxwell Macmillan Canada.

Special Committee on Non-Medical Use of Drugs. (2002). *Policy for the new millennium: Working together to redefine Canada's drug strategy.* Ottawa, ON: Public Works and Government Services Canada.

Spek, V., Cuijpers, P., Nyklicek, I., Riper, H., Keyzer, K., & Pop, V. (2007). Internet-based cognitive behaviour therapy for symptoms of depression and anxiety: A meta-analysis. *Psychological Medicine, 37*(3), 319–328.

Spielmans, G., & Parry, P. (2010). From evidence-based medicine to marketing-based medicine: Evidence from internal industry documents. *Journal of Bioethical Inquiry, 7*(1), 13–29.

Spinella, M. (2001). *The psychopharmacology of herbal medicine: Plant drugs that alter mind, brain, and behavior.* Cambridge, MA: MIT Press.

Spoth, R., & Redmond, C. (2000). Research on family engagement in preventive interventions: Toward improved use of scientific findings in primary prevention practice. *The Journal of Primary Prevention, 21*(2), 267–284.

Sproule, B. (2004). *Pharmacology and drug abuse* (2nd ed.). Toronto, ON: Centre on Addiction and Mental Health.

Sproule, B., Brands, B., Li, S., & Catz-Biro, L. (2009). Changing patterns in opioid addiction: Characterizing users of oxycodone and other opioids. *Canadian Family Physician, 55*(1), 68–69.

Srisurapanont, M., & Jarusuraisin, N. (2005). Naltrexone for the treatment of alcoholism: A meta-analysis of randomized controlled trials. *The International Journal of Neuropsychopharmacology, 8*(2), 267–280.

Srivastava, A., & Kahan, M. (2006). Buprenorphine: A potential new treatment option for opioid dependence. *Canadian Medical Association Journal, 174*(13), 1835.

Standing Committee on National Health and Welfare. (1987). *Booze, pills and dope: Reducing substance abuse in Canada.* Ottawa, ON: Queen's Printer for Canada.

Stapleton, J. (2009). Do the 10 UK suicides among those taking the smoking cessation drug varenicline suggest a causal link? *Addiction, 104*(5), 864–865.

Statistics Canada. (2014). *Sales of alcohol beverages by volume, value and per capita 15 years and over, fiscal years ended March 31.* Retrieved from www5.statcan.gc.ca/cansim/a26?lang=e ng&retrLang=eng&id=1830006&paSer=&pattern=&stByVal=1&p1=1&p2=31&tabMo de=dataTable&csid=

Stein, U., Greyer, H., & Hentscehl, H. (2001). Nutmeg (myristicin) poisoning: Report on a fatal case and a series of cases recorded by a poison information centre. *Forensic Science International, 118*(1), 87–90.

Steinglass, P. (1992). Family systems approaches to the alcoholic family. In S. Saitoh, P. Steinglass, & M. Schuckit (Eds.), *Alcoholism and the family* (pp. 155–171). New York: Brunner/Mazel.

Stevens, A. (2010). *Drugs, crime and public health: The political economy of drug policy.* New York: Routledge-Cavendish.

Stimson, G. (1995). AIDS and injecting drug use in the United Kingdom, 1987–1993: The policy response and the prevention of the epidemic. *Social Science Medicine, 41*(5), 699–716.

Stockwell, T., Bolt, E., & Hooper, J. (1986). Detoxification from alcohol at home managed by general practitioners. *British Medical Journal, 292*(6522). doi:http://dx.doi.org/10.1136/bmj.292.6522.733

Stockwell, T., Bolt, L., Milner, I., Pugh, P., & Young, I. (1990). Home detoxification for problem drinkers: Acceptability to clients, relatives, general practitioners and outcome after 60 days. *British Journal of Addiction, 85*(1), 61–70.

Stockwell, T., Pauly, B., Chow, C., Vallance, K., & Perkin, K. (2013). *Evaluation of a managed alcohol program in Vancouver, BC: Early findings and reflections on alcohol harm reduction* (CARBC Bulletin #9). Victoria, BC: University of Victoria.

Stockwell, T., Zhao, J., Macdonald, S., Vallance, K., Gruenwald, P., Ponicki, W., Holder, H., & Treno, A. (2011). Impact on alcohol-related mortality of a rapid rise in the density of private liquor outlets in British Columbia: A local area multi-level analysis. *Addiction, 106*(4), 768–776.

Stohl, M. (1988). The case of the missing gene: Hereditary protection against alcoholism. *Alcohol Health and Research World, 12*(4), 130–136.

Strohschein, L. (2007). Prevalence of methylphenidate use among Canadian children following parental divorce. *Canadian Medical Journal, 176*(12), 1711–1714.

Stuart, P. (1998). Home detox reaches more women, older adults. *Addictions News for Professionals, 27*(2), 6.

Substance Abuse and Mental Health Services Administration (SAMHSA). (2008). *Participation in self-help groups for alcohol and illicit drug use: 2006 and 2007.* Rockville, MD: SAMHSA.

Substance Abuse and Mental Health Services Administration (SAMHSA). (2013). *The DAWN report: Emergency department visits involving accidental ingestion of drugs by children aged 5 or younger.* Rockville, MD: SAMHSA.

Sumnall, H., Woolfall, K., Cole, J., Mackridge, A., & McVeigh, J. (2008). Diversion and abuse of methylphenidate in light of new guidance. *British Medical Journal, 337*, a2287. doi:http://dx.doi.org/10.1136/bmj.a2287

Sun, H., Li, X., Chow, E., Li, T., Xian, Y., Lu, Y., ... Zhang, L. (2015). Methadone maintenance treatment programme reduces criminal activity and improves social well-being of drug users in China: A systematic review and meta-analysis. *BMJ Open, 5*, e005997. doi:10.1136/bmjopen-2014-005997

Surrey Now. (2008). Daytox "breaks down barriers." *Canada.com.* Retrieved from www.canada.com/story.html?id=acb1f36d-764b-472f-8a94-d056aa92b28c

Syal, R. (2009, December 13). Drug money saved banks in global crisis, claims UN advisor. *The Guardian.* Retrieved from www.theguardian.com/global/2009/dec/13/drug-money-banks-saved-un-cfief-claims

Szasz, T. (2007). *The medicalization of everyday life.* Syracuse, NY: Syracuse University Press.

Tang, J., & Dani, J. (2009). Dopamine enables in vivo synaptic plasticity associated with the addictive drug nicotine. *Neuron, 63*(5), 673–682.

Tannenbaum, C., Paquette, A., Hilmer, S., Holroyd-Leduc, J., & Carnahan, R. (2012). A systemic review of amnestic and non-amnestic mild cognitive impairment induced by anticholinergic, antihistamine, GAGAergic and opioid drugs. *Drugs and Aging, 29*(8), 639–658.

Tayler, P. (2003). *The heart of the community: The best of the Carnegie Community Newsletter.* Vancouver: New Star Books.

Ternes, J., & O'Brien, C. (1990). The opioids: Abuse liability and treatments for dependence. *Advances in Alcohol and Substance Abuse, 9*(1-2) 27–45.

Thacker, E., O'Reilly, S., Weisskopf, M., Chen, H., Schwarzschild, M., McCullough, M., ... Ascherio, A. (2007). Temporal relationship between cigarette smoking and risk of Parkinson disease. *Neurology, 68*(10), 764–768.

Thapar, A., Fowler, T., Rice, F., Scourfield, J., van den Bree, M., Thomas, H., ... Hay, D. (2003). Maternal smoking during pregnancy and attention deficit hyperactivity disorder symptoms in offspring. *American Journal of Psychiatry, 160*(11), 1985–1989.

Thavorncharoensap, M., Teerawattananon, Y., Yothasamut. J., Lertpitakpong, C., & Chaikledkaew, U. (2009). The economic impact of alcohol consumption: A systematic review. *Substance Abuse Treatment, Prevention, and Policy, 4*(20). doi:10.1186/1747-597X-4-20

Therrien, F., & Markowitz, J. (1997). Selective serotonin inhibitors and withdrawal symptoms: A review of the literature. *Human Psychopharmacology, 12*(4), 309–323.

Thomas, G. (2005). *Harm reduction policies and programs for persons involved in the criminal justice system.* Ottawa, ON: Canadian Centre on Substance Abuse.

Thomas, G. (2008). Alcohol policy in Canada 1988–2008: Ongoing efforts to reduce harm. *Action News, 18*(4), 4.

Thomas, J. (1989). An overview of marital and family treatments with substance abusing populations. *Alcoholism Treatment Quarterly, 6*(3-4), 91–102.

Thombs, D. (2009). Moral model. In G. Fisher & N. Roget (Eds.), *Encyclopedia of substance abuse prevention, treatment, & recovery.* Thousand Oaks, CA: Sage.

Thomson, J., Draguleasa, M., & Tan, M. (2015). Flowers with caffeinated nectar receive more pollination. *Arthropod-Plant Interactions, 9*(1), 1–7.

Thorberg, F., & Lyvers, M. (2006). Attachment, fear of intimacy and differentiation of self among clients in substance disorder treatment facilities. *Addictive Behaviors, 31*(4), 732–737.

Thornton, C., Gottheil, E., Weinstein, S., & Kerachsky, R. (1998). Patient-treatment matching in substance abuse: Drug addiction severity. *Journal of Substance Abuse Treatment, 15*(6), 505–511.

Thorsteinsson, E., & Davey, L. (2014). Adolescents' compulsive Internet use and depression: A longitudinal study. *Open Journal of Depression, 3*(1), 13–17.

Tice, P. (1992) *Altered states: Alcohol and other drug use in America.* Rochester, NY: The Strong Museum.

Ticku, M. (1990). Alcohol and GABA-benzodiazepine receptor function. *Annals of Medicine, 22*(4), 241–246.

Timmons, S. (2010). A Christian faith-based recovery theory: Understanding God as sponsor. *Journal of Religion and Health, 51*(4), 1152–1164.

Timoshenko, G., Van Truong, M., & Williams, B. (1996). *Ontario profile, 1996: Alcohol and other drugs.* Toronto, ON: Addiction Research Foundation.

Tintera, J. (1966). Hypoglycaemia and alcoholism. *Journal of the American Geriatric Society, 16*(2), 28–34.

Tobacco and Genetics Consortium. (2010). Genome-wide meta-analyses identify multiple loci associated with smoking behavior. *Nature Genetics, 42*(6), 441–447.

Tobler, N. (1993). *Meta-analysis of adolescent drug prevention programs: Results of the 1993 meta-analysis.* Albany, NY: State University of New York.

Tobler, N. (2000). Lessons learned. *The Journal of Primary Prevention, 20*(4), 261–274.

Tobler, N., & Stratton, H. (1997). Effectiveness of school-based drug prevention programs: A meta-analysis of the research. *The Journal of Primary Prevention, 18*(1), 71–128.

Todd, T. (1991). Evolution of family therapy approaches to substance abuse. *Contemporary Family Therapy, 13*(5), 471–495.

Tomie, A., Grimes, K., & Pohorecky, L. (2008). Behavioral characteristics and neurobiological substrates shared by Pavlovian sign-tracking and drug abuse. *Brain Research Reviews, 58*(1), 121–135.

Toomey, T., Williams, C., Perry, C., Murray, D., Dudovitz, B., & Veblen-Mortenson, S. (1996). An alcohol primary prevention program for parents of 7th graders: The Amazing Alternatives! Home Program. *Journal of Child and Adolescent Substance Abuse, 5*(4), 35–53.

Topalli, V. (2005). When good is bad: An explanation of neutralization theory. *Criminology, 43*(3), 797–827.

Tragler, G., Caulkins, J., & Feichtinger, G. (2001). Optimal dynamic allocation of treatment and enforcement in illicit drug control. *Operations Research, 49*(3), 352–362.

Trescot, A., Datta, S., Lee, M., & Hansen, H. (2008). Opioid pharmacology. *Pain Physician, 11*(2S), S133–S153.

Trimpey, J. (1992). *The small book.* New York: Delacorte Press.

Tsilajara. H., Noda, K., & Saku, K. (2010). A randomized controlled open comparative trial of Varenicline vs nicotine patch in adult smokers. *Circulation Journal, 74*(4), 771–778.

Tuckman, B., & Jensen, M. (1977). Stages of small-group development revisited. *Groups and Organizational Studies, 2*(4), 419–427.

Turner, W. (2000). Cultural considerations in family-based primary prevention programs in drug abuse. *Journal of Primary Prevention, 21*(2), 285–303.

Turner, W., Wieling, E., & Allen, W. (2004). Developing culturally effective family-based research programs: Implications for family therapists. *Journal of Marital and Family Therapy, 30*(3), 257–270.

UKATT Research Team. (2005). Cost effectiveness of treatment for alcohol problems: Findings from the randomised UK alcohol treatment trial. *British Medical Journal, 331*(7516), 544. doi:http://dx.doi.org/10.1136/bmj.331.7516.544

Ulmer, R. (1977). Behaviour therapy: A promising drug abuse treatment and research approach of choice. *The International Journal of the Addictions, 12*(6), 777–784.

Unger, J., Baezconde-Garbanati, L., Shakib, S., Palmer, P., Nezami, E., & Mora, J. (2004). A cultural psychology approach to "drug abuse" prevention. *Substance Use & Misuse, 39*(10-12), 1779–1820.

United Nations Office for the Coordination of Humanitarian Affairs. (2008). *Cambodia: Ecstasy labs destroying forest wilderness.* New York: United Nations.

United Nations Office on Drugs and Crime. (2002). *2001 world drug report.* New York: United Nations.

United Nations Office on Drugs and Crime. (2004). *Schools: School-based education for drug abuse prevention.* New York: United Nations.

United Nations Office on Drugs and Crime. (2005). *Drug treatment courts work!* Vienna: United Nations. Retrieved from www.unodc.org/pdf/drug_treatment_courts_flyer.pdf

United Nations Office on Drugs and Crime. (2008). *2007 world drug report.* New York: United Nations.

United Nations Office on Drugs and Crime. (2009). *Guide to implementing family skills training programmes for drug abuse prevention.* New York: United Nations.

United Nations Office on Drugs and Crime. (2011). *Estimating illicit financial flows resulting from drug trafficking and other transnational organized crimes.* Vienna: United Nations.

United Nations Office on Drugs and Crime. (2013). *International standards on drug use prevention.* Vienna: United Nations.

United Nations Office on Drugs and Crime. (2014). *2014 world drug report.* Vienna: United Nations.

United Nations Office on Drugs and Crime. (2015). *Chronology: 100 years of drug control.* Retrieved from www.unodc.org/documents/timeline_E_09.pdf

United States Department of Health and Human Services. (2014). *National Survey on Drug Use and Health, 2013.* Ann Arbor, MI: Inter-university Consortium for Political and Social Research.

United States Department of Justice. (2003a). *Rohypnol (flunitrazepam).* Washington, DC: National Drug Intelligence Center.

United States Department of Justice. (2003b). *GBL (gamma butyrolactone).* Washington, DC: National Drug Intelligence Center.

United States Department of Justice. (2003c). *Methamphetamine.* Washington, DC: National Drug Intelligence Center.

United States Department of Justice. (2003d). *LSD (d-lysergic acid diethylamide).* Washington, DC: National Drug Intelligence Center.

United States Department of Justice. (2003e). *Psilocybin mushrooms.* Washington, DC: National Drug Intelligence Center.

United States Department of State. (2008). *International narcotics control strategy report.* Washington, DC: US Department of State.

Vakalahi, H. (2001). Adolescent substance use and family-based risk and protective factors: A literature review. *Journal of Drug Education, 31*(1), 29–46.

Valentine, M., Waring, D., & Giuffrida, D. (1992). Competency and treatment refusal in psychiatric hospitals. *Canada's Mental Health, 6*(1), 19–24.

Valverde, M. (1998). *Diseases of the will: Alcohol and dilemmas of freedom.* New York: Cambridge University Press.

van den Berg, N. (1995). *Feminist practice in the 21st century.* Washington, DC: National Association of Social Workers Press.

van den Bree, M., Johnson, E., & Neale, M. (1998). Genetic analysis of diagnostic systems of alcoholism in males. *Biological Psychiatry, 43*(2), 139–145.

van der Vorst, H., Engels, R., & Burk, W. (2010). Do parents and best friends influence the normative increase in adolescents' alcohol use at home and outside the home? *Journal of Studies on Alcohol and Drugs, 71*(2), 105–114.

van Ours, J., & Williams, J. (2009). Cannabis use and mental health problems. *VOX: CEPR's Policy Portal.* Retrieved from www.voxeu.org/article/cannabis-use-and-mental-health-problems

Van Wijhe, C., Schaufeli, W., & Peeters, M. (2010). Understanding and treating workaholism: Setting the stage for successful interventions. In R. Burke & C. Cooper

(Eds), *Risky business: Psychological, physical and financial costs of high risk behavior in organizations* (pp. 107–134). Aldershot, UK: Gower Publishing.

van Wormer, R., & van Wormer, K. (2009). Non-abstinence-based supportive housing for persons with co-occurring disorders: A human rights perspective. *Journal of Progressive Human Services, 20*(2), 152–165.

Vanderplasscheen, W., Rapp, R., Wolf, J., & Broekaeert, E. (2004). The development and implementation of case management for substance use disorders in North America and Europe. *Psychiatric Services, 55*(8), 913–922.

Vandrey, R., Budney, A., Hughes, J., & Liguori, A. (2008). A within subject comparison of withdrawal symptoms during abstinence from cannabis, tobacco and both substances. *Drug and Alcohol Dependence, 92*(1-3), 48–54.

Vasilaki, E., Hosier, S., & Cox, W. (2006). The efficacy of motivational interviewing as a brief intervention for excessive drinking: A meta-analytic review. *Alcohol and Alcoholism, 41*(3), 328–335.

Vedel, E., Emmelkamp, P., & Schippers, G. (2008). Individual cognitive-behavioral therapy and behavioral couples therapy in alcohol use disorders: A comparative evaluation in community-based addiction treatment centers. *Psychotherapy and Psychosomatics, 77*(5), 280–288.

Vertefeuille, J., Marx, A., Tun, W., Huettner, S., Strathdee, S., & Vlahov, D. (2000). Decline in self-reported high-risk injection-related behaviors among HIV-seropositive participants in the Baltimore needle exchange programs. *AIDS & Behavior, 4*(4), 381–388.

Vimpani, G. (2005). Getting the mix right: Family, community and social policy interventions to improve outcomes for young people at risk of substance misuse. *Drug and Alcohol Review, 24*(2), 111–125.

Vogt, I. (1989). Drug use in historical perspective: Continuities and discontinuities. *Contemporary Drug Problems, 16*(2), 123–139.

Volpicelli, J., Alterman, A., Hayashida, M., & O'Brien, C. (1992). Naltrexone in the treatment of alcohol dependence. *Archives of General Psychiatry, 49*(11), 876–880.

Virani, A., Bezchlibnyk-Butler, K., & Jeffies, J. (2009). *Clinical handbook of psychotropic drugs* (18th ed.). Ashland, OH: Hogrefe & Huber.

Wagenaar, A., Salois, M., & Komro, K. (2009). Effects of beverage alcohol price and tax levels on drinking: A meta-analysis of 1003 estimates from 112 studies. *Addiction, 104*(2), 179–190.

Wagenaar. A., Tobler, A., & Komro, K. (2010). Effects of alcohol tax and price policies on morbidity and mortality: A systematic review. *American Journal of Public Health, 100*(11), 2270–2278.

Wagner, E., Tubman, E., & Gil, A. (2004). Implementing school-based substance abuse interventions: Methodological dilemmas and recommended solutions. *Addiction, 99*(S2), 106–119.

Wahba, M., & Bridgewell, L. (1976). Maslow reconsidered: A review of research on the need hierarchy theory. *Organizational Behavior and Human Performance, 15*(2), 212–240.

Waiters, S., Clark, M., Gingerich, R., & Meitzer, M. (2007). *Motivating offenders to change: A guide for probation and parole.* Washington, DC: National Institute of Correction.

Waldorf, D., Reinarman, C., & Murphy, S. (1991). *Cocaine changes: The experience of using and quitting.* Philadephia, PA.: Temple University Press.

Waldron, H., & Kaminer, Y. (2004). On the learning curve: The emerging evidence supporting cognitive-behavioral therapies for adolescent substance abuse. *Addiction, 99*(2), 93–105.

Walsh, S., Nuzzo, P., Lofwall, M., & Holtman, Jr., J. (2008). The relative abuse liability of oral oxycodone, hydrocodone and hydromorphone assessed in prescription opioid abusers. *Drug and Alcohol Dependence, 98*(3), 191–202.

Walter, J., & Peller, J. (1992). *Becoming solution-focused in brief therapy.* New York: Taylor & Francis.

Walters, G. (2000). Spontaneous remission from alcohol, tobacco, and other drug abuse: Seeking quantitative answers to qualitative questions. *The American Journal of Drug and Alcohol Abuse, 26*(3), 443–460.

Wampold, B., Mondin, G., Moody, M., Stich, F., Benson, K., & Ahn, H. (1997). A meta-analysis of outcome studies comparing bona fide psychotherapies: Empirically, "All must have prizes." *Psychological Bulletin, 122*(3), 203–215.

Wand, G., Mangold, D., El Deiry, S., McCaul, M., & Hoover, D. (1998). Family history of alcoholism and hypothalamic opioidergic activity. *Annals of General Psychiatry, 55*(12), 1114–1119.

Watkin, J., Rowe, W., & Csiernik, R. (2010). Prevention as controversy: Harm reduction approaches. In R. Csiernik and W. Rowe (Eds.), *Responding to the oppression of addiction: Canadian social work responses* (2nd ed., pp. 19–36). Toronto, ON: Canadian Scholars' Press.

Watt, W., Saunders, S., Chaudron, C., & Soden, T. (1988). *Detox in Ontario.* Toronto, ON: Addiction Research Foundation.

Watters, E. (2010). *Crazy like us: The globalization of the American psyche.* New York: Free Press.

Webb, A., Lind, P., Kalmijn, J., Feiler, H., Smith, T., Schuckit, M., & Wilhelmsen, K. (2011). The investigation into CYP2E1 in relation to the level of response to alcohol through a combination of linkage and association analysis. *Alcoholism: Clinical and Experimental Research, 35*(1), 10–18.

Wechsler, H., Lee, J., Kuo, M., & Lee, H. (2000). College binge drinking in the 1990s: A continuing problem—results of the Harvard School of Public Health 1999 College Alcohol Study. *Journal of American College Health, 48*(5), 199–210.

Weegman, M. (2002). Motivational interviewing and addiction: A psychodynamic appreciation of psychodynamic practice. *Psychodynamic Practice, 8*(2), 179–185.

Weil, A. (1978). Coca leaf as a therapeutic agent. *American Journal of Drug and Alcohol Abuse, 5*(1), 75–86.

Weinberg, B., & Bealer, B. (2001). *The world of caffeine: The science and culture of the world's most popular drug.* London, UK: Routledge.

Weldy, D. (2010). Research letter: Risks of alcoholic energy drinks for youth. *Journal of the American Board of Family Medicine, 24*(4), 555–558.

Werb, D., Kerr, T., Zhang, R., Montaner, J., & Wood, E. (2010). Methamphetamine use and malnutrition among street-involved youth. *Harm Reduction Journal, 7*(5). doi:10.1186/1477-7517-7-5

Werb, D., Rowell, G., Guyatt, G., Kerr, T., Montaner, J., & Wood, E. (2010). *Effect of drug law enforcement on drug-related violence: Evidence from a scientific review.* Vancouver, BC: International Centre for Science in Drug Policy.

Werch, C., Owen, D., Carlson, J., DiClemente, C., Edgemon, P., & Moore, M. (2001). One-year follow-up results from the STARS for Families alcohol prevention program. *Health Education Research Theory & Practice, 18*(1), 74–87.

West, S., & O'Neal, K. (2004). Project D.A.R.E outcome effectiveness revisited. *American Journal of Public Health, 94*(6), 1027–1029.

WestEd. (2007). *California healthy kids survey.* Sacramento, CA: State of California.

Westover, N., & Nakonezny, P. (2010). Aortic dissection in young adults who abuse amphetamines. *American Heart Journal, 160*(2), 315–321.

Whitaker, R. (2005). Anatomy of an epidemic: Psychiatric drugs and the astonishing rise of mental illness in America. *Ethical Human Psychology and Psychiatry, 7*(1), 23–35.

White Bison (2002). The Red Road to wellbriety: In the Native American way. Colorado Springs: CoyHis Publishing.

White, D., & Pitts, M. (1998). Educating young people about drugs: A systematic review. *Addiction, 93*(10), 1475–1487.

White, I., Altmann, D., & Nanchahal, K. (2002). Alcohol consumption and mortality: Modelling risks for men and women at different ages. *British Medical Journal, 325*; doi:http://dx.doi.org/10.1136/bmj.325.7357.191.

White, M. (1995). *Re-authoring lives: Interviews and essays.* Adelaide, Australia: Dulwich Centre Publications.

White, M., & Epston, D. (1990). *Narrative means to therapeutic ends.* New York: W. W. Norton.

White, W. (1998). *Slaying the dragon: The history of addiction treatment and recovery in America.* Bloomington, IL: The Lighthouse Institute.

White, W. (2012). The history of Secular Organizations for Sobriety—Save Our Selves: An interview with James Christopher. Retrieved from www.williamwhitepapers.com/pr/James%20Christopher%20Interview%202012.pdf

White, W., Boyle, M., & Loveland, D. (2002). Alcoholism/addiction as chronic disease: From rhetoric to clinical reality. *Alcoholism Treatment Quarterly, 20*(3), 107–129.

White, W., Kurtz, E., & Acker, C. (2001). *The combined addiction disease chronologies of William White, MA, Ernest Kurtz, PhD, and Caroline Acker, PhD.* Retrieved from www.williamwhitepapers.com/pr/2001Addiction%20as%20Disease%20Chronology.pdf

White, W., & McLellan, A. (2008). Addiction as a chronic disease: Key messages for clients, families and referral sources. *Counselor, 9*(3), 24–33.

White, W., & Miller, W. (2007). The use of confrontation in addiction treatment: History, science and time for change. *Counselor, 8*(4), 12–30.

White, W., Sanders, M., & Sanders, T. (2006). Addiction in the African American community: The recovery legacies of Frederick Douglass and Malcolm X. *Counselor, 7*(5), 53–58.

Whitehead, P., & Harvey, C. (1974). Explaining alcoholism: An empirical test and reformulation. *Journal of Health and Social Behavior, 15*(1), 57–64.

Whitten, L. (2005). Disulfiram reduces cocaine abuse. *NIDA Research Findings, 20*(2), 1–4.

Wicki, M., Kuntsche, E., & Gmel, G. (2010). Drinking at European universities? A review of students' alcohol use. *Addictive Behaviors, 35*(11), 913–924.

Wicks-Nelson, R., & Israel, A. (1991). *Behavior disorders of childhood.* Englewood Cliffs, NJ: Prentice-Hall.

Wieland, D., Halter, M., & Levine, C. (2012). Bath salts: They are not what you think. *Journal of Psychosocial Nursing and Mental Health Services, 50*(2), 17–21.

Wildman, R. (1997). *Gambling: An attempt at an integration.* Edmonton, AB: Wynne Resources.

Wilkinson, A. (1998). Addiction is a brain disease, but we need more research. *The Journal, 27*(4), 5.

Wilkinson, A., Spitz, M., Prokhorov, A., Bondy, M., Shete, S., & Sargent, J. (2009). Exposure to smoking imagery in the movies and experimenting with cigarettes among Mexican heritage youth. *Cancer Epidemiology, Biomarkers & Prevention, 18*(12), 3435–3443.

Williams, B., Single, E., & McKenzie, D. (1995). *Canadian profile: Alcohol, tobacco and other drugs.* Ottawa, ON: Canadian Centre on Substance Abuse.

Williams, S. (2001). Introducing an in-patient treatment for alcohol detoxification into a community setting. *Journal of Clinical Nursing, 10*(5), 635–642.

Wills, F., & Sanders, D. (2013). *Cognitive behaviour therapy: Foundations for practice.* Thousand Oaks, CA: Sage.

Wilsnack, S. (1973). Sex role identity in female alcoholism. *Journal of Abnormal Psychology, 82*(2), 253–261.

Wilsnack, S. (1974). The effects of social drinking on women's fantasy. *Journal of Personality, 42*(1), 43–61.

Wilsnack, S., & Beckman, L. (1984). *Alcohol problems in women.* New York: Guilford Press.

Wilson, G. (1988). Alcohol use and abuse: A social learning analysis. In C. Chaudron & D. Wilkinson (Eds.), *Theories on addiction.* Toronto, ON: Addiction Research Foundation.

Wilson, G. (2000). Eating disorders and addiction. *Drugs and Society, 15*(1-2), 87–101.

Winkelman, M. (2003). Complementary therapy for addiction: "Drumming out drugs." *American Journal of Public Health, 93*(4), 647–651.

Winn, J., Shealy, S., Kropp, G., Felkins-Dohm, D., Gonzales-Nolas, C., & Francis, E. (2013). Housing assistance and case management: Improving access to substance use disorder treatment for homeless veterans. *Psychological Services, 10*(2), 233–240.

Wiseman, C., Sunday, S., Halligan, P., Korn, S., Brown, C., & Halmi, K. (1999). Substance dependence and eating disorders: Impact of sequence on comorbidity. *Comprehensive Psychiatry, 40*(5), 332–336.

Witbrodt, J., Bond, J., Kaskutas, L., Weisner, C., Jaeger, G., Pating, D., & Moore, C. (2007). Day hospital and residential addiction treatment: Randomized and nonrandomized managed care clinics. *Journal of Consulting and Clinical Psychology, 75*(6), 947–959.

Witkiewitz, K., & Bowen, S. (2010). Depression, craving, and substance use following a randomized trial of mindfulness-based relapse prevention. *Journal of Consulting and Clinical Psychology, 78*(3), 362–374.

Wolkstein, E., & Spiller, H. (1998). Providing vocational services to clients in substance abuse rehabilitation. *Directions in Rehabilitation Counseling, 9*(1), 65–78.

Woloshin, S., Schwartz, L., & Wlech, H. (2008). The risk of death by age, sex and smoking status in the United States: Putting health risks in context. *Journal of the National Cancer Institute, 100,* 845–853.

Womack, S. (1980). "I haven't stopped drinking, I just changed my brand." *Journal of Drug Issues, 8*(4), 301–310.

Woo, A. (2014, November 22). Vancouver addicts soon to receive prescription heroin. *The Globe and Mail.* Retrieved from www.theglobeandmail.com/news/british-columbia/vancouver-heroin-addicts-authorized-to-get-drug/article21717642/

Wood, E., Kerr, T., Montaner, J., Strathdee, S., Wodak, A., Hankins, C., ... & Tyndall, M. (2004). Rationale for evaluating North America's first medically supervised safer-injecting facility. *The Lancet Infectious Diseases, 4*(5), 301–306.

Wood, E., Kerr, T., Small, W., Li, K., Marsh, D., Montaner, J., & Tyndall, M. (2004). Changes in public order after the opening of a medically supervised safer injecting facility for illicit injection drug users. *Canadian Medical Association Journal, 171*(7), 731–734.

Wood, E., Tyndall, M., Lai, C., Montaner, J., & Kerr, T. (2006). Impact of a medically supervised safer injecting facility on drug dealing and other drug-related crime. *Substance Abuse Treatment, Prevention, and Policy, 1*(13). doi:10.1186/1747-597X-1-13

Woods, J. (1978). Behavioral pharmacology of drug self-administration. In M. Lipton, A. DiMascio, & K. Killam (Eds.), *Psychopharmacology: A generation of progress.* New York: Raven Publishing.

Woods, J., & Schuster, C. (1971). Opiates as reinforcing stimuli. In T. Thompson & R. Pickens (Eds.), *Stimulus properties of drugs.* New York: Appleton-Century-Crofts.

Woody, G. (2003). Research findings on psychotherapy of addictive disorders. *The American Journal on Addictions, 12*(1), 19–26.

Worcel, S., Green, B., Furrer, C., Burrus, S., & Finigan, M. (2007). *Family treatment drug court evaluation: Final report.* Portland, OR: NPC Research.

World Health Organization (WHO). (1964). *Thirteenth report of the WHO Expert Committee on Addiction-Producing Drugs.* Geneva: WHO.

World Health Organization (WHO). (2004). *Global status report on alcohol 2004.* Geneva: WHO.

World Health Organization (WHO). (2011). *Global status report on non-communicable diseases 2010.* Geneva: WHO.

World Health Organization (WHO). (2014). *Global status report on alcohol and health 2014.* Geneva: WHO.

Yalom, I. (2005). *The theory and practice of group psychotherapy* (5th ed.). New York: Basic Books.

Young, L. (2007). Sowing the seeds of health: Plants and clients thrive with horticultural therapy. *Crosscurrents, 10*(4), 4–5.

Young, M. (2011). *CrossCanada report on student alcohol and drug use.* Ottawa, ON: Canadian Centre on Substance Abuse.

Young, N., Wong, M., Adkins, T., & Simpson, S. (2003). *Family drug treatment courts: Process documentation and retrospective outcome evaluation.* Irvine, CA: Children and Family Futures.

Young-Wolff, K., Enoch, M., &. Prescott, C. (2011). The influence of gene–environment interactions on alcohol consumption and alcohol use disorders: A comprehensive review. *Clinical Psychology Review, 31*(5), 800–816.

Younger, B. (1991). The Drug-Free Workplace Act of 1988: Government intent and employer responsibility. *Employee Assistance Quarterly, 7*(2), 15–40.

Zakzanis, K., & Young, D. (2001). Ecstasy use and long term memory loss. *Neurology, 56*(7), 966–969.

Zalewska-Kaszubska, J., & Obzejta, D. (2004). Use of low-energy laser as adjunct treatment of alcohol addiction. *Lasers in Medical Science, 19*(2), 100–104.

Zaric, G., Brennan, A., Varenbut, M., & Daiter, J. (2012). The cost of providing methadone maintenance treatment in Ontario, Canada. *The American Journal of Drug and Alcohol Abuse, 38*(6), 559–566.

Zaridze, D., Brennan, P., Boreham, J., Boroda, A., Karpov, R., Lzarev, A., ... Peto, R. (2009). Alcohol and cause-specific mortality in Russia: A retrospective case—control study of 48 557 adult deaths. *The Lancet, 373*(9682), 2201–2204.

Zarkin, G., Dunlap, L., Hicks, K., & Mamo, D. (2005). Benefits and costs of methadone treatment: Results from a lifetime simulation model. *Health Economics, 14*(11), 1133–1150.

Zemore, S., & Kaskutas, L. (2008). Services received and treatment outcomes in day-hospital and residential programs. *Substance Abuse Treatment, 35*(3), 232–244.

Zgierska, A., Rabago, D., Chawla, N., Kushner, K., Koehler, R., & Marlatt, A. (2009). Mindfulness meditation for substance use disorders: A systematic review. *Substance Use, 30*(4), 266–294.

Zhang, S., Lee, I.-M., Manson, J., Cook, N., Willett, W., & Buring, J. (2007). Alcohol consumption and breast cancer risk in the Women's Health Study. *American Journal of Epidemiology, 165*(6), 667–676.

Zhao, Z., Gao, Y., Sun, Y., Zhao, C., Gereau, R., & Chen, Z. (2007). Central serotonergic neurons are differently required for opioid analgesia but not for morphine tolerance or morphine reward. *Proceedings of the National Academy of Sciences, 104*(36). doi:10.1073/pnas.0705740104

Zinn, L. (1997). The home detox alternative. *Behavioral Health Management, 17*(6), 24–27.

Zubieta, J., Heitzeg, M., Smith, Y., Bueller, J., Xu, K., Xu, Y., ... Goodman, G. (2003). COMT [val158] met genotype affects μ-opioid neurotransmitter responses to a pain stressor. *Science, 299*(5610), 1240–1243.

COPYRIGHT ACKNOWLEDGEMENTS

CHAPTER 1

Table 1.2: "Comparison of per capita opioid consumption in morphine equivalence among lowest and highest consumption countries, 2011" from *World Drug Report 2014*, by the United Nations Office on Drugs and Crime, copyright © 2014 United Nations. Reprinted with the permission of the United Nations.

Table 1.6: "Changes in Afghanistan farm-gate prices of select licit and illicit crops, 2009–2013" adapted from The *Report of the International Narcotics Control Board for 2013*, by the International Narcotics Control Board, copyright © 2014 United Nations. Reprinted with the permission of the United Nations.

CHAPTER 2

Figure 2.2: "Medical Model Process of Alcohol Abuse and Recovery" from "Group Therapy in Alcoholism", by M. M. Glatt in *British Journal of Addiction*, copyright © 1958 Society for the Study of Addiction. Reprinted with the permission of Wiley Publishing.

Figure 2.4: "Skinner Box" from *Psychology: From Inquiry to Understanding, Second Edition*, by Scott O. Lilienfeld, Steven J. Lynn, Laura L. Namy, and Nancy J. Woolf, copyright © 2011 Pearson Education. Printed and electronically reproduced by permission of Pearson Education, Inc., New York, New York.

CHAPTER 3

Figure 3.2: "Benzodiazepine Equivalence to 10 mg Diazepam (Valium) Source" from *Benzodiazepines: How They Work and How to Withdraw*, by Heather Ashton. Available at http://www.benzo.org.uk/manual/bzcha01.htm#24, copyright © 1999–2013 Professor C. H. Ashton, Institute of Neuroscience, Newcastle University. Reprinted with the permission of Heather Ashton.

Figure 3.3: "Trend of coca cultivation in the Andean Region, 1990–2011" from *The Drug Problem in the Americas (2013)*, by the General Secretariat, Organization of American States. Obtained from the World Drug Report. Available at www.oas.org/documents/

INDEX

opioids, 125–138; alternative terms for, 125; antagonists, 103, 128–129, 136–138; brain neurochemistry and, 127; clinical features of, 138; as CNS depressants, 25; codeine, 128, 129; duration of compared with morphine, 138; effects of, 105; elimination of, 126; endorphins and, 28; excretion of, 126; global use of, 36; half-life, 128; historical uses of, 125–126; illicit use, physical complications from, 126–127; licit vs. illicit use of, 37–38; metabolization of, 126; natural opioids, 103, 128, 129–130; opioid substitution therapy, 204–205; overdose risks, 127, 128; pain management and, 103, 126; physical dependency, 20, 127; physiological effects, 126; during pregnancy, 127; prescription opioid use, 41–42, 128; psychological dependency, 127; pulmonary complications, 126–127; relapse rate, 127; as relapsing condition, 204; respiratory depression, 127, 128; semi-synthetic opioids, 103, 128, 130–134; student past-year drug use, 44–45; synthetic opioids, 103, 128, 134–136; therapeutic uses, 126; tolerance, 127; transdermal administration of, 34; use of in Canada, 41–42, 128, 372–373; withdrawal, 127–128

opioid substitution therapy, 204–205; methadone treatment and maintenance, 240–242

opion, 126

opium, 130; administration methods, 126; cultivation of for licit pharmaceutical use, 126; dependency, 130; in drug substitution therapy, 204; farm-gate prices, licit/illicit crops, 49–50; as natural opioid, 128; slang for, 130; tolerance, 130; use of in China, 87

Opium Act (1908), 335

Opium and Narcotic Act, 335

opium gum, pharmaceutical, 95

opium poppy cultivation, 38, 94, 95

oppositional defiant disorder, 190

oral administration, drug absorption and, 32, 34

oral cancers, 33

organizational skills of addiction counsellors, 357

Osmond, Humphrey, 364

outpatient programming, 287–288

outreach, 355

overdose risks: alcohol, 125; barbiturates, 107; bath salts, 151; buprenorphine, 131; caffeine, 163; heroin, 132; hydromorphone, 132; ketamine, 179; methadone, 136; naloxone, therapeutic use of, 136; non-barbiturate sedative-hypnotics (NBSH), 109–110; opioids, 127, 128; OxyContin, 133

Overeaters Anonymous, 261, 304

oxazepam, 111, 114

Oxford House approach, in recovery homes, 291

oxycodone, 128, 133–134

OxyContin (oxycodone HCl controlled-release), 28, 133–134, 241; administration, altered method of, 133; as "hillbilly heroin", 91; marketing of, 133–134; overdose risks, 133; physical dependency, 133; potency of compared to Percocet, 133; slang for, 133; student past-year drug use, 44–45

oxymorphone, 138

OxyNeo, 133; student past-year drug use, 44–45

Pain Management (textbook), 134

pain management, opioids and, 103, 126

pain relievers, caffeine content, 159

Pakistan: per capita opioid consumption, 38; as transit hub, 95

Palladone, 132

Panama, as transit hub, 95

pancreas, effect of alcohol on, 123

Papaver somniferum (Asian poppy), 126

Paraguay, cannabis cultivation in, 37, 96

paraldehyde, 109

paramethoxyamphetamine (PMA). *See* PMA (paramethoxyamphetamine)

paranoid psychosis: cocaine and, 141; khat and, 149

parasthesia, 128

parental skills workshops, 324

parenting sessions, 303

Parest (methaqualone), 109

Parke Davis, 177–178, 179

Parnate, 191

paroxetine, 187, 191

Pavlov, Ivan, 227

Pavlovian sign-tracking behaviour, 73

Paxil, 29, 187, 191

PCP (phencyclidine), 26, 104, 165, 167, 177–179; brain, effect of on, 178; cardiovascular complications, 178; long-term effects, 178–179; physiological effects, 178; slang for, 177; student past-year drug use, 44–45; tolerance, 179; withdrawal, 179

Peele, Stanton, 16–17, 61, 271

peer group strategies, 313

penalties, drug offences, 337–341

pentazocine: as agonist-antagonist, 137; with Ritalin, 137; slang for, 137; tolerance, 137; with tripelennamine hydrochloride, 137; withdrawal, 137

pentobarbital (Nembutal), 106, 108

Pentothal (thiopental), 108

Peram, 186

perceived harm education, 313

perception, effects of hallucinogens on, 104